COOKING
DATA

CRITICAL GLOBAL HEALTH
Evidence, Efficacy, Ethnography
A SERIES EDITED BY VINCANNE ADAMS
AND JOÃO BIEHL

COOKING DATA

Culture and Politics in an African Research World

CRYSTAL BIRUK

Duke University Press · Durham and London · 2018

Printed and bound by CPI Group (UK) Ltd, Croydon, CR0 4YY
Designed by Heather Hensley
Typeset in Arno Pro by Westchester Publishing Services

Library of Congress Cataloging-in-Publication Data
Names: Biruk, Crystal, author.
Title: Cooking data : culture and politics in an
African research world / Crystal Biruk.
Description: Durham : Duke University Press, 2018. |
Series: Critical global health: evidence, efficacy, ethnography |
Includes bibliographical references and index.
Identifiers: LCCN 2017039419 (print)
LCCN 2018000301 (ebook)
ISBN 9780822371823 (ebook)
ISBN 9780822370741 (hardcover : alk. paper)
ISBN 9780822370895 (pbk. : alk. paper)
Subjects: LCSH: Medical anthropology—Malawi. | AIDS
(Disease)—Research—Malawi—Methodology. | HIV
infections—Research—Malawi—Methodology.
Classification: LCC GN296.5.M42 (ebook) | LCC GN296.5.M42
B57 2018 (print) | DDC 306.4/61096897—dc23
LC record available at https://lccn.loc.gov/2017039419

Cover art: Boxes of completed surveys in LSAM field office storage
room. Photo by Joshua Wood.

For my families, *everywhere*

CONTENTS

ACKNOWLEDGMENTS

Cooking up this book has not been easy; the labor of turning raw curiosity, excitement, and ideas into words was helped by many people and things along this book's life course.

Zikomo kwambiri to colleagues and friends at the University of Malawi (Chancellor College and College of Medicine) and the Centre for Social Research for giving me such a warm welcome in the past and the present, especially Agnes Chimbiri, Ephraim Chirwa, Mike Kachedwa, John Kadzandira, James Kaphuka, Wapulumuka Mulwafu, Alister Munthali, and the late Pierson Ntata. I am grateful to have had the chance to teach medical anthropology at Chancellor College in 2008 under the mentorship of Dr. Munthali. Thanks to Paul Kakhongwe at the Centre for Social Research's Documentation Unit, and to staff at the Chancellor College Library, the National Statistics Office, the Malawi National Archives, and the National AIDS Commission for help navigating their archives and collections. For Chichewa lessons and friendship, thank you to Arnold Mboga, and for research assistance, thanks to Andy Mguntha, Enalla Mguntha, and Tasneem (Thoko) Ninje. For allowing me to tag along with them in the field, I am grateful to all of the researchers, fieldworkers, and supervisors I spent time with between 2005 and 2009, some of whom are anonymously represented herein. For friendship, guidance, stimulating conversation, and billiards games at various times in Malawi since 2005, many thanks to Davie Chitenje, Abdallah Chilungo, Augustine Harawa, Hastings Honde, Sheena Kayira, Sydney Lungu, James Mkandawire, Evans Mwanyatimu, James Mwera, Joel Phiri, Daud Rashid, and Harry Samiton. I feel very lucky that Susan Watkins initially invited me after a happenstance meeting in 2005 to join demographers in the field for a summer; since then, she has been an unflagging source of encouragement, a sharp reader of my work, and expert at connecting me to those whom I need to talk to. I am grateful, as well, to Kathleen Beegle, Shelley Clark, Ernestina Coast, Hans Peter Kohler, Teri Lindgren, Michelle Poulin, and Sally Rankin for support and feedback on my project in its earlier stages. At various times during my trips to Malawi since 2005, the following folks have provided friendship, community, and/ or intellectual inspiration, usually over Greens or boxed wine: jimi adams, Mrs. Anderson, Phil Anglewicz, Jessi Bishop Royse, Jacobus de Hoop, Kim Deslandes, Kim Yi Dionne, Anne Esacove, Pete Fleming, Emily Freeman, Lauren Gaydosh, Stéphane Helleringer, Laura Ivey, Rose Kadende-Kaiser, Paul Kaiser, Wanja Ngure, Michelle Poulin, Joey Power, Georges Reniers, Keshet Ronen, Gil Shapira, Karolin Stahl, Gift Trapence, Jenny Trinitapoli, Cathy van de Ruit, Megan Vaughan, Anna West, Anika Wilson, and Joshua Wood. Finally, I am so thankful that my path crossed with Zoe Groves's one fateful day in the Malawi National Archives; she has been an important interlocutor, dear friend, and enthusiastic travel companion since then.

I began research for this book as a doctoral student in the Department of Anthropology at the University of Pennsylvania. My adviser, Sandra Barnes, is the kind of mentor graduate students dream of. Sandra models the sensitive and rigorous relationship to anthropological thinking, research, and writing I aspire to embody. From my first meeting with Sandy in 2003 up until today, she is my most trusted and honest reader, always encouraging me to stay grounded in the ethnographic and not to lose sight of what really matters. I admire her humble confidence and commitment to her students. I hope I have made her proud with this first book. Kathy Hall is a tireless supporter of my work and her mentorship and friendship continue to be invaluable to my scholarly and personal development. Thanks to Adriana Petryna, who arrived at Penn after I had finished coursework, but became an important mentor, reader, and interlocutor when I returned from the field and into the present. Fran Barg and I first met when I enrolled in one of her medical anthropology courses as an undergraduate; I credit her with sparking my interest in the subfield. She encouraged me to study anthropology at the graduate level and welcomed me to Penn and on to her research project at the University of Pennsylvania hospital in my early graduate career; my interactions with Fran, Joe Gallo, and Marsha Wittink through that work helped solidify my commitment to learning, conversation, and empathy across disciplines and fields of study. Courses, reading groups and/or conversations with David Barnes, Lee Cassanelli, Ali Dinar, Steven Feierman, Rebecca Huss-Ashmore, Paul Kaiser, Heather Love, Ritty Lukose, Christiaan Morssink, Brian Spooner, John Tresch, and Greg Urban were all influential on my intellectual development.

I am especially thankful to Deborah Thomas, who has continued to be an important source of inspiration, advice, and mentorship through my junior faculty years, and kindly hosted me as a visiting scholar at Penn during my junior research leave.

At the University of Pennsylvania and in the city of Philadelphia, I thank the following individuals who constitute a group of chosen family and friendly critics that made my graduate school years the perfect mix of work and play, and provided feedback on earlier versions of this work: Raquel Albarrán, Josh Berson, Bryan Cameron, Elise Carpenter, Christa Cesario, Amanda Chudnow, Megan Cook, Brian Daniels, Kristin Doughty, Kerry Dunn, Selma Feliciano-Arroyo, Michael Joiner, Rabia Kamal, Greta LaFleur, Adam Leeds, Kirt Mausert, Michael McLaughlin, Melanie Micir, Lauren Miller, Amy Paeth, Jeremy Pine, Dana Prince, Christy Schuetze, Savannah Shange, Julia Switzer, Cathy Van de Ruit, and Thomas Ward.

At Oberlin College, I am grateful for my dear friendship and intellectual exchanges with Erika Hoffmann-Dilloway and for excellent colleagues who support my well-being and scholarship, especially Grace An, Ann Cooper Albright, Judi Davidson, Jennifer Fraser, Jason Haugen, Daphne John, Carol Lasser, Amy Margaris, Greggor Mattson, Anu Needham, Gina Perez, Baron Pineda, and Danielle Terrazas Williams. Thanks to Tim Elgren for his ongoing support of and interest in my work. I would also like to thank the numerous scholar-friends who have passed through Oberlin since I arrived, variously enriching my life and scholarship in important ways: Jacinthe Assaad, Chris Barcelos, Allison Davis, Meiver de la Cruz, Bridget Guarasci, Vange Heiliger, Julie Keller, Julie Kleinman, Chelsea Martinez, Sabia McCoy-Torres, Lani Teves, and especially Sarah Waheed. I am lucky to teach at Oberlin, where my students always keep me on my toes and make me a better scholar.

In 2011–2012, I was fortunate to spend a productive year as a postdoctoral fellow at Brown University's Pembroke Center for Teaching and Research on Women, with my wonderful co-postdocs, Joe Fischel and Poulomi Saha. I learned so much from the folks in and around the Consent seminar: Rina Bliss, Bianca Dahl, Denise Davis, Igor De Souza, Paja Faudree, Pablo Gómez, Donna Goodnow, Hunter Hargraves, Maud Kozodoy, Madhumita Lahiri, Eng-Beng Lim, Moshi Optat Herman, Tom Roach, Ralph Rodriguez, Suzanne Stewart-Steinberg, Kay Warren, Elizabeth Weed, Debbie Weinstein, and many others.

I have had the good fortune to present work from this project in many forums: the Department of Anthropology, Brown University; Wits Institute for Social and Economic Research (WISER), University of the Witwatersrand;

Council on African Studies, Yale University; Holtz Center for Science and Technology Studies, University of Wisconsin-Madison; Critical Global Health Seminar, Johns Hopkins University; Program of African Studies, Northwestern University; Department of Anthropology, University of Virginia; and the Department of Women's, Gender, and Sexuality Studies, University of Cincinnati. Many thanks to the folks who invited me and to the audiences whose critical feedback improved portions of this book. Fellow panelists and audience members generously engaged my work in progress over the years at American Anthropological Association (AAA) meetings, African Studies Association (ASA) meetings, at the "Dreaming of Health and Science in Africa Conference" in Hinxton, U.K. (2015); at the "Africanizing Technology" Conference at Wesleyan (2015); at the Northeastern Workshops on Southern Africa (NEWSA) meetings; at the Social Science Conference at the University of Malawi (2014); at Society for Cultural Anthropology (SCA) meetings; at American Ethnological Society (AES) meetings; and at the Roundtables on Transnationality in Berlin (2010).

At various stages between 2007 and 2016, research and writing for this book were supported by an International Dissertation Research Fellowship from the Social Science Research Council; a Wenner Gren Dissertation Fieldwork Grant; National Science Foundation Doctoral Dissertation Improvement Grant no. 0719987; a summer writing residency at the School for Advanced Research in beautiful Santa Fe; and dissertation research and dissertation completion fellowships from the University of Pennsylvania. Oberlin College's Grants Office and the Dean's office provided funds for travel, a junior research leave year that permitted me to complete this book and funds for indexing. Some text and ideas in chapters 3 and 4 appeared in articles titled "Seeing Like a Research Project: Producing High Quality Data in AIDS Research in Malawi" and "Ethical Gifts?: An Analysis of Soap-for-Information Transactions in Malawian Survey Research Worlds," published in *Medical Anthropology* and *Medical Anthropology Quarterly*, respectively. I thank the editors and reviewers of those articles for their feedback.

I have found a rich community of scholars interested in health, medicine, global health, African studies, science studies, and topics further afield. For general encouragement, reading or teaching my work, and critical generosity, I thank Vincanne Adams, Nikhil Anand, On Barak, Naor Ben-Yehoyada, Adia Benton, Sarah Besky, João Biehl, Brooke Bocast, Marian Burchardt, Timothy Burke, Catherine Burns, Brenda Chalfin, Jennifer Cole, Johanna Crane, Ashley Currier, Bianca Dahl, Denielle Elliot, Susan Erikson, Elsa Fan, Kirk Fiereck, Ellen Foley, Inderpal Grewal, Zoe Groves, Laurie Hart, Cassandra

Hartblay, Saida Hodžić, Jim Igoe, Lochlann Jain, Bea Jauregui, Diana Jeater, Patricia Kingori, Julie Kleinman, Jennifer Liu, Julie Livingston, Rob Lorway, Dan Magaziner, Ramah McKay, Marissa Mika, Pierre Minn, Alex Nading, Abby Neely, Kalala Ngalamulume, Adeola Oni-Orisan, Melissa Pashigian, Julie Peteet, Rebecca Peters, Anne Pollock, Peter Redfield, Juno Salazar Parreñas, Thurka Sangaramoorthy, Salla Sariola, China Scherz, Jesse Shipley, Dan Smith, Harris Solomon, Harrod Suarez, Noelle Sullivan, Ann Swidler, Karl Swinehart, Matthew Thomann, Helen Tilley, Laura Ann Twagira, Claire Wendland, Anna West, Luise White, and many others.

I am fortunate for the support provided by my family, given and chosen. Thanks to my parents, Karen and John, for nurturing my curiosity and helping me see beyond the confines of the Jersey Shore, and thanks to Aunt Linda, always, for conversation, friendship, and wine. Shirley Marziali, thank you for your encouragement in the past few years. Thanks, as well, to my grandmother, Else, the most spry ninety-year-old I know! I am grateful for friendship and laughs with my sister Laureen, and also for her careful work with the figures and illustrations in this book.

I thank the editors, reviewers, and readers for their feedback as this project came to fruition, and João Biehl and Vincanne Adams for their initial faith in the project. My deepest thanks to Elizabeth Ault, my editor at Duke University Press, for her encouragement and careful attention to the project. I am also grateful to Lisa Bintrim at Duke, and to David Martinez for his work compiling the index. Vincanne Adams and Claire Wendland showed remarkable generosity, care and insight in helping shape the book.

Finally, Lyndsey Beutin is my treasure, my gem, and my brilliant coadventurer. Her ethnographer's heart inspires me daily, and I am proud to build a world with her that is queer, intentional, and playful, and centers other people's stories.

It is from all of you mentioned here—and others I surely have overlooked—that I have learned the importance of practicing compassionate critique in life, love, and scholarship. May academia and the many other institutions and social spaces we navigate show you the same generosity you have gifted me.

It was . . . necessary to be sure the African chosen would undertake his work efficiently and successfully, as with a period of only a few days to be employed, he might be tempted to sit under a banana tree and write the first figures which came into his head [on the census forms]. —C. J. Martin, "The East African Population Census, 1948"

AN ANTHROPOLOGIST AMONG THE DEMOGRAPHERS
Assembling Data in Survey Research Worlds

In 1948, C. J. Martin (1949, 315), director of the East African Statistical Department, speculated that African data collectors for the census in Uganda, Kenya, and Tanzania might invent the data they were meant to record. In mid-June 2008—sixty years later—I sat with a group of Malawian data collectors in a minibus parked in a village in central Malawi where they were administering household-level surveys for an American-led longitudinal cohort study, the Longitudinal Study of AIDS in Malawi (LSAM).[1] They had finished their work for the day and were conversing about one of their colleagues as he sat under a tree nearby, pencil in hand and head bent over a survey questionnaire. As he checked the questionnaire to ensure that each question had been answered by the respondent, those in the van jokingly accused him of "cooking data" (*kuphika madata*). Soon after the conversation, the minibus hurried back to the LSAM field office nearby, where the team's completed questionnaires were deposited in cardboard boxes until the information they contained would be carefully entered into a growing database by a data entry team.

DATE OF INTERVIEW	[__I__][__I__] (Day, Month)	
TIME STARTED	[__I__][__I__] (24 HOUR TIME)	
INTERVIEWER NAME	[_____]	
INTERVIEWER NUMBER	[__I__I__]	

RESPONDENT'S IDENTIFICATION

Village name and number_____ [__I__I__]

Headman's name_____

Head of compound_____

Respondent's name and Respondent ID_____ [_____]

Respondent's other names/nicknames_____ #living children _____

Respondent's level of education (circle and fill in level): (0) No school (1) Primary-Level____ (2) Secondary-Level____ (3) Higher

Respondent's birthplace (District and Village)_____

Respondent's father's name_____

Respondent's age (estimate if respondent doesn't know) [__I__] Check if age was estimated by interviewer [__]

Respondent's marital status 1....MARRIED   33...NEVER MARRIED   44...SEPARATED   55...DIVORCED   66...WIDOWED

Husband's name_____

Husband's other names/nicknames_____

Husband's birthplace (District and village)_____

Number of other wives that husband has_____

Husband's level of education (circle and fill in level): (0) No school   (1) Primary-level___   (2) Secondary-level___   (3) Higher

	SUPERVISOR	LOGGED BY	CHECKED BY	ENTERED BY
INITIALS	_____	_____	_____	_____
DATE	_____	_____	_____	_____

FIGURE I.1. LSAM questionnaire, 2008.

Cooking data refers to fabricating, falsifying, or fudging the information one is meant to collect from survey respondents in a standardized and accurate manner. Martin's fears that enumerators might "write the first figures which came into [their] heads" on their forms reflect his stakes in the first endeavor to accurately map African populations in the territories his office oversaw, express racialized hierarchies of suspicion, and illustrate how data collectors' practices in the field might spoil census data that would later be analyzed in the office. Meanwhile, in 2008, the phrase "cooking data" operated among Malawian fieldworkers as playful commentary on colleagues' work performance, indicating that they had come to articulate and embody the habits, investments, and standards central to the collection of high-quality data, as imparted to them by American demographers during intensive pre-fieldwork training sessions. These two accounts point to the tensions between standardization and improvisation, and concerns about data quality that are at the core of this book and continue to preoccupy those who administer surveys in sub-Saharan Africa today. Amid demographers' interest in measuring and quantifying population-based phenomena—such as HIV/AIDS and other health issues—surveys like the ones administered by LSAM's fieldworkers are a major source of health-related evidence in sub-Saharan Africa. They act as localized sensors of a global system by feeding the demand for numbers on which to base evidence-based policy and practice (Cartwright and Hardie 2012; Adams 2013; Geissler 2015a, 15).

Cooked data are a specter that has long haunted survey projects by invoking ways in which data's future certainty and value as evidence might be unraveled by human error or deviations from the standards or recipes governing their collection. Adjectives such as "cooked" versus "raw" and "dirty" versus "clean" figure across multiple scales of data talk in survey research worlds: fieldworkers, demographers, data entry clerks, policy makers, and statisticians alike employ such terms to comment on the quality of quantitative data at various stages of their collection, analysis, and storage. While we tend to think of data as abstract and intangible, these vivid descriptors draw attention to their materiality and life course. Numbers, of course, come from somewhere. A careful consideration of the social lives of numbers, rather than viewing them as stable and objective measures of reality, provides crucial context for interpreting quantitative evidence that we often deem too big or too technical to wrap our heads around. As an ethnography of the production of quantitative data, this book encourages its readers to be a little bit less in awe of numbers by understanding them as "creatures that threaten to become corrupted, lost, or meaningless if not properly cared for" (Ribes and Jackson 2013, 147). It also considers how the activities of data collection not only produce numbers but shape personhood, sociality, and truth claims.

Cooked data conjure their culinary opposite: raw data. Data are units of information (such as a number, response, or code written into a box on a survey page by a data collector) that, in aggregate form such as LSAM's public-use database of survey data collected since 1998, might become evidence for policy making, public health interventions, academic analysis, or medical practice by government, nongovernmental organizations (NGOs), scholars, and other institutions in Malawi. Whereas actors in survey research worlds take raw data to be transparent or naked—that is, prior to analysis or interpretation— cooked data have been subjected to processes that shape or transform them in two main ways. In the first sense—the "cooking data" mentioned by the fieldworkers and Martin above—raw data become deformed, dirty, or useless through bad data practices and human error or other contingencies in the field. The most egregious—and mythologized—form of cooking data in the field occurs when a fieldworker fabricates numbers or fills out a survey willy-nilly.[2] In the second sense, cooked data are raw data that have been processed, organized, and analyzed according to demographic standards and norms; this form of cooking is codified and validated by experts and mostly takes place in the office once data arrive from the field.[3] Talk of raw and cooked data recalls Lévi-Strauss's (1969) classic study *The Raw and the Cooked.* He argues that the interplay between the categories raw and cooked is the building block of hundreds of myths found across many cultures and therefore forms the basic structure of human thought. Raw and cooked are heuristics that allow humans to differentiate what comes from nature and what is produced in and by human culture, including data.

An extensive literature authored by statisticians and survey researchers has aimed to diagnose, document, and mitigate instances of cooking or data fabrication by data collectors, both during and after collection (Crespi 1946; Finn and Ranchhod 2013; Waller 2013; Kennickell 2015), with a more recent contribution suggesting that data fabrication by fieldworkers might function as critical commentary on inequalities inherent to research projects in low-income countries or as an expression of low morale (Kingori and Gerrets 2016). However, accounts of data practices in the field take for granted a fundamental difference between raw and cooked data, a binary that I hope this book destabilizes. In titling this book *Cooking Data,* my intention is not to suggest that the data produced by survey projects are fabricated or falsified, nor is it to provide advice to researchers about how to mitigate cooking among fieldworkers. This book shows how all data—even that verified as clean by demographers—are cooked by the processes and practices of production.

I view survey research worlds as embedded in a heterogeneous social field inhabited by people whose practices, rhetoric, and relations are informed by epistemic conventions that underlie what the collection of good, clean data is supposed to be. I suggest that it is in the field where surveys are administered—rather than in researchers' offices—that we can gain insight into what research means for the people who are tasked with collecting data by asking respondents questions and for those who have to answer the questions, as well as what kinds of worlds and persons it brings into being. In Malawi, this book shows, the effort to render the AIDS epidemic and its context visible and knowable to a demographic or global health gaze is constitutive of, and entangled with, attempts by fieldworkers and research subjects to achieve their own interests as members of a research world.

As an explicit expression and validation of underlying disciplinary norms or virtues, data talk and the units of information it comments on are not unlike Lévi-Strauss's myths. Data and myths are both anonymized artifacts of collective labor and seem to "come from nowhere" (Lévi-Strauss 1969, 18); consider how the wide circulation of statistics as the collective currency of policy makers and statisticians reinforces a kind of mythology that takes information as objective, free-floating, abstract, and universal (Poovey 1998, xii; Bowker 2005, 73). Take, for example, the claim made by two demographers who analyzed LSAM's survey data in an article published in a major HIV/AIDS research journal that "only 15.6 % of women and 8.1 % of men did not share their HIV test result with their spouse" (Anglewicz and Chintsanya 2011). This statement paints a particular picture of Malawian social life and garners legitimacy not only from the numbers it cites, but also from the respectable and long-standing data set from which the numbers are extracted. How did these numbers get all the way from the field in Malawi into the pages of a journal? What is their life story? This book demystifies data by tracing their life course and travels amid and with human and nonhuman actors whose heterogeneous work constitutes caring for data. *Cooking Data* foregrounds the social transactions that characterize survey research worlds all the way from the collection of raw data to the presentation of evidence in policy.

I borrow the phrase "cooking data" from my informants—both Malawian fieldworkers and survey researchers—to open an analytical space for the central questions of this book: How do raw units of information—numbers written onto a questionnaire by data collectors—acquire value as statistics that inform national AIDS policy and interventions? How do on-the-ground dynamics and practices of survey research cultures mediate the production of numbers? Finally, how are quantitative health data and their social worlds coproduced and with what consequences for local economies, formulations of expertise, and lived experience? In attempting to answer these questions, I draw theoretical inspiration from science and technology studies and critical medical anthropology to illustrate how the lives of data and the lives of those who produce it in one of the poorest countries of the world are impossible to disentangle; data reflect and cohere new social relations, persons, practices, forms of expertise, and expectations. Following recent scholarship in postcolonial science studies, in this book I track how the survey project—a particular kind of socioscientific assemblage—travels; I also consider what matters to whom about research conducted in resource poor contexts. Finally, I show how survey projects, following a long legacy of scientific and development projects dating from the colonial period, are inevitably messier and less comprehensive endeavors than we might expect (Tilley 2007, 2). The blank first page of LSAM's 2008 questionnaire that precedes this introduction invites future respondents' answers; likewise, I invite the reader to join me as I track the travels of data in survey research worlds.

Demographers' Dreams: The Assembly Line of Data

The chapters that follow explore the everyday relations between persons, data, technologies, and infrastructures that temporarily transform parts of Malawi into a field of demographic health research. Foreign survey researchers— demographers, economists, and sociologists such as those affiliated with LSAM—working in Malawi necessarily share responsibility for the quality of data collected with many collaborators, all with different interests in research: Malawian research partners, fieldworkers, HIV testing and counseling teams, data entry clerks, and research participants, for example. As is elaborated in chapter 4, raw information collected by workers in the field may be edited to remove assumptions and ambiguity as it is assembled, making data seem better or more certain than it actually is and enhancing its performative capacity and citability (Latour and Woolgar 1979; Bledsoe 2002, 130; Espeland and Stevens 2008, 421–422; Sana and Weinreb 2008, Tichenor 2017). In their polished form, data reflect the capacity and expertise of all of their handlers, even if epistemic rhetoric and metrics for good data tend to obscure the degree of uncertainty absorbed by data in their travels (March and Simon 1958, 165).

Survey research entails long periods of data collection in the field and confronts epistemic threats from start (survey design) to finish (good numbers ensconced in a database): mistranslation of questionnaires, poorly trained interviewers, respondents who lie, respondents who refuse to participate or who cannot be found, poor weather conditions, inaccurate data entry, and lost data. Making quantitative data demands designing and implementing a material and human infrastructure—a machinery of knowledge production—that requires managing the unruly people, places, and things that characterize fieldwork, a messy outdoor scientific activity (Kuklick and Kohler 1996; Knorr-Cetina 1999; Ribes and Jackson 2013). These efforts are costly in time and money; in 2008, for example, data collection activities, including data entry, took 70 percent of the survey-based Marriage and Youth Project's (MAYP, discussed below) total project budget. Efforts at standardization and harmonization symbolized by the creation of a streamlined survey script to be administered by fieldworkers serve the goal of clean and high-quality data: data that are accurate, reliable, efficiently and ethically collected, and representative of sufficiently large and bounded samples over time. Indeed, survey researchers employ the term "quality assurance" to consider ways that data processes align or depart from predefined operational standards (Usten et al. 2005; Lyberg and Biemer 2008). As we will see in chapter 1, survey researchers endorse a shared set of epistemic virtues that ensure the data they collect will be deemed objective, clean, and consumable (Daston and Galison 2010).

Throughout, the book foregrounds data's materiality and social lives as they move along what demographers imagine to be an assembly line of human and nonhuman actors. Survey researchers themselves take interest in the many stages of a survey, typically bookended by establishing the structure of the study at its birth (usually in a proposal for funding) and ending with the dissemination of findings drawn from the data (Pennell, Levenstein, and Lee 2010). They determine how to best document the production of data at all stages to help data users assess data quality, defined as the degree to which data conforms to requirements agreed upon by producers and users. While demographers may idealize data activities as a kind of assembly-line process that produces identical widgets or units of information, this book shows that survey research activities and data production look more like a life course in practice—where any individual datum results from an unfolding series of transactions, experiences, and relations.

The assembly line—associated with Henry Ford's introduction of the continuously moving technology to mass produce standardized goods—is a compelling image for thinking through and tracing data's travels. First, the Fordist assembly-line process subordinated human skill or creativity by training workers at one station to do the same repetitive task over and over again; the prefieldwork training sessions for Malawian fieldworkers discussed in chapters 2 and 4 likewise aim to harmonize the practices and procedures that constitute the data collection phase of research, characterized by administration of the same survey in the same manner to different respondents over and over again. Indeed, demographers and survey researchers in other disciplines generally view fieldworkers as a liability, harboring suspicions about the ability of the fieldworkers to do the work well and their potential to mess up data collection by cooking or fabricating data (True, Alexander, and Richman 2011). Fieldworkers across time and space are consistently framed by survey researchers as unreliable, as prone to cheating or cutting corners when collecting data, and as suspicious, thus requiring close surveillance to prevent unwanted edits to data in the field (Crespi 1946; AAPOR 2003; Biemer and Lyberg 2003; Sana and Weinreb 2008; Spagat 2010; Finn and Ranchhod 2013).

Yet, even as project design tools and survey instruments predetermine and limit the actions of fieldworkers, these individuals improvise, reinvent, and improve upon standards as they implement them in the field, far from the researchers' eyes and ears. As this book shows, making good data requires creativity and tinkering as much as it does harmonization and consistency. One major interest in writing this book is to present fieldworkers—often cast as unskilled laborers—as central actors in the story of the production of data. Intermediary local actors such as these have long been eclipsed in accounts of (post)colonial science that cast heroic scientists and Western experts as drivers of knowledge production, though anthropologists and historians have aimed to foreground the maneuverings, knowledge practices, and experiences of a wide variety of middle men and invisible technicians, including fieldworkers (Shapin 1989; Schumaker 2001; Raj 2007; Watkins and Swidler 2012; Bank and Bank 2013; Kingori 2013; Molyneux et al. 2013; Graboyes 2015; Maes 2015; du Plessis and Lorway 2016; Jacobs 2016).

Data collectors have long been portrayed as interchangeable with one another, and often do the grunt work or dirty work of survey research, including trudging from house to house in the field, collecting information, stool, urine, or blood samples, and so on. This book demonstrates that it is the creative and innovative tactics of fieldworkers that ensure that data collection proceeds smoothly, and their artful negotiation between top-down standards and bottom-up particularities—a kind of cooking data—that produces clean data as arbitrated by survey research standards. For this reason, three of the book's five empirical chapters center on the practices and interests of fieldworkers, taking the knowledge work they perform on a daily basis seriously as a form of expertise that emerges from their interactions with data and experience in the field—the spatial anchor from which much global health knowledge today emerges. Not unlike its construction in anthropology, the demographic field is the practical basis of analytical discourse (Fabian [1983] 2002, 21).

Researching Research in Malawi

This book is an ethnography of survey research projects that were collecting household-level data in Malawi in 2005 and 2007–2008. Driven by demand for current and detailed demographic and socioeconomic data on households in developing countries, and on the characteristics of those who live in those households, the data collected by these projects are a key source of evidence for economic and social policy analysis, development planning, program management, and decision making. The household survey has become the predominant mechanism for collecting information on populations in such contexts. I spent time with four projects working across the southern and central portions of the country in five districts. The book draws principally on fieldwork conducted with two projects: LSAM and MAYP. Both were collecting survey data and HIV tests in multiple waves from samples of thousands of Malawians, most of whom live in rural areas. Data from LSAM have tracked demographic, socioeconomic, and health conditions in rural Malawi, and MAYP data track a sample of young adults as they transition to marriage. As the longest-standing cohort study in the sub-Saharan African context, LSAM's data set begins in 1998, the first year it undertook field research in-country; since then, there have been six more survey waves, the last in 2012. From 2007–2009, MAYP collected data in three waves.

The book also incorporates ethnographic insights drawn from my fieldwork with two other projects: the Girls Schooling Intervention Project (GSIP) and the Religion and Malawi (RAM) project. A cash-incentives experimental study targeting girls of school-going age, GSIP also collected survey data and conducted HIV tests. The other, RAM, was a snowball-sampling-driven project collecting qualitative (interview and focus groups) and quantitative (questionnaire) data from religious leaders and church and mosque members in periurban southern Malawi that sheds light on the role of religious leaders in educating members of their churches and mosques about HIV/AIDS. While the bulk of ethnographic data in the book draws from the time I spent with LSAM and MAYP, some anecdotes and insights, as noted in the text, come from my time with GSIP and RAM. (See table I.1.)

In 2005, I first spent three months as a graduate student research assistant to LSAM, where my primary work was aiding with everyday research tasks

TABLE I.1 Survey Project Information

Project	Sample Size and Characteristics	Data Collected
LSAM	4,036 (2,361 women, 1,675 men)	Survey data, HIV tests, anthropometric data (height, weight, BMI)
MAYP	1,185 (598 women, 587 men)	Survey data, interview data, HIV tests
GSIP	3,810 young women	Survey data, interview data, HIV tests, health facility assessments, school and market surveys
RAM	620 men and women (80 religious leaders, 508 members of religious groups, 32 people living with HIV/AIDS, and 24 focus groups with religious leaders and religious group members)	Survey data, interview data, focus group discussion data

Source: Compiled by the author.

and overseeing a side project headed by a Malawian demographer that aimed to inventory cultural practices and their relationship to HIV risk across three districts in Malawi. I began to take interest in the culture and politics of survey research worlds and to formulate the research questions that animate this book. My relationships with LSAM principal investigators and Malawian researchers then led me to the other projects that agreed to host me in 2007–2008. American and European demographers headed LSAM, MAYP, and GSIP in collaboration with Malawian coprincipal investigators. All aimed to collect data that would shed light on social and economic trends over time relevant for understanding the trajectory of Malawi's AIDS epidemic, one of the most severe in the world. The fourth study, RAM, was led by two American researchers with PhDs in nursing whose work and institutional affiliations were aligned with global health nursing and who sought to understand what kinds of information religious leaders disseminated to their congregations about HIV/AIDS. All four projects employed Malawian fieldwork supervisors, data collectors, and data entry clerks for the duration of their fieldwork periods.

I participated in all aspects of fieldwork including survey design meetings, the recruitment and training of project staff, everyday fieldwork practices such as checking questionnaires with data collection teams, evening social events, trips to the airport to collect shipments of HIV test kits or other equipment, mapping exercises, data entry, and transcribing interviews. During data collection for each project, I lived alongside or with members of research teams. I spent the most consecutive time in the field with and around LSAM (three months in 2005 and then five months in 2008) and MAYP (three months in 2008). In addition to being a participant-observer during data collection, I also spent an extra month living in LSAM's and MAYP's sampling areas (Balaka and Salima, respectively) after the projects had departed in order to interview people living in recently surveyed households with my research assistant. While I initially planned to spend time only with LSAM, my broad interest in the politics of collaborative research and data collection led me to include the other projects in my research design so as to provide comparative context and to capitalize on the different tempos and data collection schedules of each project, all of which spent at least a few months engaged in fieldwork during the time span I was in Malawi. When I was not in the field with survey teams, I attended AIDS conferences and workshops where AIDS policy was discussed as well as interviewing a wide range of people involved in the world of AIDS research in Malawi, including research participants, chiefs and other traditional authorities, researchers, policy makers, government ministers, institutional review board (IRB) members, NGO staff, and district officials. Finally, I spent time in the Malawi National Archives reading documents, correspondence, and papers related to survey projects implemented in colonial Nyasaland. These censuses, surveys, and other enumerative efforts administered since the 1930s in Malawi provide useful historical context for my discussions of present-day surveys.

Throughout the book, I use the term "demographer" to refer to the core American, European, and Malawian researchers who were involved with LSAM, MAYP, and GSIP. Of those I interacted with most (thirteen), six held or were pursuing MAs or PhDs in economics, two in sociology, and five in demography. What unifies these researchers is their investment in the survey as a key tool in collecting data that will shed light on population dynamics, economic trends in rural Malawi, health issues, and the effects of the HIV epidemic on each of these. The questionnaire—in its imperative to collect standardized information that can be converted into numbers—is the base of these researchers' future analysis of a clean quantitative data set, to be followed by the dissemination of their results through journal articles, books, conferences, and other venues.

Demographers who were in academia at the time of this research were based at population studies or global health centers at the University of Malawi or American universities or, since few universities give degrees in demography, in other social science departments, primarily economics and sociology (Riley and McCarthy 2003; Cordell 2010). Three of the demographers were based at the World Bank at the time of my research in 2007–2008. Chapter 1 elaborates on how demographers render the statistical household to communicate differences in populations across time and space, an agenda I suggest is at the core of the discipline and unifies the researchers and others who produce and utilize the data sets discussed in this book (see appendix 2 for a sample household roster page from LSAM's 2008 survey that is representative of the same tool as implemented by MAYP and GSIP, as well). In the section that follows—and in chapter 1—I sketch an ideal-type demography that fails to capture the complexity and diversity of persons trained in this discipline, but nonetheless provides a heuristic sense of the general commitments of demographers for the reader; in this endeavor, I find Susan Watkins's (1993) term "the culture of [demography]" and Saul Halfon's (2006) term "population-based epistemic community" useful entry points. While culture(s) are unstable and dynamic, one can nonetheless extract patterns via ethnographic study of a discipline's thought, practices, and products.[4]

Demography and HIV/AIDS in Southern Africa

By 1998, more than two-thirds of the people living with HIV resided in sub-Saharan Africa, and by 2002, HIV/AIDS had become the leading cause of death for both men and women aged fifteen to fifty-nine globally (Carael and Glynn 2008, vii). Once it was realized that there was an AIDS epidemic and that it was worst in southern Africa, where Malawi is located, international organizations flooded into the region to attempt to stem the tide of the epidemic. Researchers contributed to these efforts by producing and disseminating knowledge of the ways that HIV can be prevented, treated, and contained. Rural Malawians widely associate the term "AIDS" with the Chichewa term for research (*kafukufuku*, notably used also to mean survey), pointing to the history of efforts since the 1990s, usually by outsiders, to document and thus contain the HIV virus through the collection of information, anthropomorphic data, and bodily fluids.

Approximately 10 percent of Malawi's population of 16.9 million is HIV positive, and it is ranked 173 of 188 countries on the Human Development Index (UNDP 2015). The mostly rural population engages in small-scale farming and depends heavily on rain-fed agriculture to grow maize to prepare the staple food dish, *nsima*. Subsistence agriculture is complemented by growing small cash crops (mostly tobacco and cotton), casual agricultural labor, and selling vegetables and secondhand clothing.

The projects discussed in this book all take up HIV/AIDS as a central indicator in the data they collect. Zuberi et al. (2003, 472) suggest that the rise in AIDS mortality is the most important feature of African population since the early 1990s, particularly in southern and eastern Africa, making population-based surveys and HIV testing important tools through which to know and measure the significant impact of HIV on rural Malawians' lives (Garenne 2011). Although Malawi's "silent epidemic" probably began before 1980— the first case was diagnosed in 1985—a strict ban imposed by postindependence life president Dr. Kamuzu Banda on discussing (or researching) family planning (until 1982) or social problems that would challenge his discourse of Malawi as his land of milk and honey prevented the topic from becoming a point of public discussion until much later (Kerr and Mapanje 2002; GoM 2003; Lwanda 2005; Illife 2006). Pushed by the Global Program on AIDS in Geneva and by Western donors, Banda did establish a short-term plan to contain AIDS by mid-1987 and set up the National AIDS Control Programme in 1989, but its mandate and objectives were impeded by political stagnancy (Wangel 1995). It was only after democratization in 1994, when Banda lost the election and newly elected president Bakili Muluzi publicly prioritized AIDS, that international organizations began unimpeded and intensive work in this arena, eventually complemented by an enhanced governmental response led by the National AIDS Commission (NAC), established in 2001 as a condition for receiving World Bank funding for AIDS (Putzel 2004). The NAC has since overseen AIDS prevention and care initiatives and coordinated the country's AIDS response.[5] Today, Malawi's AIDS budget continues to rely on international sources, with funds flowing from the World Bank, Global Fund, WHO/UNAIDS, and the President's Emergency Plan for AIDS Relief (PEPFAR), among many others.

The social sciences have played a central role in formulating policy and interventions into the AIDS epidemic in Malawi. Since the early 1990s, research has focused on assessing, among other things, AIDS-related beliefs, attitudes, and practices; determining the economic effects of HIV on the population; documenting support networks' care strategies for infected individuals; identifying a wide variety of ever-shifting risk groups (adolescent girls, truck drivers, sex workers, migrant laborers, and today's key populations, such as men who have sex with men); understanding low rates of condom use and/or family planning; and determining the feasibility and impact of HIV prevention and treatment efforts, lately male circumcision and distribution of antiretroviral therapy (McAuliffe 1994; Bisika and Kakhongwe 1995; Chirwa 1997; Illife 2006; GoM 2015).

The HIV virus interacts maliciously with tuberculosis, malaria, and bacterial infections and has significantly affected social and economic life in Africa. The impact of AIDS on social institutions in southern and eastern Africa has triggered interest in infectious disease, as manifest in the Global Fund to Fight AIDS, Tuberculosis and Malaria and several other global health initiatives. Anthropologists have documented the burgeoning projectification of the African landscape, with exceptional focus on AIDS (Nguyen 2010; Crane 2013; Dionne, Gerland, and Watkins 2013; Meinert and Whyte 2014; Prince 2014; Benton 2015; Moyer 2015); a body of excellent work in critical global health studies has examined how resource-poor settings become central sites for the rise of global health science that unfolds in clinics, trials, laboratories, and hospitals, particularly amid what Watkins and Swidler (2012) term "the AIDS enterprise."

This book builds on this scholarship but takes readers outside the wards, laboratories, and offices of global health and into the field that is the site of survey research. Understanding the population impact and dynamics of infectious disease is crucial to global health efforts to reduce morbidity and mortality and for decisions on where to best direct resources; data collected, cleaned, and analyzed by demographers plays a key role in untangling these variables and is vital to the measurement and practice of development in Africa. Indeed, many of the cooperative formations and partnerships between states, parastatals, and other organizations that fall broadly under the headings "development" and "global health" in Africa take as their main goal the achievement of indicators or targets that evaluate severity of health or economic conditions in a population over time, with AIDS as a central concern. Close scrutiny of the everyday socioscientific practices of survey research worlds can thus shed useful light on the politics of making numbers amid the rise of data-driven global health research in Africa.

An Ethnographer in Demographyland

I met with Richard Castells, a WHO epidemiologist, at Giraffe Lodge, a twenty-minute kabaza journey from LSAM's field headquarters in Balaka District. With another American epidemiologist, he has been commissioned by NAC to develop a new AIDS prevention strategy in collaboration with a local consultant. He is in Malawi for a short time to gather data from reports, interest groups, and interviews. . . . I noticed that Richard prefaced a lot of his sentences with "One thing I've noticed just from looking at the data . . ." I think this works to give him a kind of numerical authority that helps to obscure the fact that he has spent little to no time in Malawi, but lots of time amid numbers and statistics from "Malawi."[6]

A close reading of this excerpt from my field notes illuminates the enduring chasm between anthropology and the more quantitative applied and practical sciences. Richard, by virtue of his disciplinary training as an epidemiologist, holds intellectual interests and commitments very different from my own. Even in the semiprivate genre of field notes, I perform a boundary between Richard and myself: I have been in Malawi for a long time, Richard for a short time. I make clear that I took a local form of transportation to the lodge (*kabaza*, bicycle taxi), and leave unmarked that Richard likely traveled there in an air-conditioned suv from the capital. I view our meeting as potential data (e.g., "I noticed that . . . ," the act of recording field notes soon after the meeting), whereas Richard likely did not write up field notes after we parted. Richard, too, nods to our difference when he implies a contrast between his "*just* . . . looking at the data" and the kind of things I have been up to for over a year at this point in Malawi. Finally, my prose emphasizes the difference between an anthropological approach to Malawi (spending time in-country) and a demographic, expedient one (spending "lots of time amid numbers and statistics" that, in my view, will only ever capture a partial and scare-quoted "Malawi").

In 2007–2008, as an ethnographer of survey research worlds in Malawi, I came to identify as an anthropologist among the demographers, playing on Bernard Cohn's (1987) elaboration of the differences between the culture, forms of expertise, and even modes of dress of "Anthropologyland" and "Historyland." Like Cohn, I recognized myself as a sympathetic outsider to practitioners and thinkers from a discipline whose goals were at odds with the tenets anthropologists hold dear. I did not become a demographer, even if I did learn better how to see and think like one. I "played the stranger" to the culture of demography by "adopting a calculated and informed suspension of [my] taken-for-granted perceptions" of demographic practice and its products (Shapin and Schaffer 1985, 6). My own distrust of numbers aligned unexpectedly with some (certainly not all) demographers' explicit recognition that their data are fraught with limitations. The acknowledgment of uncertainty built into demographic methods and epistemology works to grant numbers a provisional certainty within the discipline. This book is decidedly not an effort to reclaim the power of numbers—they have enough power already—but rather seeks to present a fine-grained answer to the deceptively simple question: What's in a number? This project resonates with Caroline Bledsoe's (2002) brilliant study of fertility practices in the Gambia, but whereas she seeks to understand the vital events in women's lives that numbers claim to represent (the "lives behind the numbers"), this book aims to trace the lives of numbers themselves, and the social worlds and persons they produce as they come into being. The book illustrates how producing numbers is a technoscientific endeavor that generates new kinds of knowledge, persons, and politics along the way.

So what kinds of things did I get up to as an anthropologist among the demographers? In the following vignette and ensuing discussion, I aim to demonstrate my own position in the larger infrastructure of survey research.

> I sat in the LSAM minibus, red pen in hand, checking a survey that had recently been handed in by Ephraim, a fieldworker. Upon finishing, I called Ephraim over from where he was playing bao with an elderly man. He took a quick look at the red marks on his survey and headed back to the household for his callback. From the seat behind me, Esau, a supervisor who had been looking over my shoulder, said, "Crystal, you are not strict enough with them [the fieldworkers]. You need to reprimand them more strongly when they make mistakes . . . or they will just 'cheat' you."[7]

Esau not only chastises me for being too easy on fieldworkers, but manifests a reversal of the anthropological gaze as he, one of my informants, "strains to read over [my] shoulder" a survey that will soon enter into a larger "ensemble of texts" destined to gain meaning as data for demographers (Geertz 1977, 452). His gaze embodies a question I was asked again and again, usually playfully or with a wink, by informants ranging from district health officials to researchers to survey respondents after I explained my research on research to them: "But who will research you?" For many months, I joined fieldworkers making numbers in the field. Yet even as I participated in the daily peregrinations of fieldwork—searching for sample households, checking surveys, filling in log books, and commiserating over bad weather—I was recognizably different from my fellows. Aside from my obvious status as a white person (*mzungu*), I was an anthropologist. My intentions were not purely to collect clean data for survey projects, but to study them along the way.

In the scene above, Esau solidifies a boundary between us. Though I am trained as an anthropologist, he sees me as a novice fieldworker who has not yet absorbed the skills necessary to making good data. He thinks I am more easily cheated than Malawian supervisors. As an honorary fieldworker, I have different investments and lower material stakes than he and other fieldworkers do in living from project to project (for them, a livelihood; for me, fieldwork funded by grants). Finally, in marking up a survey, I play a role in assembling data. I am complicit as I critique, in other words. My corrections to Ephraim's survey alter and affect the quality of the data that will eventually become evidence. Somewhere in Malawi, perhaps, the surveys covered in my pen marks many years ago still sit in a dusty storage room, material traces of data now transferred into databases.

It was my complicity in the larger infrastructure of survey research worlds that afforded me a deeper understanding of where and how quantitative health data come to be facts. Along the way, I learned, as well, that my critical gaze was shared by the people I was studying: some demographers, too, are well aware of the shortcomings of their numbers, but keep making them for the sake of policy, journal articles, and a faint sense that they might somehow improve the lives of rural Malawians. Like their informants who complained about the "too small" gift of soap they received after participating in a survey (see chapter 3), demographers recognized that soap is an inadequate gift for data, but kept giving it because it fit best into the ethical guidelines for human subjects research that govern their activities. Fieldworkers did not need me to tell them that their project-to-project lifestyle exploits them and articulated fine analyses of the structural effects of global health and the AIDS industry on their livelihoods and the well-being of the villagers they encountered. Rural research respondents made clear their critiques of extractive logics undergirding survey research, even if they did not dress them up in the jargon familiar to scholars, but talked about bloodsuckers instead. Policy makers told me they knew that policy was not as evidence-based as we might think and explicitly theorized the gap between themselves and researchers in their ivory towers. Tracing data's life course from survey design meetings to downstream sites reveals a diversity of actors whose practices and rhetoric reflect their position relative to the other actors in survey research worlds and to the data they are meant to collect and protect.

I took up a temporary position as an honorary fieldworker on the demographers' assembly line, likewise training my mind and body to absorb guidelines and standards for clean data. I wore a *chitenje*, proper field attire, when interacting with research subjects. I grew faster and more efficient at checking surveys as time went on. I surveilled fieldworkers to ensure they were doing what they were supposed to. With supervisors, I kept meticulous log books that tracked the outcomes of research encounters. While *Cooking Data* stands in as the primary material artifact of my fieldwork, the numbers I helped produce are delinked from me and float anonymously in databases. The I-witnessing of the anthropologist, so evident in ethnographic representations, is contrasted with the collective and anonymized labor of survey research (Geertz 1988).

As anthropologists of global health and science, it is important to consider our own role in reproducing the logics, intentions, and data of the institutions we study, even as we position ourselves as critics of them. Discussions with my disciplinary fellows indicates that we check surveys, fill out bureaucratic forms, check pulses, file papers, lead trainings, create leaflets, author grant proposals for NGOs, and so on in the field. This, too, is the labor of fieldwork today, but often remains obscured by normative definitions of critique that still require us to present ourselves as somehow "float[ing] above" our subjects and seeing what they don't, even if we long ago exchanged Malinowski's "white canvas tent . . . on a beach" for clinical wards, minibuses, and air-conditioned NGO offices (Taussig 2009, 120–121). Critique seems to rely on preserving a kind of god's-eye view whereby the objects of global health and other enumerative projects can only be seen from the outside (Haraway 1988), covering over how anthropologists make global health in the process of studying it, and continue to be as "doubly ambivalent," perhaps, as our colonial predecessors—in quiet collaboration with power and institutions even as we critique them (James 1973, 42).

Bad Numbers: Anthropologies and Histories of (Postcolonial) Quantification

Despite efforts from both sides, anthropology and demography have largely maintained their distance. In this section, I hope to elaborate this divide without valorizing anthropology (my own discipline), instead emphasizing that what are considered good data—trustworthy, valuable, and usable—in each field can help us see why the two disciplines often do not see eye to eye. This divide parallels the broader critical position that anthropology adopts relative to disciplines and projects that rely on quantitative evidence. Surveys, censuses, and other enumerative projects are key sites of biopower where vital aspects of life are enlisted into political calculation, governance, and management (Foucault [1978] 2007, 333–361). Anthropologists have shown how numbers—rather than stable or objective stand-ins for reality—are provisional and malleable entities that reflect their political and epistemological contexts (Andreas and Greenhill 2010; Lampland 2010; Erikson 2012; Hodzic 2013; Adams 2016a).

Demography, glossed as the quantitative study of human populations, with central interest in size, growth, density, migration, and vital statistics, is a positivist science rooted in the assumption that reality can be observed, measured, and counted accurately. Surveys such as those discussed in this book are at the core of the discipline's effort to successfully count, describe, and monitor people and events; as a methodological instrument, the survey claims to collect "identical data from . . . varied settings" that can be easily analyzed by statisticians who may never set foot in the geographic places—the field— where the data originated (Riley and McCarthy 2003, 55). Inevitable progress toward low fertility (which implies also progress toward modernity vis-à-vis normative interpretations of the demographic transition) is at the core of demographic thought, and a search for universal explanations for trends in population finds expression in the numerical data demographers collect and the methods they use to make knowledge (Bledsoe 2002, 19–56).

In this brief overview of demography's interests and pursuits—which are elaborated in chapter 1—we observe how far afield they seem from those of the anthropologist. Demographic approaches to human population, in general, stress the individual rational actor Homo economicus, neglect the historical and political context of demographic variables, and rely on quantitative data and methods that masquerade as objective and value neutral (Riley and McCarthy 2003, 40; Szreter, Sholkamy, and Dharmalingam 2004). Further, amid demographers' growing interest in enlisting quasi-anthropological methods into their work since the 1970s, anthropologists have been dissatisfied with their treatment and definitions of culture, viewing them as too simplistic, dated, or unreflexive (Greenhalgh 1990, 1995, 4, 13; Hammel 1990; Kertzer 1995; Kertzer and Fricke 1997; Coast 2003).[8] Leading demographers of Africa Caldwell and Caldwell's (1987) important article on the cultural context of high fertility in sub-Saharan Africa—cited 803 times at this writing— identifies the need to place fertility in a broader context than surveys can capture, yet still falls into many of the above traps and describes culture as a "seamless whole" to boot (410). Demography has looked to anthropology as a quick fix in response to critiques of its "culture blindness" from outside the discipline. From the anthropologist's perspective, meanwhile, anthropology's totem—culture—has been made profane in the course of its travels to Demographyland.

The gulf between anthropology and demography is reflected, as well, in the different orientations that the respective disciplines have toward numbers, and particularly toward the history of numbers as tools of imperial and state power. Whereas anthropologists are number averse and harbor suspicions of quantification as a mode of knowing, demographers are happily awash in numbers and consider well-collected quantitative data to accurately represent reality. Indeed, a main point of controversy between anthropologists and demographers is how they might answer the question, What is the relationship between data and the social reality it claims to represent or count? Whereas demographers invest much time and money in revealing or discovering reality, anthropologists contend that classificatory exercises such as counting or surveying create reality or "make up" people (Hacking 1986; Greenhalgh 2004).[9] Whereas the former seek to control the field even from afar, the latter remain open to the many surprises it holds; both approaches, it is important to note, carry with them different costs and benefits that underscore their investments in collecting a particular kind of good data. To oversimplify, demographers deem description and interpretation to be autonomous endeavors, while anthropologists have, since at least the 1980s, made much of their labor debunking that separation. Anthropologists, as we will see in detail in chapter 1, have thoroughly critiqued the categories, variables, and taxonomies at the heart of survey design for failing to acknowledge the diversity and dynamism of cultural contexts and definitions (Hirschman 1987; Bledsoe, Houle, and Sow 2007; Johnson-Hanks 2007; Loveman 2007; Bledsoe 2010).

Anthropologists and other scholars have shown that there has long been a link between those who measure or count population-based phenomena and those who seek to govern or control populations. Demography, in its focus on the very aspects of a population—birth, death, health, longevity, and so on—that Foucault places at the heart of governmentalized societies, is profoundly implicated in biopolitical projects (Foucault 1978 [2007]). Statistics are the "science of the state" (Foucault 1991, 96), a major tool through which the state sees and knows its citizens (Anderson 1991; Appadurai 1996; Scott 1998). The census—and its technologies, including the survey—shape the way states and other actors imagine their dominion, and its categories are key tools of power and empire in their ability to exoticize and classify citizens into moralized groupings and to affect the distribution of goods, allocations of social power, and services (Cohn 1987, 224–254; Kertzer and Arel 2002; Greenhalgh 2004; Cordell 2010; Mamdani 2012). As I show elsewhere, following James Scott (1998), demographers of Africa engage in a kind of "seeing like a research project" (Biruk 2012), and such optics produce the kinds of indicators and numbers that are at the core of global governance regimes today (Davis, Kingsbury, and Merry 2012; Gerrets 2015a).

Here it is worth noting, however, that the modern state at the core of Foucault's theorizations of biopower is an analytical category that might fail to capture the nuance of the colonial state's imagining and management of its subjugated populations and, moreover, obscure the racism and racialization constitutive of biopolitical projects in Africa today. Megan Vaughan (1991) usefully suggests that even as colonial subjects were "unitized" by enumerative practices such as censuses or taxation efforts or, for example, weighing and measuring Nyasa migrant laborers, these processes were merely preliminary to the colonial state's agenda of aggregation, producing a collective Otherness invested in the overriding difference of race. Colonial medical discourse denied the possibility that Africans were self-aware subjects, throwing a wrench into Foucault's fulcrum of biopower: the subjectified "speaking subject" (Vaughan 1991, 8–13). Indeed, we might better consider how "racializing assemblages," where sociopolitical processes—here, counting—that parsed populations into human (colonizer) and not-quite-human (colonized) were the pivot of colonial governance (Weheliye 2014); such taxonomies hinged on "cultural difference" and were the alibi of racialized violence enacted in the name of civilization or hygiene projects (Pierre 2013). Agnes Riedmann (1993) documents African demography's role, in particular, as an agent of cultural imperialism. Global governance regimes, including human rights and global health, likewise stake claims to a form of suffering predicated on racialized bodies whose difference is often depoliticized by benevolent universalizing language. As will become especially clear in chapter 4, the legacies of racialized colonial imaginings of African others persist in some of the survey tools implemented today in the name of health and development.

King (2002) suggests that the conversion logics that undergirded colonial health projects invested in replacing traditional knowledge and practices with modern biomedical and scientific thought have shifted. He argues that the defining feature of postcolonial global health is integrating local places into global networks of information exchange, an endeavor undergirded by modern projects of total surveillance (782). Demography today has inherited its slot among the human sciences as a "policy-implicated discipline" (Szreter, Sholkamy, and Dharmalingam 2004, 20). Demand for demography's products remains high, even if the focus of research is often limited by the strings attached to funding flows to policy-relevant topics. For demography's products to remain saleable, they must be quantitative, standardized, and replicable (Demeny 1988; Riley and McCarthy 2003, 77); as we will see in chapter 5, data carries with it a brand that imbues it with quality and makes some data more in demand than others.

African Demography

Demography came of age during the mid-twentieth century, largely through its institutionalization in the United States. Amid rising concern about population growth, population became central to American definitions of development, and funding from both private and government organizations for population research increased (Riley and McCarthy 2003, 61–67). The 1960s and 1970s saw the founding of a number of population studies centers based at major American universities (Michigan, North Carolina, Brown, Johns Hopkins, Penn, and Columbia) funded by institutions such as the Hewlett Foundation, Mellon, National Institute of Health and Childhood Development, and the National Institutes of Health, amid the rise of the international family planning movement and Rockefeller and Ford Foundation funding that fostered the field of demography (Demeny 1988; Cleland and Watkins 2006).

Field sites in Africa are a major source of data for the long-term demographic projects based at such population studies centers; the University of Pennsylvania's center, for example, has "always been heavily weighted toward international population research . . . with a strong ameliorative component" (UPPSC 2017). Some suggest that the relatively secure funding available for demographic research has enabled demographers to avoid critically examining their premises; as Greenhalgh (1995, 10) contends, postmodernism did not enter demography as it did the other social sciences (Riedmann 1993, 96–110). In general, these critiques suggest that demography is a field weak or thin on theory and the most matter-of-fact discipline (Desrosiéres 1998). Its main investments are methodological: improving data collection and analysis processes to collect more and better data (McNicoll 1990).

The surveys discussed herein, as legacies of technoscientific projects in the service of colonial interests, raise the specter of the exploitation, extractive logics, racism, and ethnocentrism that have underlain science in Africa, and global demography's presumed "right to invade" in the name of knowledge production (Riedmann 1993). As can be seen in chapter 3, impoverished survey participants in 2007–2008 drew on extensive past experience with research projects to evaluate whether or not to participate in a survey headed by researchers from wealthy countries that might bring them no returns; subjects were highly research conscious and expressed their suspicions or wariness of the means and ends of projects by employing resistive tactics that threatened to influence data quality. Residents across sub-Saharan Africa have by now become accustomed to projects in their midst. Diverse actors were interested in counting and enumerating Africa's population(s) even before the first official or modern census efforts. Owusu (1968) notes that precolonial head counts carried out by chiefs saw the heads of families drop articles such as grains of cereal, beads, or cowrie shells that stood in for the number of a chief's dependents, for example.

Early colonial counting practices largely entailed unscientific walking tours by district officials, estimating local populations with the help of word-of-mouth information from local people, or via simple head counts. These ad hoc techniques were likely adopted by the earliest census takers in Nyasaland in 1901 (Deane 1953, 143; Zuberi and Bangha 2006; Gervais and Mandé 2010). The first systematic attempt to describe the population dynamics of sub-Saharan Africa was Kuczynski's (1949) *Demographic Survey of the British Colonial Empire*, meant to be useful evidence to help in implementation of the Colonial Development and Welfare Act (1940), which provided for large investment in development, agricultural, and health research (Havinden and Meredith 1993). In colonial Malawi, the late 1930s saw the implementation of an ambitious nutrition survey project whose commitments and implications are elaborated in the course of this book and which was symptomatic of a mid-1930s rising colonial interest in coordinating and funding health and agricultural research initiatives in Nyasaland and the Rhodesias (CAA 1935; 1936). As Tilley (2011) documents, from the mid-1930s, the ambitious African Survey led by Lord Hailey shaped research priorities in Britain and colonial Africa, solidifying its role as a living laboratory increasingly dotted by scientific field stations. The migration of the loose discipline of population studies to Africa was somewhat coterminous with the rise of international health as a field of practice and the rise of development as a central concern (Packard 2016, 181–186).

Scholars and policy makers have paid close attention to population in Africa and the global South since World War II; the first world population conference that drew institutes, researchers, and implementers from around the globe was in 1954, and the first round of the African Census Program was initiated in the mid-1960s (Ghana held the first modern census on the continent in 1960; Malawi's first census was in 1966). Access to populations increased by the 1970s and 1980s via censuses; knowledge, attitudes, and practices surveys of fertility in the 1960s; the World Fertility Survey; and the Demographic and Health Surveys (DHS) program (Tarver 1996, 7–8).[10] In 1984, the Union for

African Population Studies—whose 2007 conference in Arusha, Tanzania, figures in chapter 5—was founded through a UN initiative to promote the scientific study of population and application of research evidence in Africa. Headquartered in Accra, Ghana, the association has convened a general conference on African population every four years since 1988 in an African country (UAPS 2017).

In the mid-1990s, the institutionalization of population studies and demography on the continent continued with the establishment of the African Population and Health Research Center (APHRC) in Nairobi, Kenya, and the Africa Centre for Health and Population Studies in South Africa, both of which play a key role in collecting field-based survey data in Africa and as collaborators with foreign researchers engaged in data collection. Likewise, increasing opportunities for training of African demographers and statisticians—some of which have been included in proposals as capacity-building activities by the projects discussed in this book—has made a dent in the huge volume of statistics and publications produced exclusively by researchers from other countries (Oucho and Ayiemba 1995, 73).[11] Nonetheless, as will become evident in chapters 1 and 5, disparities in access to data, graduate training, and statistical software and asymmetries in the material conditions of foreign and Malawian researchers poke holes in global health's dominant rhetoric of "partnership" and "collaboration" (Crane 2010b).

Rethinking Poor Numbers

The imperative to collect high-quality, clean data (terms whose precise meanings are elaborated in chapter 1) is at the core of survey research and underlies demographers' dreams of data production on a well-oiled assembly line. The harmonizing efforts of survey projects aim to combat the problems of data quality that have long plagued similar endeavors in colonial and post-colonial African contexts. Talk about data from and within Africa since the colonial period has trafficked in metaphors of scarcity, lack, and poor quality (Hill 1990). In the classic volume *The Demography of Tropical Africa*, Lorimer (1968, 3) calls for a shift from cruder sources of demographic information (such as tax registration) to more systematic efforts such as surveys or censuses, and van de Walle (1968, 13, 59) observes that the inability of Africans to know their exact ages or to identify dates without being accustomed to calendars leads to poor data quality.

Many reflections on data in Africa implicitly place responsibility for poor data quality on the figure of the African enumerator, not unlike Martin's

(1949) comments on the 1948 census. This trend dates from the colonial period. Lord Hailey, reflecting on the immense need for population statistics in the pages of his *African Survey* (published in 1938), suggested, "There is still much to be learnt of the technique of sampling in African conditions, and it must, moreover, be recognized that whatever the advance made in technique, there will remain the problem of securing enumerators who can elicit the information required" (Hailey 1957, 139). Phyllis Deane (1953, 10), in her analysis of data collected in the late 1930s on economic transactions in Northern Rhodesia (present-day Zambia) and Nyasaland, suggests that "deficiencies in data" were attributable to the lack of trained African research assistants. In the present, meanwhile, the costliness in time and money of the intensive prefieldwork training sessions for fieldworkers illustrates researchers' enduring perception that fieldworkers are likely to mess up their data.

Researchers have likewise long associated Africa itself with bad population data. Oucho and Ayiemba (1995, 44) suggest that prior to the 1970s, "the African continent was a desert in terms of availability of accurate and reliable demographic data." In an annual review article, Zuberi et al. (2003) note that understandings of Africa's demography up to the present day are based on the unsystematic analysis of data from different sources and periods. The head of the Statistics and Survey Unit at the APHRC suggests that it aims to fill a "data gap" in Africa, where the paucity of "accurate, reliable, and timely data" has constrained effective monitoring of development programs and interventions on the continent (Beguy 2016). Responding to this discourse of data scarcity and problems, economic historian Morten Jerven's (2013, 32) important book-length analysis of the poor quality of statistics pertaining to economic development in Africa is an effort to "gauge the size of errors and evaluate the direction of bias in [statistical] evidence," which are often obscured by data users' blind faith in the experts who produce or interpret numbers.

Amid a sea of poor numbers, however, it should be noted that the data collected by the survey projects described here yield—by demographic criteria—better numbers than, for example, censuses or DHS surveys, because they provide localized surveillance in a smaller area over time. Unlike the census, which aims to provide a full, comprehensive count of a nation's population for the government, or DHS surveys, which yield nationally representative data, the surveys discussed here collect responses from individual agents in a sample—a portion of the total population drawn from the same enumeration units employed by the census and DHS. Data from the surveys in this book complement census data by administering comprehensive and directed questions to a random sample.

Despite the generally critical or antagonistic relationship of anthropology to demography, the book does not endeavor to prove that demographic data fail to represent rural Malawian realities or to expose their uncertainty, but rather takes a more sympathetic tack toward quantifying projects (Colvin 2015). Rather than dismissing numbers as simply false, socially constructed, or inaccurate, the book aims to critically examine the criteria and metrics that help numbers attain their legitimacy and authority by presenting a fine-grained account of data's life course and handling by many diverse actors. Others have sufficiently critiqued the quality of Africa's poor numbers, showing how and why quantifying projects often get things wrong or miss out on what is really going on. Building on this work, I analyze in depth the social lives and cultural work that numerical data do, even before they appear as statistics. Numerical data's provisional and uncertain status, I show, is often well known to those who make it. Following Lampland (2010, 2): "Provisional and false numbers can only function if there is some sort of agreement about their status as temporary or fragile symbols" and "false numbers appear when the primary task is to learn how to deploy numbers, making the relative accuracy of the numerical sign less important than the attempt to master the logic of formal procedures." As Erikson (2012, 373) points out, even if numbers are "hollow" they enable other forms of value to be produced.

This book does not aim to determine how accurate estimates of HIV prevalence or other statistical phenomena are, but carefully considers how demographers tell (themselves and others) convincing stories about AIDS and other social, economic, and health issues in Malawi through numbers (Setel 2000, 10). These stories reveal some things clearly and hide others, not unlike the stories anthropologists tell about their field sites (Wendland 2016, 60). We should remember that, even as numbers and surveillance are at the heart of colonial and present-day governance projects of racialized bodies, they nonetheless can do important work in turning uneventful suffering into aggregate suffering and making it visible (Povinelli 2011, 14; Livingston 2012; Stevenson 2014, 186). Furthermore, being counted in an impoverished context such as Malawi might entail forms of incorporation, recognition, and support that would be otherwise unavailable (Ferguson 2015, 85).

In this sense, this book critically examines the criteria and metrics that underscore data's production and consumption. These standardizing criteria, rather than being stable, are invented, embodied, and negotiated in the everyday practices of research worlds. Like other recent work by scholars engaged in critical global health studies, this book considers how large-scale outsider-led projects in Africa are situated in and rely on local regimes of economic, cultural, and social capital. However, the emphasis is on showing how a particular set of epistemic criteria creates the human and social scaffolding for its implementation and to what ends. Importantly, it challenges the abstract universality of data unanchored from its site and relations of production by showing how Malawi and Malawians shaped it.

Scholars have shown how numbers, categories, and statistics are taken up, critiqued, or negotiated by those they claim to represent; this book contends that understanding how those who make numerical data handle and engage with it can shed new light on the politics, stakes, and unintended consequences of quantification in sub-Saharan Africa. While the book is an account of enumeration practices in academic-demographic research, my analysis of how these practices operate in the field should resonate with those involved in implementing operations research and monitoring evaluation projects—which often face more time constraints and are less well funded than the projects in this book—as well. This book reflects the potential of anthropology's commitment to "slow research" amid the value placed on speed, efficiency, standards, and comparability in global health, development, NGO worlds, and population science (Adams, Burke, and Whitmarsh 2014), but also prompts anthropologists to reflect on how our own data activities likewise cook data, with important implications for the claims it is possible to make (my own attempt to do this appears in the conclusion). A granular analysis of research worlds in a particular place at a particular time, the book suggests, encourages us to more critically engage with the kinds of evidence we too often take for granted, whether inside or outside our discipline or training.

Assembling Data: A Road Map

In chapter 1, I introduce the work that must be done before survey research projects enter the field where data will be collected. The chapter interprets survey design, the first step in assembling data, as an exercise that attempts to amalgamate the idealized categories of insider (local) and outsider (foreign) expertise. In analyzing debates between Malawian and foreign collaborators around cultural and linguistic translation and fine-tuning of survey concepts and questions, around plans for where surveys should be administered, and around what should be the objectives of research, the chapter draws attention to the different material and academic investments of foreign and Malawian researchers in data collection, which are often obscured by partnership rhetoric. Chapter 1 illustrates how demographers' dreams of an assembly line for data take shape in the office, before data collection begins in the field.

The middle three chapters of the book center their attention on data collectors, whose practices in the field determine the quality of data. Chapter 2 introduces the Malawian secondary school or college graduates employed as data collectors by research projects, unskilled middlemen who have been overlooked in accounts of science in Africa, despite their central roles in producing and handling data. Since the earliest surveys were enacted in sub-Saharan Africa, these individuals have been portrayed as menial laborers, as interchangeable cogs in the machinery, and as liabilities to the collection of good data. Chapter 2 challenges such assumptions by showing how data collectors, through serial research project jobs, acquire particular forms of expertise that ensure projects run smoothly. I describe fieldworkers' interests in maintaining ownership over the local knowledge foreign researchers expect them to possess. I also examine prefieldwork training sessions as an important site where fieldworkers are initiated into new professional identities and where social and spatiotemporal boundaries that undergird data collection are performed. Throughout, the chapter takes interest in how fieldworkers come to live from project to project, enabling them some measure of access to social, cultural, and economic capital, and producing new forms of value and expertise.

Chapter 3 examines the transactions that undergird the administration of household-level surveys. Centering the encounters between fieldworkers and their rural Malawian research subjects, it explicitly considers the value of data for different actors in research worlds. In line with international human subjects research ethics that privilege informed consent and prohibit provision of inducements that might endanger it, research participants were given bars of soap as a gift in exchange for information they provide to research teams. I interpret this standardized gift as a central site where people negotiate political, ethical, and moral questions that arise in research worlds. This standard research gift facilitates the recognition that bits of information are tangible items with a negotiable value and highlights the role of small-scale transactions in stabilizing—and potentially unraveling—data as they move through their life course. Chapter 4 argues that producing high-quality data necessitates standardization of habits, scripts, and social interactions across thousands of research encounters in the field. I employ ethnographic analysis to show how demographers' epistemic investment in clean data that is accurate, reliable, and timely not only guides the movements and agendas of survey research teams in the field but also produces categories, identities, and practices that reinforce and challenge these standardizing values.

Chapter 5, the final empirical chapter, is an ethnographic study of downstream sites where data in their clean and finished forms are performed to and consumed by audiences. It is concerned with how the kind of data repre-sented as raw (survey responses, HIV tests), discussed in previous chapters, is validated as evidence in the policy-research arena. Drawing on participant observation at a number of Malawi-based, regional, and international AIDS research conferences where quantitative health data were presented, at policy-making sessions and meetings, and on interviews with survey researchers working in multiple African contexts, I show how knowledge is made and evaluated in contingent social performances that employ scripts, props, lead-ing actors, special effects, and supporting actors. I interpret these sites as con-tingent end points in data's life story, and show how even data in their final finished form as evidence are further cooked in their re-presentations and in social relations. The chapter also critically analyzes the discourse of the policy-research gap—conceived of as a chasm of blocked communication or knowledge sharing between researchers and policy makers. I show how this gap is better analyzed as a confluence of multiple interests that determine the kinds of evidence that gain authority in the policy-research nexus, and the efficacy of its translation between the two spheres.

The book's conclusion is a meditation on the meanings, intentions, and as-sumptions embedded in the anthropological project to critique global health and other research institutions in Africa. I present vignettes from my field notes that did not make it into the empirical chapters of the book to turn the lens on the anthropologist among the demographers. I take up long-standing concerns of anthropologists—complicity, the field, and the compulsion to make our work useful—from the perspective of a contemporary ethnogra-pher of global health. The conclusion takes full circle the main interest of the book by showing how data—whether demographic or ethnographic, quan-titative or qualitative—reflect and cohere the social worlds they claim to represent.

ONE

THE OFFICE IN THE FIELD

Building Survey Infrastructures

It is market day at Mangochi turnoff in southern Malawi, and the trading center is bustling with activity. Buyers and sellers of *kaunjika* (secondhand clothes), sneakers, vegetables, printed fabrics, and batteries bargain over prices and socialize, creating a low buzz of voices against a backdrop of persistently blaring minibus horns. On a sunny June morning in 2008, I walk a short distance away from the busy trading center. Passing an open-air butcher shop where young men sit beneath a tall tree hung with two goat carcasses, I arrive at a large compound. Surrounded by walls hand painted with bright advertisements for Boom washing powder and Panadol pain relievers, a squat rest house sits back from the open gates: a favored stop for truck drivers, the rustic motel is called Mpaweni, or Other People's Place.

There is no vacancy at Mpaweni. Its rooms have been taken over by the fieldwork teams—American researchers and graduate students and Malawian fieldworkers, data entry clerks, and drivers—of the Longitudinal Study of AIDS in Malawi (LSAM), a cohort study that has collected demographic data in villages nearby since 1998. For the next two months, fieldworkers will survey and HIV test about a thousand Malawians. From a vantage point in the dirt courtyard, a visitor might not notice that one of the motel's conference rooms has been converted into a makeshift field office. Data entry teams tap at the keyboards of LSAM-owned laptops, manually transferring data codes from the dusty pages of completed surveys administered the day before to a growing database. Boxes of Lifebuoy body soap and Sunlight laundry soap are piled neatly around the periphery of the room, gifts that will compensate research participants for answering the questions that make up this year's twenty-five-page survey. A photocopier and printer whir quietly, printing off endless copies of questionnaires, consent forms, and log forms that will soon be filled in with data and information. Electrical cords snake underfoot, ending in overworked power strips that protect the electronic devices in the room from the periodic power surges and outages so common in Malawi. Parked helter-skelter around the compound are minibuses that carry fieldworkers to the project's sample villages, all within an hour's drive of Mpaweni: one by one, fieldworkers will visit the households where the members of the study sample live.

Mpaweni is the temporary headquarters for LSAM for the duration of data collection fieldwork. In the words of local residents who notice the visitors around town, "Akafukufuku abweranso! [The researchers have come again!]"

. . .

The scene at Mpaweni hints at the massive human and material infrastructure that must be built in order for large-scale survey research to be carried out in a corner of Malawi far from LSAM's home office in the Population Studies Center at an elite research university in the United States. Reams of paper, laptops, and extension cords must be carried to the field from abroad or from Lilongwe; minibuses must be rented to ferry field teams to and from rural households; fieldworkers must be hired; housing must be found for researchers and fieldwork supervisors for the duration of data collection; and green bricks—in 1,000-kwacha increments rubber-banded together—must be withdrawn periodically from cash points to pay the salaries and per diems of fieldworkers employed by the project. Trips to the airport to pick up arriving researchers or imported items, such as weight scales to collect anthropomorphic data and HIV test kits to collect samples from respondents, were a weekly occurrence. Sometimes items such as the test kits would get tied up in customs bureaucracy, necessitating complex efforts to free them. Building the temporary infrastructure of people and things necessary to carry out peripatetic survey research in one of the poorest countries in the world is a Herculean task.

This chapter shows how planning and designing field survey projects entails imaginative work on the part of researchers who aim to translate standards—conjured in the office—into clean, high-quality data produced in the messy space of the field. Adopting the position of an anthropologist among the demographers, as discussed in the introduction, I first elaborate how the human infrastructure for survey research, made up of foreign and Malawian experts who bring different expertise to the table, is built in difficult conditions. I draw attention to the disparate material and academic investments of foreign and Malawian researchers in data collection, often obscured by the discourse of partnership or collaboration central to development, humanitarian, and global health worlds today (Mercer 2003; Crane 2010b; Watkins and Swidler 2012; Kenworthy 2014; Thoreson 2014; Brown 2015; Gerrets 2015b). In the second half of the chapter, I articulate the epistemological dreams and standards that call into being the infrastructure for data collection in the field. In analyzing debates between Malawian and foreign collaborators around cultural and linguistic translation and the fine-tuning of survey concepts, instruments, and questions, around plans for where surveys should be administered, and around what should be the objectives of research, the chapter excavates the multiple interests and forms of expertise that coalesce in the pages of a survey, even before it is administered to the first household in the field.

The survey questionnaire is the tool at the core of data production and operates as a framing device that aspires to make Malawi visible and intelligible as data or numbers that circulate among demographers or policy makers: "The world appears to the observer as a relationship between picture and reality, the one present but secondary, a mere representation, the other only represented, but prior, more original, more real" (Mitchell 1991, 60). The survey—as the key mechanism of ordering, counting, and framing the division between real and represented—plays a central role in effecting what demographers experience as a good-enough representation of the really real: data. As I show, the questionnaire itself and data practices in the field reflect a fundamental distrust of data on the part of the most diligent demographers, who recursively ask themselves and others, Are the data good? Is this the right question to answer our research problem? Are people lying? Are fieldworkers cooking the data? These questions arise in the prefieldwork meetings discussed in this chapter, but, more importantly, they are a quality of data themselves. If one assumes one can collect data that transcend these questions and the uncertainty they signal, posing such questions indicates that uncertainty is inherent to data themselves. This chapter's central interest is in how questions, standards, and tools that eventually produce quantitative data that are devised in the office are translated into and for the field. I theorize translation as an ongoing and improvised practice that privileges the epistemic investments of those who design the survey, one that betrays their shared imagination of a cultural Other who will answer their questions, leaves the culture of demography itself unmarked, and prefigures the nature of data to be collected.

From the Office to the Field: The Spatial Politics of Data Production

I sometimes get depressed when I come to Malawi. I'm used to sitting in my office crunching numbers and having the categories be anonymous, not personified. . . . But I'm pretty wedded to coming to check up on things. . . . If you don't come now and then you have no idea what is going on in the field if you don't hover over people's shoulders there. —Dr. Jones, economist and MAYP coprincipal investigator, September 20, 2007

The way you enter the village the first time, will remain in the minds of the people and will also determine the success or failure of your objectives. . . . As a fieldworker [you] should know that the [villagers'] culture has been there for ages. . . . To effectively work with the community you also have to be participative in the community, attend funerals, attend village meetings to show you are not just there to work, but you are one of them. However . . . attending political rallies [is not advised]. . . . You might only be a part of one group thereby losing the other. . . . Refrain from any political gatherings or debates to be part of the whole community. —LSAM Fieldwork Manual 2008

Reading these two texts alongside each other—the first an excerpt from an interview with a Marriage and Youth Project (MAYP) researcher and the second an excerpt from a fieldwork manual designed by Malawian supervisors working with LSAM for many years—I am struck by their shared construction of a place called "the field." Dr. Jones sets up a clear contrast between being in her office "crunching numbers" and being in the field. Implicit in this contrast is an assumption that the office is a clean space for data analysis and tinkering with numbers while the field is a messy place where numbers become people. In the office, it is easy to "forget that the numbers once represented people with real communities and real histories and complex genealogies" (Jain 2013, 36), but this becomes more difficult when researchers like Dr. Jones confront poverty and suffering firsthand on a visit to Malawi.

Jones acknowledges, however, the importance of visiting the field now and then to check up on the activities transpiring there, hinting at their potential influence on the data that wind up in the office. Although when we met she had been in Malawi for only a few days, she asserted her difference from other economists who never set foot "on the ground" (in the field). Her insinuation that things might go awry in the field if one doesn't "hover over people's shoulders" connotes epistemological and structural hierarchies that characterize survey projects: she looks over the shoulders of potentially unreliable Malawian fieldworkers on the front lines of data collection, implicitly acknowledging their ability to mess up or dirty the data to be ferried to the office.

Finally, the distinction she draws between anonymous numbers and categories and personified realities indexes the interest of this chapter in how abstract standards and ideals for clean data translate into the field and hints at how subjective practices in the latter might erode the objective status often granted to statistical data. Across a large body of published work on guidelines, methods, and survey design across cultural contexts, the construction of the field as a place of "difficult geographic topography" rife with "weather and seasonal impediments" and "danger[s]" that threaten to "bungle" a survey is consistent (Pennell, Levenstein, and Lee 2010; see also Bulmer and Warwick 1983). "The field" compels the translation work needed to link standard survey methodology and procedures to "environments of stringent budgetary constraints in countries with widely varying levels of survey infrastructure and technical capacity" (Yansaneh 2005, 5). To manage impediments to smooth and timely data collection in remote or rustic locales, survey projects sometimes selected the sites for their data collection based on their proximity to the office. For example, MAYP's research proposal notes that researchers selected Salima District to administer its surveys because working in only one district (as opposed to several) would allow the field staff to monitor data quality. As an added benefit, Salima is close to the national capital, thus reducing project transport and infrastructure costs. Even before the first survey is administered, then, behind-the-scenes decisions determine and delimit the nature and quality of data to be collected, in this case, via convenient bounding of the sample area.

The Malawian supervisors who authored the fieldwork manual (cited above) meant to provide guidelines to fieldworkers implementing LSAM's 2008 survey similarly construct the field as a place of difference, distance, and complexity. They cast it as foreign to the fieldworkers who will enter it for the first time and attempt to prepare the teams for the culture they will find there, presumably more pronounced, dense, traditional, visible, and different than their own culture, which, of course, is not recognized as such. Fieldworkers are advised to walk a fine line between being participative and maintaining proper distance from the villagers they will interact with in the field. They are encouraged, for example, to attend funerals and community meetings for the duration of data collection, but discouraged from getting involved in local politics, which might serve to alienate some research subjects and make them less willing to answer survey questions. For Dr. Jones and fieldworkers alike, the field is a place whose uncertainties and stumbling blocks must be imagined prior to fieldwork such that their influence on data quality can be minimized. The talk and practices of researchers and fieldworkers make the field intelligible by inventing it, facilitating their ability to imagine themselves and the data collection tools they employ as translators between the field and the office (Wagner 1981).

Holding steady a vision of the field as container of data facilitates the collaborative effort to assemble high-quality data. Whereas chapter 2 explores this imaginative labor and its entailments specifically from the perspective of fieldworkers, this chapter focuses on how the field undergirds and directs the efforts of researchers in the office to design survey questions, tools, and research plans that self-consciously aim to manage the messiness and unpredictability of the field. Before data are collected, this chapter shows, rural Malawi and its residents must be recast as "the field" and "research participants," respectively, enabling researchers to translate their epistemological dreams into a contained—and manageable—space of difference.

Demographers leading survey projects in Malawi were very clear about the simultaneously marginal and core role that the field played in their research efforts. On the one hand, they agreed that survey researchers "rarely, if ever, step foot in the field" and don't see the fieldwork component of research as important to their work.[1] Dr. Payson, MAYP demographer, suggested that her disciplinary kin tend to "parachute in and out of countries," echoing critiques by anthropologists and others that "the demographer could study a society without . . . knowing much of anything about it. . . . Visits to the country, if required at all, could be confined to short stays in western luxury hotels" (Kertzer and Fricke 1997, 11).[2] Payson suggested that for those who work on survey projects in Africa, doing fieldwork is actually detrimental to furthering one's career in academia: disciplinary norms—and, by proxy, tenure expectations—see a researcher being too heavily involved in the field side of things as a waste of time that could be instead directed toward writing new research proposals, publishing results, or analyzing data.[3] She was frustrated that her investment in qualitative methods and longer-term fieldwork as accompaniments to collecting numbers was squashed by disciplinary norms and structures. Dr. Canton, a Canadian social demographer leading projects in Burkina Faso, Kenya, and South Africa, echoed Payson's claim that the disciplinary norms of demography disallow long-term fieldwork: "Fieldwork is seen as a vacation; its point is not understood at all."[4]

In such disciplinary renderings, the field becomes a distant and exotic site that is hierarchically situated far beneath the space of calculation, intellect, and analysis that is the office. This spatialization likewise grafts on to the actors who are expected to populate each of these spaces: fieldworkers and villagers in the field and expert demographers crunching numbers in the office. Indeed, the space between these two sites is crucial to producing the kinds of knowledge expected by the epistemic community of demographers: dispassionate, objective, and universally circulating numbers. Dr. Matenje, a Malawian demographer based in South Africa, emphasized the ways in which number crunching simultaneously made him aware of harsh on-the-ground realities and made him feel helpless: "As a demographer, when I started analyzing the DHS data, I realized what was killing people was AIDS. . . . I understand how important that data is, but it just incapacitated me. I couldn't do anything about [the people dying]."[5] Matenje, like Dr. Jones, suggests that crunching numbers in the office—the everyday labor of the demographer—necessitates an emotional distance between himself and distant realities, one that nonetheless compels him to consider the moral implications of his work. Numbers, as portable placeholders for people themselves and stand-ins for human suffering, operate to make realities appear as taken-for-granted givens to be measured or enumerated rather than structurally produced inequalities and suffering to be meaningfully ameliorated.

Other researchers spoke about how their multiple and competing commitments made spending time in the field virtually impossible: those based at academic institutions, for example, suggested they found it difficult to escape for too long from committee work, teaching, or obligations such as chairing their home departments. Researchers based at the World Bank and academic institutions alike mentioned, as well, the difficulty of spending good chunks of time in one field when you have so many fields (and projects) ongoing across sub-Saharan Africa, reinforcing the notion of the field as a bounded and interchangeable data container, delinked from politics, geographic specificity, textured local life, or people themselves (Justice 1986; Pigg 1996). This, of course, departs starkly from the anthropologist's affective attachment to his or her field site, often cast in disciplinary rhetoric as a peopled site of mean-ingful friendships and obligations, a lifelong other home, and a place one is po-litically, morally, and epistemologically invested in. While in both the anthro-pological and demographic disciplinary imagination, the field is constructed as a distant, different place of roughing it, for the former, the field, and specifi-cally the long time an anthropologist spends there, are central anchors in his or her claim to disciplinary legitimacy (Gupta and Ferguson 1997). In con-trast, time spent in the field is, for demographers, largely a liability to career advancement or a pursuit incompatible with their expertise.

At the same time that researchers heading data collection efforts across sub-Saharan Africa acknowledged that the field was a place they rarely, if ever, had the opportunity to travel to, they well understood the important effects that the practices and processes that constituted fieldwork could have on the quality of data collected: hiring "bad" fieldworkers or turning a completely blind eye to fieldwork activities on the ground would result in messy, cooked, or bad data, from their perspective. Researchers invested time and money, then, in putting in place mechanisms that would enable them to monitor data collection activities: short-term visits to Malawi to check up on field-work themselves, assigning Malawian research collaborators this surveilling role, and implementing intensive training sessions meant to standardize field-workers' behaviors and practices.

While the last of these is examined in detail in chapters 2 and 4, in what follows I show how hierarchies of expertise and structural inequalities inform the kinds of work performed by those who occupy different levels in survey research infrastructure. The metaphors and rhetoric employed by researchers hint at the unequal division of labor: being on the ground in the field has the largest effect on data but—from the perspective of researchers—the activi-ties of fieldworkers are framed as menial labor performed by easily replace-able and interchangeable individuals (see chapter 4). Between the office—here coded as the office at one's home university or the World Bank in the United States, Canada, or Europe—and the field, however, lies the liminal space occupied by Malawian researchers collaborating with foreign-led sur-vey projects. While these individuals by no means visit individual households to ask survey questions, they are expected to more regularly check up on the progress of data collection activities in the field and to manage logistical, technical, and social issues that come up in the course of field research. The local expertise they offer, then, is not in designing research or writing propos-als but comes as an additive to a project conceived in a distant office. The hierarchy of the field and office maps on to the kinds of work those at different levels of research projects are expected to contribute. These hierarchies are embedded in political-economic structures that privilege the knowledge work that is the purview of Western academic researchers over the so-called unskilled labor performed by fieldworkers. Meanwhile, as we will see, Malawian research collaborators occupy a middle space that is both constructed by and fraught with power and economic inequalities.

Recruiting Necessary Collaborators:
Hierarchies within Partnership

In Malawi at the time of my research, the National Health Sciences Research Council (NHSRC) and the College of Medicine Research and Ethics Committee (COMREC)—both local ethics boards discussed in further detail in chapter 3—mandated that research proposals submitted for local review by foreign researchers list a Malawian coprincipal investigator and include a detailed letter of affiliation to a local institution. Research guidelines also provided clear instructions to guide coauthorship of articles produced by research. The contract for collaboration between foreign and Malawian researchers has a wider sweep whereby benefits or resources also flow to the institution where the latter is based.[6] The acting head of the National Research Council of Malawi explained that national review boards were increasingly vigilant about ensuring that proposals submitted by foreign projects put in place solid plans for genuine collaboration; for example, Dr. Jones described how MAYP's initial proposal did not pass review because NHSRC claimed that the institutional collaboration between the American team and a Malawian university was "not meaningful."[7] In response, the team secured a Malawian economist as a collaborator and created a memorandum of understanding (MOU) with a Malawian university that, among other things, specified the number of computers to remain in Malawi once fieldwork ended.

Also, LSAM incorporated capacity-building activities into their proposals: in October 2007, I attended a presentation by a graduate student affiliated with LSAM to a group of thirty-five students and faculty at the University of Malawi's Chancellor College. In addition to providing a PowerPoint tour of LSAM's activities and data collection in-country since 1998, she also emphasized how the continued collaboration between the university and LSAM would benefit the students, including access to LSAM data, a resource center near the university, access to libraries online, an Internet hot spot, and training courses in STATA, a statistical software package. During LSAM fieldwork in 2008, graduate students overseeing data collection in the field led smaller-scale activities to enrich the skill sets of field supervisors. Field supervisors were invited to wake up before dawn to attend workshops on preparing a curriculum vitae, becoming competent with STATA, writing a cover letter, and so on. Due to the long and grueling hours of fieldwork days, however, many supervisors preferred to sleep during these sessions.

Despite the detailed scripts and guidelines meant to guide collaboration in Malawi, collaborators from both the North and the South generally agreed that collaborative relationships were unequal and imperfect when measured against global health's prevailing rosy rhetoric of partnership. In interviews with researchers based in Malawi and other locations in the global South, it was clear that they recognized their expedient and instrumental—rather than substantive—role as a rubber stamp on foreign-led projects (see also Crane 2010a, 852).

A Malawian demographer and collaborator with both the LSAM and MAYP survey projects, Dr. Kamwendo, put it this way: "I think these days a typical research group is you have one group in the North, maybe someone in the South, but the person in the North brings money to the person in the South. But, the people in the North cannot get the money in the first place without the collaborator in the South."[8] In Kamwendo's words, we note how North-South collaborations often find their connective tissue in money: only if Northern projects secure a local collaborator can they access grant monies and the field in which data will be collected. The general model for sourcing a collaborator—consistent across the four projects at the center of this book and others in 2007–2008—is to make contact with a Malawian researcher who is invited to collaborate; if the researcher agrees, his or her name is printed in the blank space left for "Malawian co-PI" on the cascade of forms to be submitted to NHSRC or COMREC. Importantly, though this process produces Malawian or Southern collaborators as autonomous actors who engage foreign researchers and institutions out of free and rational choice, it also obscures the relative inequalities between the two parties (Geissler 2013b). Prior to the establishment of a relatively informative and comprehensive website to guide foreign researchers, the role of a local collaborator early in the project especially entailed guiding foreign researchers through ethical review procedures and other bureaucracies to be navigated before setting foot on Malawian soil to implement projects. Barring any real objections to the plans for the project outlined in the proposal, the Malawian co-PI takes up a role as a kind of local expert. Notably, however, the co-PI usually takes up this position long after the research study has been conceived and sometimes after it has already been funded.

Following successful ethical review, foreign researchers may make a short visit to Malawi to meet local collaborators face to face and to work with them on prefieldwork tasks such as tweaking the survey, translating questions, or choosing suitable research sites (the second portion of this chapter discusses survey design in more detail). In the contracts drawn up between collaborators, Malawian researchers are granted payment in return for specific kinds of expertise itemized in the budget appended to a proposal: participating in meetings with local research gatekeepers, selecting project supervisors and fieldworkers, assisting in translation and back-translation of questionnaires, spending at least a few days supervising data collection fieldwork on the ground, and generally providing oversight to the foreign researcher.[9] In this list of activities, Malawian coinvestigators are called upon to perform a middleman role. Yet despite their more consistent proximity to the field of data collection for the duration of fieldwork, Malawian researchers often shirk their duty to visit the field sites of projects, a fact bemoaned by foreign collaborators and interpreted as a case of the former failing to live up to their end of the bargain.

Malawian researchers, meanwhile, attributed their inability to participate more meaningfully in collaborative projects to being overworked and overextended by the work of collaboration itself. For example, some collaborators on survey projects were academics based in departments at the University of Malawi or at the Centre for Social Research (CSR), an institutional arm of the university, established in 1965, with its own budget—funded by UNICEF until it was taken over by the government in 1982—whose main function is to house rotating faculty from the university who oversee collection of data for research projects in the national development interest (interpreted loosely). The imperative to undertake policy-relevant research today finds historical corollary in postindependence rhetoric of research in the national development interest. At the conferral of the first degrees earned at the University of Malawi, then-president Kamuzu Banda said in his speech, "Malawi has no time for ivory tower speculation. . . . What the country needs is the commitment of its academic elite to the solution of practical problems in Malawian life" (quoted in Joffe 1973, 517; Hunnings 1981). A 1982 report on CSR's activities, meanwhile, noted that the "Centre has done very little in the way of basic research since staff [faculty members] have been busy with commissioned . . . research projects" ("Centre for Social Research," CSR/16/82) a trend that has been exacerbated by the global health boom. Dana Holland (2006, 128) argues that the creation of centers for the study of poverty or education in Malawi tend to align with donor interests and are major culprits in drawing academic social scientists further away from the traditional university via de-institutionalization, an observation borne out by my own findings.

In 2007–2008, three faculty affiliates to CSR were each collaborators on upward of ten projects at one time, including, for example, monitoring and evaluation research for UNICEF-funded community-based child care centers, a UN Food and Agriculture Organization study on rural aging and livelihood, and an assessment of how Malawian farmers experienced input subsidies in 2006–2007. As Malawian academics explained it, they accumulated these collaborations because of the small size of the country, the small number of people holding master's or PhD degrees in Malawi, and the high density of research networks through which collaborations were forged.[10] One might argue, in fact, that a rite of passage for academics working in universities in sub-Saharan Africa is becoming skilled at finding those opportunities (conferences, consultancies, workshops) outside the university's walls that can most supplement normatively meager salaries with handsome consultancy fees, per diems, and travel to foreign locations. During dinner at a conference held in Zomba, Malawi, sponsored by a foreign African studies institute in late 2007, the young African academics in attendance—mostly PhD students or junior scholars at African universities—complained that the sponsoring institution had not provided them with pocket money or per diems. A young Zimbabwean historian gave a passionate monologue:

> We live off per diems! We search the Internet for conferences to attend constantly. We make money that way. A number of us are familiar with this one man who presents almost the exact same paper every time he goes to a conference in slightly different form. . . . This guy is a real expert at rewriting his abstract again and again. He tones his topic [drought] toward whatever are the larger interests of the conference in question. Drought and HIV/AIDS orphans, drought and global warming, drought and development [everyone laughs]. That man makes money, let me tell you![11]

This account of a character familiar to others at the dinner hints at the central importance of per diems as supplemental income for African academics, which only intensifies as one moves up through academia from graduate student to faculty member and requires money to raise a family, support less wealthy rural kin, and so on. Living off per diems entails intensive labor that distracts academics from their research and writing, symbolized in the repackaged drought paper delivered at multiple conferences by the character described above. Amid the rise of per diems as income supplements in global health and research worlds in sub-Saharan Africa (Lwanda 2005; Heimer 2007; Ridde 2010; Conteh and Kingori 2010; Vian et al. 2012), Malawian collaborators on projects such as the surveys are often unable to spend time on the ground as laid out in their contracts. A Malawian demographer and frequent collaborator to foreign-led survey projects, Dr. Chirwa, described why she enjoyed traveling to conferences outside the country: "It is nice to have respite from people knocking on my office door constantly and some time when I can just read my e-mails in peace!"[12] However, as another Malawian collaborator pointed out, constant travel takes a toll on one's mind, body, and intellect. He described 2008 as his "worst [year] yet" amid traveling once or twice a month to diverse locales to interface with collaborators: Pretoria, Johannesburg, London, Norway, Uganda, Geneva, and the United States.[13]

The socioeconomic asymmetries that produce lopsided collaborations between institutions and researchers from abroad and within Malawi were a recurrent theme in interviews I conducted with Malawian researcher-academics, who largely suggested that partnership is little more than a performance (Mercer 2003, 759). A senior faculty member at the University of Malawi and collaborator on survey and other projects, Dr. Mponda, articulated the multiple demands he faces:

> One of the major problems we face is, quite simply, our low salaries. . . . How can I pay for groceries, fuel, my children's school fees? It happens that many older people spend all their time doing consultancies instead of building a solid academic foundation in this country by publishing and researching and teaching. . . . I feel that if we got a little more money we would be more devoted professors to our students and do original research and stop moonlighting on consultancies. . . . We cannot compete for research money at a global level. . . . Proposals for consultancies I've mentioned [e.g., for evaluation of NGO and government projects], on the other hand, are not as comprehensive. If you submit a [proposal] in country, you hear in two weeks [whether you were successful], get the money, and life goes on. The research may not be intellectually stimulating but it pays.[14]

Senior Malawian academics such as Mponda earned a salary at the time of around $500–600 per month; consultancies paid hundreds of dollars per day at the time (Holland 2009). Moonlighting becomes less a distraction than a norm, leaving research collaborators stretched thin and unable to develop their own research interests, especially in a university climate that is not invested in faculty research, and largely devalues the social sciences, except when mobilized toward applied and technical ends (Swidler and Watkins 2009).[15] To make ends meet, they have become savvy at marketing themselves as experts in multiple capacities; as Holland (2006, 2009) points out, however, their entrepreneurial success is likely inversely related to their academic success.

Thus, while Malawian collaborators are key ingredients in establishing a research infrastructure on the ground, they, not unlike their foreign counterparts, tend to play only a minimal role in the field phase of research, making the labor of Malawian fieldworkers and supervisors central to everyday data collection. Nonetheless, both foreign and local researchers invest much time and energy in creating the recipe or template in the office that will guide and—in their imagination—standardize and harmonize the collection of clean data by fieldworkers in the field. Data need to be imagined as data to exist and, as such, close attention to how they are imagined before the fact can shed light on their material forms as culturally coded rather than given: there are no data behind the various practices that do data (Law and Lien 2012, 366).

Survey design meetings and discussions are a central site in which we can observe how the culture of demography emphasizes and instantiates modes of knowledge production that privilege the comparability of concepts over space and time and the harmonization of methods and modes of data collection (Randall, Coast, and Leone 2011, 220). After briefly describing the nature and intentions of a survey, this chapter considers the politics of translation. While I am attentive to the translation of words and concepts from source (English) into target (e.g., Chichewa) languages, I also analyze survey instruments, concepts, and questions to show that a focus on how respondents will hear or interpret them necessitates the invention of a cultural Other and allows the culture of demography itself to go unremarked.

What Is a Survey?

"Survey" operates as both noun and verb, and, notably, the Chewa term for research is likewise the term for survey (kafukufuku). A survey is, in the first sense, a tangible collection of papers with questions compelling responses (a questionnaire) and, in the second, a method whereby information is gathered from a sample of individuals who are surveyed. A survey questionnaire is a systematic, organized method of gathering quantitative data from a sample of individuals, and survey methodology is largely seen by demographers as a science, where surveys derive data to test hypotheses (de Leeuw, Hox, and

Dillman 2008). Unlike a census—which also relies on face-to-face encounters between an interviewer and a respondent—a survey does not endeavor to measure or count all members of the population, but rather extracts data from a population of interest, the sample.

A sample, or group of people "living at a specific time in a defined region, belonging to a specific societal stratum, sharing specific characteristics, etc." (Mohler 2006, 11), is the anchor for data quality because it is incorporated into algorithms and calculations that determine whether a given data set is good or bad. The quality of data is arbitrated by calculations that measure construct validity, measurement error, sampling error, nonresponse error, processing error, and so on (Anderson et al. 1979; Groves 1989; Hansen et al. 2010). The point of sampling is to economize resources but also to draw inferences from the sample to a larger population of concern through the application of statistical tools that ensure ahead of time that data will be good enough to do so. A larger sample means smaller sampling error, but in places like Malawi, there are often cost and time constraints that act to limit sample size. Further, developing valid constructs and minimizing error enables the standardization of information across countries and regions (Adams 2016b, 28). As an axiomatic category of demographic analysis, the sample must be imagined as a bounded container or a closed population, demographic abstractions or workable imaginaries that make data collection possible (Adams and Kasanoff 2004).[16]

Demographers are invested in rendering complex entities such as the family or the household into standard sets of categories to communicate and enumerate difference across time and space. As will be seen in chapter 4, these standard categories, not unlike the data talk mentioned in the introduction, are part of the cultural parlance of demographers, and, for this reason, intensive training sessions for fieldworkers function to entrain them into a new linguistic and cultural community whose core preoccupation is collection of high-quality data (Higgs 2004). Fieldworkers not only follow a script by reading it off the survey pages to their respondents but must also understand the aim of each question and the meanings of terms and concepts that may be foreign to them as nondemographers.

Ample critiques of enumeration show that counting is never a straightforward, neutral activity; depending on who is doing the counting and why, people may be allocated to different categories, left uncounted, and so on (Prohmmo and Bryant 2004, 245). Analyses and comparisons of different data sets for the same country illustrate this well. For example, UN and WHO projections and household survey-based estimates of the fraction of children aged below fourteen years who are maternal, paternal, or double orphans in Malawi differed significantly in the early 2000s (Grassly et al. 2004, 210). In Malawi, HIV prevalence differs depending on whether one consults LSAM data or Malawi government data (Thornton 2008). Further, we often overlook the fact that numbers about health in Africa are based on estimates, rather than real counts (Wendland 2016, 65–67). At a finer-grained level, demographers recognize the powerful influence that individual data collectors—their practices, biases, behaviors, and intentions—may have on the numerical output of enumeration efforts even within a single project, as is evident in chapters 2 and 4.

Latour and Woolgar (1979, 49–50) show how, in the space of the laboratory, samples extracted from rats undergo a radical transformation into paper sheets containing figures, graphs, and so on. Designing surveys entails a similar transformation of the real into representation, where responses provided to data collectors become pencil marks on a page and then data points in databases. The survey form, even as it aspires to collect raw data, is a framing device whose apparent objectivity hides its cultural story and commitments (Gitelman and Jackson 2013, 5–6). The finalized field-ready survey is the key actor in an ontological choreography that features demographers' efforts to make data in the same way over and over again amid unpredictable human and nonhuman actors in the field (Thompson 2005).

Survey design is a negotiation constrained by a number of factors: financial resources, the capacity of the organization that will implement the survey, and the willingness of household members to provide the desired information, for example. As they translate survey questions and negotiate the final form of the survey, those present at survey design meetings have in the back of their minds a number of questions: How many households will be sampled and how long will a fieldworker need to spend at each? What will be the costs of training fieldworkers, particularly if the survey employs a large number of complex sections or questions? How long can the survey be before participants grow tired of answering questions? What information will respondents be reluctant to provide or unable to recall? These queries point to how the questionnaire itself can introduce error into the data collection process: Information collected can be ambiguous, not well defined, or inconsistent. The order of questions may affect responses gathered, and as Bledsoe (2002, 330) shows, the thematic order of a questionnaire betrays the chronological naturalism and logics of its designers. Open-ended versus closed-ended questions may produce different results. Even the actual, aesthetic look of a questionnaire may affect the interviewer's mind-set and ability to administer it in a clean fashion.

As implied above, designing a survey with the target population in mind entails tensions between reducing errors of all sorts and the cost of reducing these errors. In this sense, the survey—and data themselves—incorporate uncertainty: their final forms are merely good enough. The next section analyzes survey design sessions to illustrate how demographers' shared notions of good data inform the survey questionnaire, and how the questions and translations aim to predict and mitigate human and other forms of error in the data set.

Designing Surveys: The Politics, Perils, and Possibilities of Translation

On the covered verandah of a lodge in Zomba, Malawi—colonial Nyasaland's capital and the present-day site of the University of Malawi—a team of MAYP researchers sits together on a Saturday evening in mid-January 2008, heads bent over piles of survey papers. As rain pours down, we work late into the night to give a final polish to the questionnaires that will be piloted in a few days. The main purpose of this meeting is to make sure the survey questionnaires are field ready, so we painstakingly review the questions one by one, considering the quality of translation from English to Chichewa and the precision and clarity of the queries. Present at the meeting are a diverse group of MAYP's research collaborators: the American principal investigator, Dr. Payson (a sociologist); a graduate student in economics at a Dutch university heading data collection for a related World Bank project in Zomba; a graduate student in economics at an American university who will oversee data collection for this project; two faculty members from the University of Malawi (Dr. Mponda, an anthropologist, and Dr. Kalenga, an economist); Chifundo (a Malawian fieldwork supervisor); and myself.[17]

Our discussions not only center on accurate linguistic translation from English into Chichewa; we also speculate about how survey respondents will hear (interpret) the questions. Demographers understand translation as a multifaceted endeavor and concern themselves with semantic equivalence across language, conceptual equivalence across cultures, and the ability of a translated text to adapt to local social norms. The imperative to ensure questions are heard in the same way by all respondents to a survey takes form in survey design meetings as collaborative wordsmithing, where changes to the literal words on the page or to the questionnaire structure are imagined to improve the accuracy of the answers to be solicited and the validity of numerical data. As the late Etienne van de Walle (1993, 124), longtime demographer of Africa, suggests, "small differences in phrasing of survey or census questions can yield extraordinary differences in [meaning]," with implications for data quality down the line. The perils of inaccurate translation are borne out by research suggesting that close attention to standardized translation of surveys, despite its costs, often pays off in the form of higher-quality data (Weinreb and Sana 2009), though some suggest that thoughtful selection and intensive training of interviewers is just as important as translation (Bignami-van Assche, Reniers, and Weinreb 2003). Translation of survey questions from English into Malawi's three primary languages—Chewa, Yao, and Tumbuka—is necessary, as well, to ensure that project interviewers will read each question exactly as written in the local language, increasing reliability of data collected and decreasing noise in the data.

For example, we deliberated over how participants might interpret a question inserted into the section of the survey titled "Social Capital" by Dr. Payson: "Are you comfortable walking to the market alone?" She explained that the question was meant to examine respondents' experiences of intentionality, community, and security; her interest in this measure reflects rising interest in the link between health outcomes and social networks and support in international health research (Harpham, Grant, and Thomas 2002). Chifundo and Drs. Kalenga and Mponda immediately raised concerns, suggesting that a person could go to the market multiple times per week and in a different fashion each time, and, further, that going to the market could never be something one does entirely alone since each time one goes, one meets many people along the way. The question would be misheard by respondents, they cautioned, and generate dirty data resulting from its confusing construction. Ultimately, this question was made more precise by providing respondents with a hypothetical scenario: "If you wanted to go to the market during the day and no one was available to go with you, would you walk alone?" Here, the rephrasing of the question built confidence among the researchers that the answer generated would be more reliable and accurate than the answer elicited by the previous version of the question, which, according to the Malawians at the table, did not make sense culturally, regardless of its linguistic translation.

A few hours later, all of those present at the meeting grew weary after a lengthy discussion about a section of the survey that focused on religion— the Malawians at the table suggested we clarify a question on religious identification because of people's tendency to switch religions. One of the graduate students argued that we should move on from such "small points": "It's not as if Malawians change their religions enough to warrant all this discussion," he suggested. At this, the Malawian researchers laughed, and Dr. Kalenga explained, "Malawians change their religions all the time! Constantly. We need to spend more time here [on this set of questions] for sure." The elite Malawians present proceeded to joke about how rural Malawians will strategically join different faiths and churches without much thought if they hear that there are benefits (bread, blankets, etc.) to such conversion. Later, Chifundo, longtime fieldwork supervisor, reinforced Kalenga's claim: "When you are talking in English, these things can be straightforward, but in Chichewa [they are not]." Dr. Kalenga's claim not only contests the foreign graduate student's knowledge claim, but also enacts a kind of boundary work that points to his lack of local knowledge and naïveté about Malawi and Malawians (Gieryn 1999). Survey design meetings foreground how the survey frames and contingently aligns the interests of demographers from across geographic and cultural contexts in a form that attempts to mitigate and anticipate deviations or modifications in its translation into the field.

The scene on the verandah foregrounds not only the implicit culturally shared disciplinary norms of demographers, all of whom are invested in collecting data that will achieve the epistemic standards and virtues held in common, but also the different roles of the multiple experts present at the meeting. As indicated above, Malawian research collaborators contribute nominally, if at all, to research proposals or plans. It is when foreign researchers arrive on the ground in Malawi that they take up their primary role on the project as translators who are meant to reassure foreigners that survey questions will make sense to an imagined rural research subject. The expertise they offer entails not only translating English tokens into local vernacular, but also ensuring that the survey itself will act as a sufficiently good recipe to collect the clean and accurate data disciplinary norms dictate.

The roundtable of experts who tinker with the survey design and translation is a presurvey administration ritual in which hierarchical forms of expertise and knowledge are expressed in the debates and discussions of the specific items that constitute the instrument. Mohler (2006, 13) argues that such ritualized meetings often feature the principal investigator acting as "Machiavelli's Principe" with the final say, although in my experience the degree to which this was true depended on the topic being discussed; when it came to questions around linguistic translation, Malawian collaborators were often the chief arbiters, for example. In what follows, I examine how demographers' commitments to clean data—defined as data that are accurate and reliable, efficiently collected, and collected from sufficiently large, representative samples—are embodied in the categories, queries, and form of the survey itself. Indeed, the final version of the survey that becomes the recipe for data collection is the outcome of a process in which hundreds of decisions—with high stakes for data quality—are made (Glewwe 2005a, 36; Kasprzyk 2005). The questionnaire tool itself carries the dreams and ambitions of researchers into the field and plays a leading role in determining the quality of data collected down the line.

Visualizing Wealth and Health: The Steps Instrument

One question—included in the questionnaire by economists—asked survey respondents to locate themselves on a set of steps (depicted visually on the survey page) based on their perception of their relative wealth within their community (*gulu*) (figure 1.1).[18]

Respondents could indicate verbally or by pointing with a finger whether their family belonged on step 1 (the poorest), step 6 (the wealthiest), or somewhere in between (figure 1.2). This exercise acts as an indicator of an individual's broadly defined quality of life, which encompasses perceived or felt relative wealth. Researchers employ a psychometric tool to convert the subjective judgment or feelings of a respondent (e.g., "I am very poor") into a form suitable for statistical analysis ("I am very poor" becomes 1).

As we considered the merits of this question, Kalenga, Mponda, and Chifundo raised concerns about the translation of the word "community," suggesting that respondents would interpret the term in its current form (gulu) inconsistently and undo both the reliability and validity of the data collected. They argued that the question should be narrowed—that community should be written instead as village (*mudzi*)—so as to elicit the most precise responses and avoid respondent confusion. The Malawians' suggestion to replace "gulu" with "mudzi" was taken up in the version to be read to respondents by fieldworkers. Whereas the former Chewa word refers loosely to a group (used conventionally in forms such as *gulu la akuba* [gang of thieves] or *gulu la anthu ambiri* [a crowd or group of lots of people]), "mudzi" aims to anchor the question in a specific and clear location: the people who live in the area a respondent designates as "his or her village." In fact, the translation that was finally settled upon aimed to specify even further the spatial unit for comparison: *mudzi mwanu **muno*** (my emphasis) tacks on the emphatic demonstrative pronoun used to denote precise locality across Bantu languages:

Imagine six steps, where on the bottom, the first step, stand the poorest people in your community, and on the highest step, the sixth, stand the rich in your community.		
SHOW THE PICTURE OF THE STEPS.		
5. On which step are you today?	6. On which step are most of your neighbors today?	7. On which step are most of your friends today?

FIGURE 1.1. The steps question from the MAYP questionnaire, 2008.

"Your village, the one *here.*" One might read the elevation of the Malawians' translation as best—and its inclusion in the final draft of the survey—as a moment when local expertise trumps or eclipses that of the foreign experts. However, it is important to note that the survey form traveled to Malawi in drafted whole form, underpinned primarily by the theoretical interests of the Western collaborators; linguistic wordsmithing becomes the genre of additive, rather than substantive, expertise proferred by Malawians who are likewise trained as demographers. The expertise they offer in the survey design meeting, however, is logistical and linguistic and manifests in the genre of "add culture and stir," whereby the cultural knowledge of local collaborators is expediently, rather than substantially, incorporated into a fully formed survey questionnaire as well as the research project more broadly.

In its technical nature, it is hierarchically subordinate to the intellectual, theoretically informed expertise that produced the survey in its given form; further along data's life course, the Malawians likewise rarely earn a spot as lead author on journal articles resulting from data analysis. As we will observe in the next chapter, close attention to local expertise in survey design meetings or everyday fieldwork practices helps destabilize presumptions that it is an entity of local origin or implies mastery of the local. Indeed, the rise of a global health apparatus produces a particular kind of commodified local expertise that presumes its context of emergence: lopsided global-local partnerships and collaborations. The production of this form of expertise, in fact, relies on the spatialized difference between the field and the office rooted as it is in imperial geographies of knowledge.

While the content of the question about wealth (its linguistic translation) was deemed a worthy object of discussion in the survey design meeting, the form of the question went unremarked. Neither the Malawian nor the foreign researchers at the meeting questioned the fundamental validity of the steps visual aid or speculated how respondents might react to or interpret the instrument itself. In this sense, among the demographically minded experts

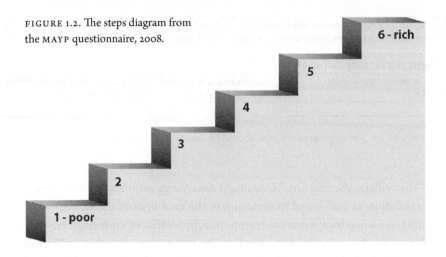

FIGURE 1.2. The steps diagram from the MAYP questionnaire, 2008.

6 - rich

5

4

3

2

1 - poor

at the table, a shared image of the ideal-type villager set a consensual basis for the form of the question, one that makes clear their own interpretation of the steps as a translation tool appropriate to the target population, takes for granted its validity as an instrument, and foregrounds their focus on linguistic rather than conceptual equivalence (Bowden and Fox-Rushby 2003, 1299). This shared imaginative labor on the part of survey designers—conjuring the villager who will respond to their question—resembles the ways in which filmmakers who produced colonial health education films in Nyasaland and Northern Rhodesia relied on the imagined creation of an audience who would view them (Vaughan 1991, 196). The scalar or metric equivalence of the steps instrument—that is, whether the act of ranking the self on a spectrum is consistent across cultures—is presumed and largely untheorized (Herdman, Fox-Rushby, and Badia 1997, 243). The steps instrument becomes a stabilized fact whose origins and history are obscured by demographers' tacit knowledge that it is a well-functioning, familiar, and routinized metric whose dimensions are not necessary to discuss explicitly each time it is included in a survey (Latour 1987, 43). The steps attain a kind of universal validity through their importation into surveys whose designers hold steady a shared conception of the low-literacy research subject.

The steps exercise likewise embeds certain assumptions about its target audience of low-literacy, largely rural respondents. The question aspires to field readiness in its provision of a visual, rather than textual, prompt. The imperative to imagine a cultural other entails producing forms of difference and ways to manage them that recall imperial, racialized hierarchies of intelligence. Namely, visual-analogue survey tools such as the steps presume text to be read by enumerators is too complicated to be heard properly by respondents, recalling Carothers's (1953, 87) claim in his ethnopsychiatric study *The African Mind in Health and Disease* that the "African mind" lacked logic and capacity for abstract thought. Visual or pictographic scales are often preferred for use in surveys because, as demographers suggest, they are "easy to understand and to handle by the respondents" and carry "low cognitive load" for respondents.

The steps exercise resembles many other nonverbal scales, including visual questions and image-based responses used in clinical and research settings, such as thermometers, ladders, truncated pyramids, symbols, and figures (Smith 2002, 74–76). The most familiar of these visual scales to the reader is likely the FACES pain scale—first developed for pediatric use—that ranges from a smiling to crying face associated with no pain and extreme pain, respectively (Tomlinson et al. 2010). In international research, pictographs and scales such as empty and full pill bottles have been used to measure adherence to HIV drug regimens, and feeling thermometers are used to measure subjective health status. Bolton and Tang (2002, 538) suggest that standard instruments developed in Western countries (such as the Work and Social Disability Scale, WSDS) contain too many "culture bound" questions that are difficult to adapt, citing questions on a respondent's ability to climb stairs or go shopping as examples. To address this, they substituted a nonverbal response card using sketched images of a woman in local dress carrying an increasingly heavy sack and clearly burdened to elicit the same constructs as the WSDS in rural Uganda and Rwanda (539).

Also, LSAM used a pictograph—a health state thermometer—on the last page of a questionnaire administered by its voluntary counseling and testing (VCT) team (see figure 1.3).[19] The accompanying question asked respondents to draw a line to a point on the thermometer that best captured their health status ("indicate how good or bad your own health is today, in your opinion"). The thermometer, however, caused some confusion in the field. For example, respondents sometimes pointed to their weight instead of their felt relative health (e.g., pointing to 50 to capture a weight of 50 kg), leading interviewers to double-check responses to this instrument by asking probing questions or confirming the respondent's choice.[20] The thermometer tool carried with it intertextual references to other contexts in which respondents had encountered scales, thermometers, or measuring devices related to health and well-being, meanings that had the potential to interfere in the collection of clean data.

Similarly, the steps visual aid falls prey to an absolutist concept of wealth as the same across the world (Herdman, Fox-Rushby, and Badia 1997). In the field, the steps exercise faced difficulties—not because people did not understand the words on the page, but because the question of how to define wealth generated confusion. Respondents struggled to pinpoint their location on a continuum of relative wealth, often deliberating aloud about how to assess whether a neighbor was richer or poorer than he: Does he own land? Do his relatives have jobs, and what kind? Did he have a good crop this year? The steps instrument carries with it assumptions that come into tension with Malawian notions of wealth as socially distributed and potentially obscures how having "long legs" or many associates and patrons—wealth in people—might mean a respondent is poor and rich at the same time (Barnes 1986, 78). Further, as Elias Mandala (2005, 14) has shown, rural Malawians do not see feast and famine as mutually exclusive and are well aware that some people are always full and others often go hungry, perhaps confounding some of the questions elsewhere in the questionnaire regarding food stocks and famine. Similarly, in the Gambian context, Bledsoe (2002, 95) shows that survey questions about whether or not women use contraceptives embed assumptions that contraceptive use could only ever function toward limiting fertility, obscuring the tactical ways in which Gambian women use contraceptives as a form of birth spacing oriented toward having the largest number of healthy children.

Analysis of the steps and thermometer instruments embedded in the MAYP and LSAM surveys, respectively, sheds light, first, on how survey designers imagine their research subjects and, second, on how translating surveys is concerned primarily with linguistic dimensions of conversion and with ensuring that tools make cultural sense—from the perspective of researchers—in a local context of administration. Despite demographers' best efforts to predict how questions will be heard (or seen) by respondents, their administration in the field brings many surprises (Nations and Rebhun 1988, 32–33). Yet, even as misunderstanding abounds, the tools themselves retain their status as valid instruments that expediently collect data from respondents. Even if they appear to fail from the perspective of individual interview encounters observed by the author, they succeed from the perspective of demographers whose standards for data already ensure such tools will work. The steps tool, for example, collects a certain number of 1 responses entered into a database down the line that tell us the percentage of a sample of Malawians who identify as very poor. Missing from the number, of course, is the thought processes and discussions that manifest in the interview encoun-

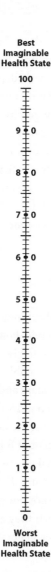

Best Imaginable Health State

100

9 ● 0

8 ● 0

7 ● 0

6 ● 0

5 ● 0

4 ● 0

3 ● 0

2 ● 0

1 ● 0

0

Worst Imaginable Health State

FIGURE 1.3. The health thermometer tool from the LSAM VCT questionnaire, 2008.

ter, or attention to how the fundamental construct (wealth) is interpreted in the Malawian context. In losing sight of these things—in excising them as nondata—the statistical claims enabled by the thousands of data points linked to this instrument become facts and evidence.

Clean data—well-collected raw numbers—contain within them thousands of stories of their messy contexts of production that remain silenced by the narrow definition of demographic data as codes recorded on a page and transferred to a database. Considering the politics of translation in action, it is notable that rhetoric presumes that original survey tools, technologies, and methods need to be altered for or adapted to both the field and to the low-literacy respondents they will measure. In the meantime, the culture of demography, reflected in its tools and instruments, is unmarked, presumed to be the natural origin or starting point from which translation into an Other's space, language, or culture is compelled. Assuming demography to be naked of culture upholds the fiction, as well, that raw or clean data exist. In casting itself as the acultural original or source language for survey knowledge production, demography obscures, specifically, the deeper tracks that carry data from the field to the office and convert it into fact. As Latour (1983, 155) observes, "scientific facts are like trains, they do not work off their rails." Quantitative evidence collected by surveys takes for granted the existence and validity of one important epistemological anchor: the household.

Statistical Household as Epistemic Anchor

For demographers, the statistical household is the unit of enumeration underlying censuses, DHS surveys, and the surveys discussed herein. Finding and interviewing members of this unit is the primary labor of fieldwork. "Seeing like a [survey] research project" has at its optic core this tangible, visible, and measurable category (Biruk 2012), which became the standard and ubiquitous unit of enumeration in the 1980s (Randall, Coast, and Leone 2011). A barrage of critiques anthropologists and others have leveled against the household as a standard unit of enumeration suggest that it fails to account for patterns of residence, kinship, and economic organization (Yanagisako 1979; Guyer and Peters 1987; Morphy 2007; Randall, Coast, and Leone 2011). For these critics who draw on comparative evidence, households are not bounded groups and fail to encompass networks of resources and support; they are not fixed forms but evolving, and they are differentiated by gender, generation, and so on. While some survey researchers have taken such critiques seriously and attempted to devise a notion of the household that is more capacious and flexible to its various contexts (Kriel et al. 2014; Randall and Coast 2015), demographers have, for the most part, not incorporated such critiques into survey design, even if survey researchers acknowledge that processes of household dissolution, formation, or alteration can result in changes in the representativeness of a sample over time (Deaton 1997, 20).

Van de Walle (2006, xxii) argues that the household is an expedient and preferred category because it is "obvious" to a superficial observer (fieldworkers), even if it is a "necessary evil." He suggests that "the ubiquity of the household in social, economic and even agricultural studies all over the world may reflect a lack of sensitivity to local particularities of the forms of social organization but it is a fact of life for the analyst" (xxvi). Townsend et al. (2006, 36) likewise suggest that the fact that the household has a physical location and structure presents logistical advantages for survey teams interested in counting and mapping them. Yet, as Kriel et al. (2014, 1317–1319) illustrate, fieldworkers for a household wealth survey in South Africa saw "household" as an external analytical concept developed for the survey, and struggled to translate it into their research practice and to respondents, with implications for who was included or excluded from the sample. Despite the shortcomings of the definition of the household as identified by anthropologists, then, survey researchers are invested in its demographic utility, take it as a fact of life, and require conceptually simple, relatively unambiguous flexible ways to code relations that are comparable across cultural contexts (Townsend et al. 2006, 37, 56), especially in an era when producing readily accessible and standardized forms of knowledge amid "a world of indicators" is a priority (Merry 2011; Rottenburg et al. 2015). The survey itself acts to anchor abstract epistemic standards for data to the key visible and countable unit of demographic knowledge production: the statistical household.

Even as the household determines the movements and practices of field teams, it acts as a flawed placeholder for a more complicated reality on the ground. Fieldworkers struggle to locate households. Once the proper household is found, making sure of the correct respondent is often a problem—especially when the survey is longitudinal and the same respondent needs to be interviewed in each survey wave. Some respondents hide, not wanting to spend time on the survey; others in the household of interest, however, might take the respondent's name in the hope of benefiting from the survey, as we will see in chapters 3 and 4. Naming conventions in Malawi, too, make identifying the correct respondent difficult. A person might go by Gift and Mphatso (Chichewa for gift) alike, or a respondent might take on a nickname he stops using before the next survey wave begins, or he might take on a new name following a religious conversion. And even if interviewers find the correct respondent, they have to negotiate in real time whom they will or will not list in the household roster administered by projects (see appendix). The household functioned as a top-down expedient optic tool that is imagined as a container of valuable data (consider the name "household-level survey"), with implications—discussed in chapter 4—for data quality down the line.

Survey Validity: The Fetish for Codes

Beginning with the very physical unit at which the survey tool is administered, then, anthropologists level critiques against a demographic rendering of the world: the household, they argue, is yet another "demographic category [among other] . . . western folk categories dressed in scientific garb" (Szreter, Sholkamy, and Dharmalingam 2004, foreword). This scientific garb obscures or renders unnecessary that which stands outside of the parameters, measures, and universe of possible responses that capture that which counts as data collected by a survey. Indeed, it is the ability of demographers to narrow as tightly as possible the representation of reality the survey produces that ensures data are of good quality.

The major dimension of data quality is validity, or the extent to which a test (question, instrument) measures that which it is intended to measure. In other words, how well does a question perform in the field? Validity hinges, of course, on adequate translation, as discussed above; for demographers, the objective of translation is to produce the same response from a respondent in a target population that the survey question would had it not been translated from English to Chichewa or another language. Even as this investment in equivalence presumes cultural and other forms of likeness between respondents, it speaks to the epistemic interest of researchers in devising and fine-tuning questions that correspond with what they believe is the true value of a construct: poorly designed questions, for example, may produce reliable results—meaning that all respondents hear them in the same (wrong) way—that are neither accurate nor valid. Further, as will become clear in the following chapters, the validity of a question may be undone in the field via fieldworkers' tinkering with or inconsistent administration of instruments across respondents. For example, one section of LSAM's 2008 survey included a set of ten anchoring vignettes inserted into the questionnaire by a sociologist. King and Wand (2007) and Harkness et al. (2010) describe vignettes as cameo descriptions of hypothetical situations or individuals. These allow for individual assessments to be broadened, ostensibly increasing the validity of data.[21] Vignettes have been used in over eighty countries and deemed efficacious at constructing a common scale of measurement across respondents, mitigating the differential item functioning associated with differences in how respondents understand ordinal response categories of degree (strongly disagree, disagree, etc.; King and Wand 2007).

Underlying administration of these tools are assumptions that respondents assess their own health in the same way they assess that of a fictitious

V4	On some days Grace travels to a larger market in a nearby trading center about 5 kilometers away. She enjoys this trip because there are more goods at this market and she can meet up with friends to chat. She doesn't ask his permission to go to this market because he gets suspicious if she goes to the market alone. How much power does Grace have to travel when and where she wants?	A lot Some A little None Don't know	1 2 3 4 88

FIGURE 1.4. A sample vignette from the LSAM questionnaire, 2008.

character and that scenarios presented in the vignettes are perceived in the same way across respondents. As in the case of the pictographic instruments, the vignettes, too, attempt to address potential cross-cultural incomparability in survey research. Vignettes are meant to describe someone like the respondent, evident in the names assigned to these fictitious individuals (see figure 1.4). In LSAM's case, the skeleton version of an anchoring vignette used to measure women's travel autonomy stages a particularly Malawian scene: a woman named Grace, markets, and a suspicious male lover. In addition to making respondents hear the question correctly, the wide inclusion of these instruments across cultural contexts enables comparability of constructs previously deemed incomparable. In the process of rewriting the bare-bones form of a question—imported to the LSAM survey from external contexts—researchers invent culture as manifest in local names and locally resonant scenarios. Paradoxically, then, vignettes aim to make commensurate the seemingly incommensurable, in line with the culture of demography's emphasis on the comparability of concepts over space and time and their harmonization (Randall, Coast, and Leone 2011, 222). Comparability becomes an end in itself.

Demographers and field teams place the burden of blame for poorly functioning questions on themselves; as Andrews, longtime LSAM field supervisor, told a new crop of interviewers in training: "In research we don't blame the respondent."[22] This phrase was often repeated during training sessions, reinforcing the assumption that researchers (in the office) and fieldworkers (in the field) have control over the quality of data collected through meticulous attention to survey design and translation and standardized implementation, respectively.

Another practice that helps ensure questions' validity manifests in the preferential inclusion of closed questions, what I—an anthropologist among the demographers—in my field notes referred to as a "fetish for codes" in survey research. In LSAM and MAYP surveys, closed questions are the dominant genre of query, illustrating the presumed link between this form of question and data quality. As Glewwe (2005a, 44) advises, "questionnaires should be designed so that the answers to almost all questions are pre-coded." Precoded closed questions leave less up to the interviewer, who, in survey design guidelines and literature from the colonial era to the present, is consistently framed as unreliable, a source of error, unskilled, and untrustworthy. The familiar specter of the interviewer cooking data lurks in the imagination of researchers, informing their investment in the simplest, most easily administered questions with a clear set of possible responses. Closed questions, as well, help ensure that the appearance of a survey is "neat" and "uncluttered," ostensibly making the interviewer's work easier and faster in the field (Casley and Kumar 1988, 72). A code-based survey, however, requires an appendage packet of questionnaire codes to go along with some questions, which in LSAM's case was seven pages long. As demographers are well aware, these codes stand in as representative of a respondent's answers; indeed, the interviewer's action of recording a code on the survey page is the act in which information is transformed into data. Nancy Luke (2006) points to what is lost in this conversion. She examines Kenyan census data from 1989, looking specifically at questions that asked respondents to choose their marriage status from among six possibilities. In western Kenya, where *ter* or widow inheritance—whereby a widow is "inherited" by her deceased husband's brother—is very common, she shows how the expectation that inherited women would self-identify as married was misguided; considering the attention given to ter by policy makers and public health programming, the data, then, likely are not very useful (Luke 2006, 209–210).

Echoing Luke's critique of closed questions, I noted instances across a number of interviews in which the codes provided for LSAM interviewers in the coding packet did not sufficiently cover the responses given by respondents. Section 4 (page 8 of 25) of the LSAM survey "Investment in Children's Education" contained one question that was exemplary in this regard. The section began with the interviewer recording the full names of all children of school-going age living in the household on a roster. Following this step, the interviewer proceeded to ask a series of eleven closed questions—each with corresponding possible codes—about each child named. The last of these questions (D13) asked respondents to mention what they expected each child

```
Codes for Question D13

    1= Monetary help
    2= A place to live
    3= Medical expenses
    4= Food
    5= Other
    6= Nothing
```

FIGURE 1.5. Codes to accompany question D13 from the LSAM questionnaire, 2008.

to provide them with when they were old ("When you are very old do you expect this child to provide you with:"). Interviewers were instructed to record
up to three responses, drawing from the numerical codes in the accompanying code guide (see figure 1.5).

After the interviewer asked question D13, respondents often laughed,
rather than providing a response. For example, during one interview in central Malawi in June 2008, Grace, the interviewer, struggled to deal with her
respondent Esther's response to D13. Upon hearing the question, Esther
laughed loudly and said, "Eeee, they are my children!" She implied that Grace
knew already that her children should provide her with "everything," which
she later said explicitly: "Everything! [Zonse!] They are my children after all."
Grace awkwardly attempted to get Esther to narrow her response such that it
would correspond to one of the codes itemized in figure 1.5, but to no avail.
In this case, Grace followed the advice she had been given in prefieldwork
training sessions: she best approximated her respondent's answer with the
possible codes, listing 5 among two others to capture "everything" by adding
in "other," despite researchers' continual advice that interviewers use "other"
as a code only sparingly across all closed questions. In this research encounter, then, it is through cooking up an answer not mentioned by Esther that
Grace embodies her role as a good interviewer adherent to standards for data
collection. In the field, we note that even the most closed questions—meant
to mitigate the influence of fieldworkers on data collected—rely on improvisation and creativity on fieldworkers' part. Whereas in the field, "Other"
becomes a kind of saving grace for interviewers who struggle to convert
the words of their respondents into preset codes, in the office, it is the least
desirable form of data because as a catchall, it encompasses too much to be
useful in data analysis.

Conclusion

In mid-2008, I witnessed a debate about survey translation during a training session for HIV VCT counselors working with LSAM in a district in central Malawi. A few of the interviewers objected to the way that a "circumcised person" was referred to in Chichewa on the questionnaire (*mdulidwe*, or one who has been cut), claiming that people in central Malawi—where cultural male circumcision is infrequent—would not know how to respond or would be confused. This debate, which interrupted the flow of the training for half an hour, indicates that even after surveys have been pored over in survey design meetings, they undergo negotiation and alteration as they travel out of the office. One interviewer suggested, "In Balaka [a Yao and predominantly Muslim area further south], people might know because it [circumcision] is their culture and tradition, but here in Mchinji [central Malawi], we will find people don't know. . . . People would only know it from the Bible, or just say to us, 'The Yaos do that, not us.'" As people nodded in agreement, another interviewer suggested that the current translation made it appear as if the man was naked, making a very personal question even more embarrassing to ask. Eventually, the group came to the consensus that instead of translating circumcision as "mdulidwe" (personified, "he who has been cut," from *kudula*, to cut), it should be referred to as *jando*, a Chiyao word that refers to the circumcision ritual experienced by male Yaos. Even in Christian areas, people know that Muslims practice jando. Thus, the group concluded, referring to circumcision as jando would ensure that data collected were consistent and accurate. For this particular question, field teams found both English and Chichewa inadequate, borrowing instead a word from Chiyao to ensure a question was as straightforward as possible.[23]

Notably, the final version of the VCT questionnaire—following deliberations about this point between Malawian supervisors and foreign researchers—employed the verb *kukotola* (close to the original kudula, "to cut," also "to strip from") dismissing both of the earlier translations. This vignette about translating the term "circumcision" depicts many of the themes this chapter has explored. First, it highlights that translation entails not mere conversion of words from one language into another: in this case, interviewers agree that the best token to capture the meaning of the word comes from neither the source nor the target language but another altogether. They also enact a kind of imaginative labor that mirrors that of the demographers who penned the initial question: they conjure an ideal-type respondent who, for example, on cultural or other grounds might be offended by the original token used to discuss circumcision. Finally, the instability of the word on the page itself as the survey travels into the field is a metaphor for the instability of the data the question later collects. The interviewers who debate the question have absorbed and legitimated researchers' epistemic investments in straightforward questions that will generate the best possible data, even if their position in the apparatus means their suggestions to researchers are rarely acted on.

The disciplinary culture of demographers, statisticians, and survey professionals encompasses international standardization, households as sampling frame, investments in clean data, and comparability. This chapter has traced the important role of translation in the early stages of survey research in places like Malawi. Demographers first conjure an other space—the field—that informs survey design enacted in the office. In the process, they enlist local experts who provide knowledge about Malawi that is instrumental in planning survey fieldwork, even as this knowledge and its forms reflect structural and material inequalities between foreign and Malawian experts obscured by partnership rhetoric. Finally, ethnographic analysis of the processes and relations embedded in the survey as a recipe for data collection indicates the important role that translation plays in assuring validity and quality of survey data as it travels its life course, even as it carries into the survey unremarked assumptions held by those who design it. It is these assumptions that ensure ahead of time the quality of data.

The translative efforts on the part of both past and present survey administrators in the African context foreground how relations across cultural distance bring the original into the translator's purview and stoke the translator's desire to make meaning commensurate (Pratt 1991). In the late 1930s, the Nyasaland Survey Unit noted difficulties with translating qualitative food schedules administered as part of the Nyasaland Nutrition Survey:

> One of the chief difficulties found in eliciting information for filling in these ... schedules has been the native's interpretation of the term "food." The answers to the question, "Have you eaten to-day?," or "Have you cooked to-day?," will be yes if they have eaten a main meal consisting of porridge made from the staple foodstuff, maize or other cereal or cassava, together with some side dish or dishes. A reply in the negative does not mean that no food at all has been eaten, but that the informant has not had what he considers to be a proper meal. (Berry and Petty 1992, 27)

Translation's primary connotation invokes its ambitions to determine linguistic equivalence: for survey researchers, correctly chosen word tokens carry potential payoff in the form of better, more valuable data. Whether in the case of the Nyasaland Survey Unit anticipating discrepancies between the token (food) and its interpretation by the "natives" or in the debates about translation among survey design teams introduced above, translation attempts to process the knowledge and practices of one society into the context of another. In this conversion, we note the contradiction between making apprehensible and preserving cultural difference, as rooted in epistemological and economic hierarchies that commodify translation: from words themselves, data (and value) are produced. Yet, neither the English original nor the vernacularized translation are fixed and persisting tokens; they lack essential quality and are continually transformed in space and time. Nonetheless, the claim that words can be made commensurate through careful translation and attention to the probable thought processes of an imagined low-literacy research subject betrays the epistemic commitments of researchers that define the criteria by which data are evaluated and valued. Translation is a technology that produces the subject positions and epistemological relations necessary to making bits and pieces of knowledge into valuable data.

In participating in survey design sessions and prefieldwork meetings as an anthropologist among the demographers, I was especially attentive to deployments and investments in the term "culture," that intangible and slippery aspect of human realities that anthropologists guard as their own. The invention of culture in survey research worlds plays many roles, not least of which includes compelling the translation of survey tools, metrics, and technologies into other spaces and populations than the ones they were conjured in. For demographers, culture and the field are imaginaries that enable the planning and implementation of data collection. They facilitate the building of extensive human (local fieldworkers and supervisors) and material (makeshift field offices in rough conditions) infrastructures that are social and technological hybrids reflecting demography's normative disciplinary investments.

Much of the literature on designing, implementing, and ensuring data quality in the context of survey research in developing countries centers on the problem of translation: How do we translate dominant standards for high-quality data into foreign and remote places rife with impediments that threaten to undo data's value? How do we translate survey instruments—and their underlying constructs—from one language and one cultural milieu into another without sacrificing their validity and reliability? Notably, however, these questions at the core of demographic research in places like Malawi presume demography itself as an acultural endeavor rooted in science and in possession of objective measures and instruments with universal value for collecting clean numerical data. Recent work in critical demography, science studies, and anthropology has troubled this assumption, even if its insights have failed to migrate into survey research worlds. This body of critical literature often assumes that scientists' myopic focus on their end goals narrows their vision and causes them to overlook important local factors or miss the blind spots in their own research. In her reevaluation of the Nyasaland Survey Project's well-known failures, for example, Cynthia Brantley (2002) attributes its shortcomings to a "clash of values" between the British survey team and the African ways of life they aimed to study. Surely, they may have been "puzzled that Africans viewed wealth differently [than they did]" and possessed faith in a universalizing science that promised—but failed—to provide answers to problems (51, 58–59). However, close attention to the culture of demographers in action indicates that they come to see exactly what they want to see: the survey forecloses alternative optic possibilities so that data will be clean and valid.

In analyzing how the material and human infrastructure for survey research comes about, and how the survey—the core framing device and recipe for data collection in the field—materializes, I have shown how demographers adopt heuristic tools that require imagining their objects of study as stable, fixed, and unitary, as in the case of population or household. These tools make it possible to see and represent realities of interest, to make commensurate the incommensurable, and to measure even the most intangible and subjective of constructs in an objective manner. Returning to Ferguson's (1994) insights, the remainder of the book shows specifically how the form of discourse that is the survey and its underlying epistemic fields constructs objects of knowledge and creates an infrastructure of knowledge around those objects. From the perspective of anthropologists and other critics, this structure might be said to traffic in false pictures or oversimplified numbers. The main thrust of this book, however, is not to show that demography gets it wrong, but to show that the institutionalized production of certain ideas and measures of Malawian realities have important effects and create new social worlds and possibilities. Indeed, my question is not how can demographers do better, but how do demographers generate a particular usable representation of Malawi for themselves and others who assign it legitimacy (Ferguson 1994, 71)?

Sample and household, as we have seen, are central categories in demographic analysis, and both graft a certain false fixity onto shifting and complex human realities that far exceed the ambitions of the bounded container metaphor central to the demographic imaginary. They very much influence data collection methods and the kinds of instruments inserted into surveys. Individuals behave in uncontained ways—but demography has ways of capturing and measuring such unruly behaviors as migration, refusals to answer a survey question, death, and so on, such that they do not threaten the imagined bounded container that underlies epistemic virtues. The bounded container model incorporates well-formulated checks and balances that enable statements to be made about data's reliability. These categories are not simply objective or statistical but culturally embedded, as this book elucidates. Categories do not merely measure something out there but are symptoms of the foreclosure of other ways of seeing.

As chapter 2 illustrates, the meaning of the categories and terms enshrined in the questionnaire can only be understood in terms of the discursive processes in the forms and instructions used in the collection of data (Higgs 2004, 90). In its movement from the office discussed in this chapter into the field that is the geographic setting for the next three chapters, the survey form's standardizing, clean, and neat ambitions and dreams are threatened at every turn.

TWO

LIVING PROJECT
TO PROJECT

Brokering Local
Knowledge in the Field

In the living room of a guesthouse in Blantyre—Malawi's commercial capital—members of a research team gather around Dr. Cook, an American researcher affiliated with Religion and Malawi (RAM), who is leading a project investigating the medicinal practices and HIV-related knowledge of traditional healers. The guesthouse serves as RAM's temporary headquarters for the next several weeks, a base from which fieldwork teams will set off each day to collect questionnaires and interview data in surrounding areas, and the office where interviews will be transcribed and data entered into databases. In addition to the young college-educated Malawians who will administer the questionnaire to traditional healers in the field, John and Victor, Malawian fieldwork supervisors who have worked on many such research projects in the past, are present. After introducing the survey to her audience, Dr. Cook looks expectantly at Victor, asking, "Traditional healers are of different sorts, right? I've heard that there are different categories of healers—herbalists, witchcraft-related . . ." He answers this question concisely, one among many he fields on a daily basis about Malawi and Malawian culture from the foreign (*azungu*) researchers he works for. Later, John and Victor lead a training session to familiarize the new fieldworkers with the questionnaire. In addition to going over technical details pertinent to conducting a good interview, they provide the fieldworkers with some advice that might make their work go more smoothly. Victor explains:

> We aren't there to correct their [traditional healers'] misconceptions, just to collect them. Even if we know what they are telling us is wrong, about AIDS or whatever, don't be judgmental. . . . Know how the healers are. They want respect and can be hard to deal with, as they expect to be treated like big men even if they are no big deal at all: "Take off your shoes when you enter my house, or bow down to greet me." If they want you to take off your shoes and bangles so you don't disturb the spirits or whatnot, just do it! [Chuckles from audience.] It's the same thing with the pastors we've met [on past projects], where we pray with them before we start [the research] to connect with them.[1]

Victor brokers local knowledge to different audiences. First, he clarifies the fuzzy picture Dr. Cook holds of traditional healers in Malawi. Second, his advice to novice fieldworkers bridges a potential gap between urban-dwelling and college-educated fieldworkers and the traditional healers they will soon encounter. This scene captures some of the expectations of individuals hired as knowledge workers on survey research projects. I use the term "knowledge worker" deliberately here for two reasons. First, the term is often associated with elites who "think for a living," and falls on the "skilled" side of a modernist dichotomy between "labor of the head" and "labor of the hands" (Arendt 1958, 90). In using it to refer to fieldworkers, I trouble the assumption that fieldworkers are unskilled laborers or minor actors in survey research; in fact, knowledge production depends on their innovative work in the field. Second, the term is capacious enough to capture what I deem to be two important dimensions of fieldwork: (1) the process of producing data, tangible material units (e.g., survey responses recorded on a page) that fieldworkers help along a life course, rather than abstract statistics; and (2) the ways in which fieldworkers work to produce and claim ownership over the kinds of local knowledge researchers value (in the process, working knowledge to their benefit to protect their economic niche in a larger global health apparatus).

As middlemen, knowledge workers skillfully mediate between disparate spaces and groups of people on a daily basis. In addition to filling in gaps in the course of survey design and fieldwork, they also police boundaries between kinds of knowers and produce the forms of difference that data collection relies on. Traditional healers—often framed as repositories of medical knowledge—are, in Victor's view, saddled with misconceptions about AIDS that will soon be collected in the space of an interview encounter. In foregrounding the cultural obstacles fieldworkers might face (superstitions, traditional beliefs and customs, and inflated big-man egos), he marks the healers as Other and emphasizes the status differential between interviewers and their interviewees. Meanwhile, the fieldworkers chuckle at the thought of disturbing spirits during routine administration of a survey, making known their own disregard for such backward beliefs.

. . .

Chapter 1 illustrates how the tangible pages of a questionnaire—yet to be administered—are material manifestations of researchers' dreams and designs, a template for proper collection of data. Whereas the foreign and Malawian researchers we encountered in survey design sessions are the familiar and recognizable experts of global health in Africa, the value of survey data is constituted by the largely invisible labor performed by the hundreds of fieldworkers and supervisors—such as the one pictured in figure 2.1—in the field who are the focus of the next three chapters. Field research, even as it appears to be simply the systematic collection of information from respondents, necessitates a complex and flexible assembly line of people, equipment, technical and logistical know-how, and appropriate social and environmental conditions. The field is not just a place from which data are collected; rather, it is a constructed and negotiated space in which knowledge, value, and new kinds of relations take form (Gupta and Ferguson 1997; Schumaker 2001). The transformation of raw information into statistics that become evidence for policy or interventions is facilitated by many individuals who shape data as they travel in their life course, the large majority of whom—unskilled data collectors—have until recently been overlooked by ethnographers of global health (Kamuya et al. 2013; Kingori 2013; Molyneux et al. 2013; Engel et al. 2014; Prince and Otieno 2014; Kingori and Gerrets 2016).

Since the earliest surveys and research endeavors enacted in sub-Saharan Africa, fieldworkers have appeared in accounts as individuals whose menial labor is necessary to field research, but without any particular kind of expertise. In the Nyasaland Survey (1938–1943), for example, "native assistants" appear as an undifferentiated mass of individuals whose work entailed, for example, collecting stool and urine specimens in chip boxes and test tubes or measuring gardens by stepping out their circumference with the aid of a compass (Berry and Petty 1992, 290, 29). This chapter aims to challenge such

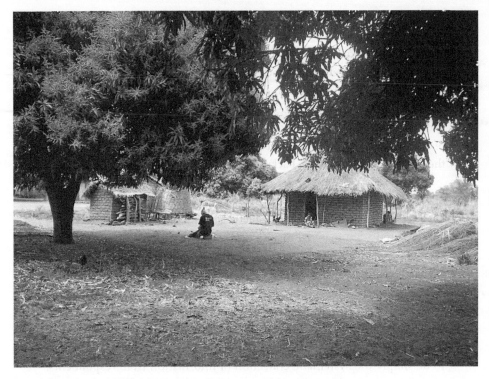

FIGURE 2.1. An LSAM fieldworker checks a survey questionnaire near the household where it was administered. Photo by the author.

depictions. The increasing expansion of markets for knowledge work amid proliferating global health projects affords Malawian fieldworkers new opportunities for social and economic mobility, however precarious or short lived those opportunities may be (Prince 2014). As this chapter illustrates, while foreign researchers tend to view local knowledge as a stable entity that streamlines everyday fieldwork, fieldworkers capitalize on the fact that their expertise is not stable or inherent but rather malleable and performative. Inspired by Lambek's (1993) classic study of knowledge in Mayotte, I consider how local knowledge is produced, distributed, and consumed, paying close attention to how the forms and techniques of knowledge in research worlds emerge from a crowded social field of diverse actors.

Reflecting on the place of local knowledge in data collection, longtime fieldwork supervisor Andrews suggested, "Researchers don't just want a tour guide; they want a Renaissance man!" Rather than a tour guide who might provide mere geographic direction in an unfamiliar place, a Renaissance man possesses diversified knowledge of a local context that is crucial to the smooth running of data collection.[2] Presuming local expertise to be embodied, relational, and improvised, this chapter argues that the local knowledge and professional identities of Malawian fieldworkers are cooked and commodified in the practices of data collection in the field. In what follows, I provide an ethnographic glimpse at some of the everyday interactions between fieldworkers, supervisors, and researchers, each of whom is differentially invested in a shared knowledge-making project.

First, I describe fieldworkers' interests in maintaining ownership over the local knowledge foreign researchers expect them to possess. I examine prefieldwork training sessions as an important site where fieldworkers are initiated into new professional identities and where the social boundaries (between knower and known) and spatiotemporal boundaries (between office and field, urban and rural, and modern and backward) that undergird data collection are performed and practiced. Following fieldworkers into the field, I then show how such tactical boundary work informs research encounters and revalues and redefines the local expertise at the core of data collection. Throughout, the chapter takes an interest in how the governing structures of research work as temporary, underpaid, and difficult—glossed by fieldworkers as living project to project—nonetheless enable them potential access to social, cultural, and economic capital and facilitate the imagining of new futures.

Recruiting Knowledge Workers

Survey research projects afford some measure of economic and social mobility to a cohort of young Malawian secondary graduates and college graduates who find temporary, contractual employment in the world of AIDS research. These individuals are hired as fieldwork supervisors, interviewers, or data entry clerks. The uncoupling of authorship of data from a singular sovereign researcher entails both possibilities and pitfalls for the kinds of knowledge produced. Table 2.1 summarizes the major daily duties of these individuals. While the table overlooks the contributions of other members of fieldwork teams (such as drivers, cleaners, and cooks), it reflects the focus of this chapter on knowledge workers, or individuals who have sustained contact with data in some form. The duties summarized here are elaborated in the course of the chapter.

Many of the college graduates employed at the time of this research were contract workers with the Centre for Social Research (an arm of the

TABLE 2.1 Fieldwork Team Members' Roles

Job Title	Summary of Duties
Fieldwork supervisor	Supervise a team of 5–10 interviewers in the field, check and monitor the progress of data collection in real time, make decisions and set agenda for daily data collection, interface between foreign researchers and fieldwork teams, attend daily meetings with foreign researchers, fieldwork trouble shooting, hiring and firing of interviewers (sometimes), provide input and feedback on the content of surveys and other data collection instruments, introduce fieldwork teams to traditional authorities and district officials
Interviewer/data collector	Work as a member of a fieldwork team, visit individual households to collect survey, HIV test, or anthropometric data, check surveys or other data before submitting to supervisors, provide input on daily logistics and fieldwork schedule
Data entry clerk	Enter survey and other data into a growing digital database as it is submitted in hard copy by fieldwork supervisors, help with organizational and office tasks as needed

University of Malawi whose history is elaborated in chapter 1) or a consulting firm. These organizations hire out ready-made teams of experienced fieldworkers and field vehicles (minibuses or SUVs), displacing much of the responsibility for survey research logistics from foreign researchers to local firms or centers.[3] Whereas MAYP, RAM, and GSIP sourced college-educated fieldworkers in this way, LSAM preferred to pick and choose its own fieldwork teams, recruiting fieldworkers locally by posting printed advertisements on trees, walls, or at the district offices some days ahead of its arrival at a field site. On interview day, hundreds of secondary school graduates from the project's sample areas turned up with their school certificates in hand. For aspiring fieldworkers, securing a temporary but stable job was a welcome and unusual opportunity. In some cases, after LSAM finished data collection in one region of Malawi, interviewers would migrate with LSAM to its next field site in a different district with the hope of securing the same position there. College graduates, too, sometimes traveled from the city to rural recruitment sites to apply for these jobs, in a reversal of the more familiar Malawian countryside-to-city labor migration path.

The relatively small number of LSAM fieldwork jobs available often engendered accusations from locals that persons selected to administer surveys in their district or village were outsiders taking their jobs. Hiring practices expressed and reified underlying stereotypes or caricatures of ethnic groups. Supervisors who interviewed potential employees lamented the paucity of educated Yao speakers (making timely administration of surveys in Yao-speaking areas difficult), and also considered Yao interviewers to be "dull[er] and slow[er]" than interviewers of other ethnic backgrounds.[4] Likewise, fieldwork teams considered Balaka District in southern Malawi their least preferred fieldwork site, complaining, "Yaos [a large, primarily Muslim ethnic group in the district] have so many spouses and so many children" (making filling in a household register on a survey an onerous task) and that Yaos are uneducated, making them more likely to accuse research teams of bloodsucking or to refuse to participate in surveys. They claimed that Yao men were difficult to find for interviews, as they were always out "doing business."[5] The construction of both Yao interviewers and respondents in research cultures enlist popular notions of Yao-ness as they play out in the Malawian national imagination and showcase the ways in which survey projects become sites where social boundaries and difference are (re)invented and performed.[6]

Swidler and Watkins (2009) term secondary school graduates in Malawi such as those who work intermittently for research projects "interstitial elites"; in a country where only a small minority achieves the status of either secondary school or college graduate, they aspire to a bright future.[7] However, because they are not sufficiently educated, for example, to be competitive for NGO jobs in the cities, these young people—like others of their generation across sub-Saharan Africa—often also find work as volunteers in donor-implemented programs or AIDS interventions (McKay 2012; van de Ruit 2012; Madiega et al. 2013; Swartz 2013; Prince 2014; Maes 2017). These positions come with benefits such as small stipends and the possibility of being hired as a paid employee in the future. Similarly, research jobs provide a temporary paid break from farming and petty trading. Many fieldworkers suggested that after a project left town, they would return home to do farming and "wait for [more] jobs from projects," and most articulated ambitions to return to school for degrees in practical fields such as computing or accounting if they saved enough money in the future. In 2008, I administered a short survey ($n=117$, response rate 98/117, 84 percent) to a cohort of fieldworkers (supervisors, data collectors, data entry clerks, and HIV test counselors) working for LSAM, MAYP, RAM, GSIP, and other survey-type projects in 2007–2008. The survey revealed that the average age of fieldworkers was 25.41 years old; 30 percent were secondary school graduates; 60 percent had also attained a postsecondary school certificate (in fields such as accounting,

VCT, or secretarial skills); and 10 percent were college graduates (percentages rounded to whole numbers).

Brokering Local Knowledge in the Field

As a fieldworker, the [HIV] counselor should . . . know that culture has been there for ages and your plan is new to them [the villagers who are participating in research] and it might also take another generation to change the culture.[8]

This excerpt from a training manual distributed to fieldwork teams by LSAM—authored by veteran Malawian fieldworkers—implicitly solidifies boundaries even as it attempts to make them permeable, much like the supervisor's words during the training session at the start of this chapter. First, it rhetorically places a boundary between the VCT counselors and their subjects, rural Malawians, by confining culture to the villages and associating the power to change culture with counselors. Likewise, in its objective to train or teach the counselors to be good fieldworkers, it draws a boundary between the project and its employees. Solidifying and emphasizing boundaries between themselves and their employers and between themselves and rural research participants enables fieldwork supervisors and interviewers to preserve ownership over local knowledge and to ensure it remains valuable. As we will see, within a survey project, it is not just data that are produced, but identities, dreams, and social boundaries as well.

TRAINING FOR THE FIELD: BOUNDARY WORK
AND THE PRODUCTION OF DIFFERENCE

During the first week or two of a fieldwork season, LSAM, GSIP, MAYP, and RAM all held extensive training sessions for their fieldworkers. These trainings took place in rented facilities (such as a teacher's college or a hotel conference room) or at the guesthouse where fieldwork teams stayed for the duration of data collection. Their purpose was to encourage bonding among the field teams, to determine before fieldwork began which fieldworkers should be let go, to familiarize fieldworkers with the survey or other instruments to be implemented, and to standardize and harmonize data collection procedures as much as possible. Becoming a competent fieldworker necessitates training as a mode of professionalization into the world of survey research. Fieldworkers are trained to transform villages into "the field," snippets of conversation into data, and rural dwellers into interviewees. Instead of initiating fieldworkers into local culture, these trainings initiate them into research culture and, in the process, facilitate new imaginings of self and other. Whereas chapter 4 shows how the epistemic virtues held by demographers come to be embodied—if imperfectly—during the administration of surveys to rural Malawians, this chapter focuses on how data collection produces new kinds of social boundaries and forms of difference and revalues local knowledge. In fact, it is in their interactions with data and standards for their collection that fieldworkers gain the local expertise they offer to foreign researchers.

Participants in the training sessions coconstructed an archetypal villager or research subject to facilitate their work in the field. Engagement with this ideal villager necessitated preparations and forethought as to proper comportment, behavior, and dress code on the part of the fieldwork teams. On day two of a joint training session for LSAM interviewers and HIV counselors in May 2008, Francis, the Malawian VCT team supervisor, provided a rapid-fire set of guidelines to his trainees: "How do we dress for the field? We put on *chitenje* [cloth wrap worn by most rural women]. We can't wear what we wear in the city. You have to suit the environment. Strong perfume can make the respondent uncomfortable. Manners affect everything. Chewing gum is rude. Don't whisper or appear to be gossiping in front of villagers."[9] The supervisor closed this session with a performance of a commonly known piece of village culture in Malawi: he clasped his hands together and thanked the trainees for their attention: "Zikomo! [Thank you!]" The gesture—Zikomo—was explained for the benefit of those who may have been unfamiliar: "Always do this if you pass someone in the village or if you wish to enter someone's compound." Instructions such as these belied an assumption on the part of LSAM's Malawian supervisors that fieldworkers must be familiarized with or acclimated to the field. As they are trained to embody a new occupational role, they are also taught that they are fundamentally different—more urbane, more familiar with international branding, more sophisticated, more open-minded—than the villagers they will be interviewing (Pigg 1996).[10] However, Francis's instructions also point to the supervisors' interest in maintaining a boundary between themselves and their trainees: they are the experts imparting accumulated fieldwork wisdom to a group of initiates (see Englund [2006] on the production of such boundaries in professionalized human rights advocacy spaces in Malawi).

Project guidelines for dress and comportment were meticulously observed by fieldworkers and monitored by fieldwork supervisors, and clothing and comportment became embodied symbols of fieldworkers' professionalism, status, and difference from rural villagers (Justice 1986, 143; Nading 2013, 98).

In June 2008, I attended training sessions for LSAM interviewers who would be administering a long survey to villagers in the coming weeks. As they prepared to enter the field for the first time to pilot the survey, a supervisor singled out a fashionably dressed male interviewer who was sporting a Kangol brand cap to drive home a lesson: "We can't be putting on hats like this one *ku mudzi* [in the village]!" A few months later, another male interviewer was sent home to change his trousers before work. His supervisor asked him, "What were you thinking coming to work with those jeans with 50 CENT [the American hip-hop artist] written on them in big letters?" Interviewers, too, commented on their colleagues' attire, often in gendered fashion, as when one woman was consistently singled out for choosing to wear "shoes meant for clubbing" in the field. Critiques of field attire such as these produce the city and the village as incommensurable places: "Blantyre is Blantyre, but Mchinji [a rural fieldwork site] . . . *ndi ena!* [The city is one thing, but the rural areas are another thing altogether!]," as Francis put it.[11]

In their effort to blend in with villagers, fieldworkers employed costumes, props, and accessories. During our daily minibus journeys to the field, I witnessed a ritualized collapse and maintenance of boundaries between the categories of field and office, and researched and researcher. At about the half-way point between the field office and the field in the mornings, the women in the van tied headscarves or bandanas around their heads and knotted colorful chitenje fabric around their waists (usually over trousers or a skirt). At the end of the day, they sighed with relief, unwrapped their heads, and removed the now dusty chitenje. Men, too, adopted certain ritualized codes of dress and mannerisms; they often referred to their older or less fashionable sneakers as fieldwork shoes and replaced them with their regular, cleaner, and more stylish shoes at the end of the day before heading into town for dinner. During downtime in the field, supervisors often shopped at weekly markets in trading centers near sample villages for low-priced field clothes. The symbolic distance between the fieldworkers and the villagers was reestablished as the minivan hurried back to the office in the evenings.

In July 2008, rituals of fieldwork dress were at the center of a discussion between Dr. Smith, an American public health researcher who was in Malawi with RAM for two weeks, and John, the supervisor for the project's data collection that summer. Dr. Smith inquired why female fieldworkers wore headscarves while in the field but not in the office. John explained that it was to foster closeness to their respondents by hiding things like expensive extensions or elaborate hairstyles village women do not have access to. "To not wear the scarf would be saying, 'I have a lot of money and I'm not from around here and I care too much about my hair.'" In practice, however, wearing scarves and *zitenje* worked to accentuate the social distance between interviewers and research subjects. Villagers could tell if a fieldworker wore her hair in extensions even if she covered them with a headscarf and knew she was dressing down. However, attempting to blend in allowed the interviewer to maintain a foothold in both the local and research worlds that she straddled. Interviewers gradually became skilled at using cultural diacritics to competently blend into the field and embody a certain cultural style by "deploying signs in a way that position[ed them] in relation to social categories" (Ferguson 1999, 96). Even if they are not fooling anyone, dressing and undressing indicates their interest in knowing and mastering the local, an endeavor at the center of their professionalization into fieldwork. Clothes and accessories may seem insignificant props in the drama of fieldwork, but they are symbolic markers of the shared investments of members of fieldwork cultures in policing the boundary between the field and the office, and the knowers and the known (Gieryn 1999). In fact, it is the shared agenda of the actors who make up the survey research project—producing clean data—that gives birth to new social hierarchies and status regimes mirrored by the spatialized narration and performance of difference.

The field was also produced as a place of difference in fieldworkers' narrations of fieldwork as an adventure, as out of the ordinary, and as a kind of roughing it. In the open-ended survey questionnaire I distributed to over one hundred interviewers and supervisors (working on survey projects including my case study projects, mentioned above), I asked respondents what they most enjoyed about fieldwork. The responses complemented conversations I had with project staff members: the field was imagined as an almost magical place that was unfamiliar and new. Most respondents mentioned that they enjoyed fieldwork because it afforded them the opportunity to travel and learn more about Malawi (77/98, or 79 percent of respondents to the survey mentioned these as the main benefits of fieldwork jobs).[12]

Fieldworkers viewed fieldwork as an opportunity to get out of familiar settings and explore new ones. They described fieldwork as "a chance to discover the world" and liked that it provided opportunities to make business or other connections, to see family in other parts of Malawi, or to eat new and different foods. While teaching at the University of Malawi from September to December 2008, I frequently socialized with research supervisors, many of whom were tired of the downtime between projects, since most data collection happens during the American or European summer (Malawi's winter). They "longed to be on the move again." Some projects took fieldworkers on short leisure trips to places like South Luangwa National Park in neighboring Zambia, to wildlife reserves near research sites, or on other special outings. All projects organized parties, often with a *braii* (barbeque), a DJ, and dancing, for employees at the end of data collection at one site. Finally, fieldworkers appreciated the intimate fictive kinship that developed in research cultures, often referring to their workmates as a "fieldwork family." Fieldwork and the field offer the same opportunities for adventure, novelty, and leisure to Malawian staff as they do to foreign graduate or undergraduate students who look forward to a summer in Africa, even if the economic investments of these parties in research may be drastically different.

Fieldworkers liked learning what rural Malawians do, being exposed to the cultural beliefs of rural people, learning about Chewa culture, playing *bao* (a traditional game of skill and strategy played on a board with pitted holes and small stones or seeds) or football with young men in trading centers, and listening to elders' stories in the villages.[13] Fieldworkers enjoyed interacting with people of different backgrounds, cultures, and beliefs, and saw fieldwork as an opportunity to understand "the real life of the people and their culture and to see what it means to be Malawian" or to see remote parts of Malawi.[14] For fieldworkers, then, as for foreign researchers, the households they visited and the villagers they met stood in for an imagined real Malawi different from what they were used to: indeed, this is the poor, undeveloped, and backward Malawi that motivates data collection in the first place. Fieldworkers also look upon and construct rural research participants nostalgically, as symbols of a nation of peasant farmers, bearers of tradition, and masters of cultural knowledge, as foils to their more modern selves.

Just as Anna Tsing's (2004, 122) Indonesian "nature lovers" learn to love nature as a modern, technical, and scientific thing, so too do fieldworkers (and anthropologists, for that matter) come to see the field as something outside their everyday worlds that must be embodied through discipline, training, and experience. Interviewers who were working in their own districts or villages (in the case of LSAM) emphasized this difference in order to lend credibility to their new role as expert interviewers and to draw attention to their belonging in a community of researchers. This role and its associated symbols (project T-shirt, badge or photo ID, clipboard, canvas bag for holding soap and surveys) gave them significant status and cultural capital among their peers, who, in cases where projects hired locally, might also be acquaintances or family members (Justice 1986, 102–103; Riedmann 1993, 47–65). Through their initiation into research culture, individuals learned to see research participants as different, even as they mastered a set of techniques to align themselves with the field.

Training sessions produced expectations and stereotypes about village culture meant to guide the actions and interactions of fieldworkers on the job. Trainings employed a cultural competency approach based on predictions of behaviors or scenarios one is likely to face when interacting with, for example, someone from a different ethnic group or gender than one's own. During the training session for LSAM's HIV counselors who would be deployed to villages to test and counsel research participants, a supervisor said, "In Rumphi, you might find that a man can have seven wives; in Balaka, there [they also have multiple wives] too."[15] Other assumptions manifested in the supervisors' explanation that men in village households do not cook or carry water and that women do not build houses. The training manuals that accompanied these lessons in cultural sensitivity presented a number of scenarios likely to happen in the field (a place described as "never short of drama, dilemma, laughter or even tears" by the veteran supervisors who authored the manual). The scenarios were followed by formulaic suggested responses to guide the counselors in real time. Throughout, the manual and the training sessions objectified culture as a stumbling block to the progress of research in the field: "Everyone is molded by culture and . . . defends his culture and it is not easy to change one's culture just by comparing to some culture practiced by some people somewhere. . . . Us [sic] as counselors are not supposed to advise but rather just give information, have a small mouth [hold one's tongue] and avoid developing anger [creating bad feelings] in the people you are working with."[16]

Interviewers at another training session were encouraged "to try not to change whatever they [villagers] might believe . . . or tell them it is wrong to believe in *afiti* [witches]." By relegating culture to the realm of the traditional, old fashioned, rural, and backward, the training sessions produce a temporal and spatial distance between the fieldworkers who are presumed to be naked of culture, and villagers (or others) who are imagined to be mired in culture. These sessions and the talk and rhetoric common to research worlds effectively make culture visible to fieldworkers by inventing it—and containing it in the field—which facilitates fieldworkers' imagination that they are links or translators between two worlds glossed as the field and the office. This recalls Wagner's (1981) argument that anthropologists invent culture as their object of study upon entering the field. Trainings further compel the imagination of a national topography characterized by field sites, pockets of stagnant culture, intersected by the paths of mobile and cosmopolitan fieldworkers; the field constructed in the space of training sessions functions to negate the coeval existence of fieldworkers and respondents (Fabian [1983] 2002). The trainings ask interviewers to black box culture in order to render it incapable of complicating or slowing down fieldwork. This black boxing plays a central role in "seeing like a research project" (Biruk 2012), where the sample is the standardized and bounded unit that acts as a tidy container for data. In inventing culture as something other, fieldworkers and supervisors shore up their own performances of objectivity, neutrality, and professionalism. Data collection is framed as a scientific, rather than a cultural, enterprise; rather than waiting to be collected, then, data are invented in the social processes that constitute survey research.

Historian of science Lyn Schumaker (2001) observes that fieldworkers associated with the Rhodes-Livingstone Institute (RLI) in its heyday came to view themselves not as mere research assistants but as researchers. The same was true in Malawi, especially among supervisors who worked for many years with projects (indeed, LSAM supervisors have been coauthors on research articles published in demographic journals). Identifying as a researcher entailed performances that theatrically emphasized the difference and distance between science and culture or between the rational and irrational. Telling jokes and sharing silly villager stories were one act in these performances. These took diverse forms, but articulated a general theme of backwardness or stubbornness about change: villagers are short sighted when they carry maize to a nearby trading center or *boma* to sell it, or villagers think maize mill owners grind children's bones into maize flour, or villagers believe in bloodsuckers, for example (see chapter 3 for an extended discussion of bloodsucker stories).[17] The conclusion of one of these stories was met with generalized agreement among a narrator and her audience that "villagers believe the craziest things!" This storytelling conjured a narrativized foil to fieldworkers charged with researching villagers and solidified their higher social status (Riedmann 1993, 33–46; Englund 2006), not least to the anthropologist in their presence.[18]

CHECKING AND CREDIBILITY STRUGGLES IN
THE FIELD: MAKING LOCAL KNOWLEDGE

Even as fieldworkers enact a social, cultural, and geographic distance from rural Malawians, they also performatively draw attention to their difference from foreign researchers or project staff. Fieldworkers stake a claim on authentic local knowledge that only they possess. This entails the maintenance of boundaries between local and global expertise that function to sequester and sacralize the former. This boundary work hinges on explicitly or implicitly identifying oneself in opposition to those who occupy different social positions in research cultures.

Well into LSAM's 2008 fieldwork season, the American researchers modified the division of fieldwork labor. The study employed numerous American and British graduate and undergraduate students. As these students framed it, they did the grunt work for the project: photocopying surveys, buying soap gifts for research participants in town, supervising data entry teams, coding qualitative data, making trips to the airport to fetch foreign team members or gear, crunching numbers, organizing databases, and so on. A few students were engaged in small projects of their own, while others were described as lazy by LSAM's principal investigators. Either way, though, the graduate students often had idle time when fieldwork teams were out in the vans for the day. After some deliberation, researchers assigned the students a new role as checkers who would leave the office to travel to the field a minimum number of times each week of their stay in Malawi. A student would accompany a team of about ten fieldworkers to the field and help supervisors check the questionnaires for completeness and errors as the interviewers submitted them during the day. This checking process, usually accomplished by the Malawian supervisors alone, is an important way to reduce the number of follow-up trips to fill in the blanks left by negligent interviewers. If errors or omissions are discovered while a team is still near a household, the interviewer is sent back the same day to correct them (this is termed a callback). If they are discovered later, the team has to make a special trip and loses valuable time and gasoline in the process.

When the project directors introduced this new plan over a late dinner of chicken and *nsima* one night, the supervisors were not enthused. They claimed that the non-Malawian checkers would "slow [them] down" and be "dead weight." In the course of the next few weeks, their fears were made manifest (in their eyes). The new checkers tended to question things that the supervisors were confident should not be questioned on the completed surveys. Each time an error or incongruence was flagged on a survey by a checker, the team had to deal with callbacks to the household in question. For instance, azungu checkers would flag questions on the survey where an interviewer had filled in the age of a child in Standard 4 as fourteen years or had written 30,000 *kwacha* (at the time, 214 USD) for the amount a rural household had saved last year. Supervisors explained that one must be Malawian in order to know basic things, and to check most of the figures and information filled into the questionnaires. They suggested that a Malawian would know that it is not unheard-of for a fourteen-year-old in a rural area to be enrolled in Standard 4, even though most pupils in that grade would be nine years old. Similarly, they said, although 30,000 kwacha is a large sum for a rural family to save up, some families run maize mills or enjoy bumper tobacco crops. Checking, then, is a form of expertise that entails having an eye for checking; checkers are able to quickly assess whether a recorded datum makes sense in the universe of possible responses to a survey question. Team members endorsed hierarchies of checking where foreign checkers were on the bottom and longtime fieldworkers possessed the greatest ability to accurately "eyeball" a survey's pages (Coopmans and Button 2014, 774).

The supervisors suggested there were specific kinds of local knowledge the survey sought that the American students were unlikely to be able to gauge for accuracy: how much cash crops like tobacco or groundnuts had fetched per kilogram the prior year, how much money a family saved or loaned in a year, or how many times a respondent reported having sex.[19] In the words of long-time research supervisor Andrews:

> That's the problem with having someone check questionnaires, like the azungu they [principal investigators] are sending as checkers to us. . . . Someone from somewhere else doesn't know the area. They are not familiar with what is happening on the ground. . . . You can have the azungu working in the field, which is proved through simple calculations, but if you are trying to study something which is . . . sort of a local thing, something unknown to them, you have to have people who know what is happening on the ground, so that your data can't be questionable. These guys don't know enough about the context, about Malawi, to be able to check a questionnaire and to correct the interviewer's work. These people just here for a few weeks just can't do that kind of work![20]

The claim that azungu checkers lack the local knowledge needed to properly check and preserve the quality of research data articulates a solid boundary between these two categories of experts, preserving certain tasks, translations, and contexts as the sole purview of the Malawian fieldworkers. Andrews casts local knowledge as possessed only by native Malawians or by those who have assimilated to the local culture. We might interpret this as an instance of what Steven Epstein (1996) terms credibility struggles. The kinds of knowledge that are second nature to Malawian local experts but alien to azungu checkers have the potential to enhance data quality, according to fieldworkers. In survey research worlds, the positions occupied by the Malawian local experts are always already relative to those occupied by non-Malawians. Fieldworkers are interested in preserving their status as purveyors and owners of local knowledge and in portraying this expertise as indispensable to the smooth operation of data collection.

It is via these kinds of boundary work that local knowledge is produced as a valuable entity. Indeed, projects such as those depicted in this book provide fruitful sites for rethinking anthropological analyses of how knowledge is defined and arbitrated, how it is justified, communicated, learned, or withheld. Anthropologists have long taken interest in hierarchies of knowledge that privilege technical, scientific, explicit, and Western knowledge at the expense of indigenous, local, tacit, or vernacular knowledge. An underlying thread in critical development and global health studies is an effort to uncover, rescue, or elevate local knowledge that is often marginalized or discredited. Local knowledge has become associated with the nuance that global designs and projects lack. Yet the example of survey project fieldworkers illustrates how, in global health worlds, "local knowledge" must carry with it the scare quotes that de-emphasize its stability and legitimacy (cf. Peters 2016). More generally, this case indicates the epistemological specificity of local knowledge: indeed, the peripatetic nature of LSAM (which took up temporary residence in three different districts in the course of three months) belies the fact that local knowledge is not something possessed, rooted in a specific place or person, but rather a set of techniques and self-presentations, a habitus (Boyer 2008, 44). Countering common representations of fieldworkers as intimately familiar with the people and places they collect data from and in, and as natural translators between global and local (e.g., Madhavan et al. 2007, 374–375), I suggest that it is through their engagement with data that fieldworkers gain local knowledge. Their expertise reflects their structural position in a research world and, predictably, often resonates with their patrons' existing assumptions (Tilley 2007, 17–19). Amid countless accounts that narrate how local knowledge is cannibalized or exploited by global projects, the case of fieldworkers in Malawi meanwhile illustrates that local knowledge comes to exist—and to gain value—because of them.

Student checkers were short-term visitors to Malawi who were unlikely to return again in the future. They had little to no knowledge of Malawi and, in some cases, could have just as easily ended up in a completely different country. To them, Malawi was a kind of undifferentiated field, a place to get research experience. Conversely, many of the Malawian research team members—as mentioned above—viewed themselves as researchers who had accumulated years of experience and wisdom about survey work in Malawi. Further, although some of the students were close in age to some of the supervisors, the longitudinal nature of these projects means that successive crops of students remain the same age while the veteran supervisors and fieldworkers grow older. The tensions around checking point to some of the frictions that arise between Malawian and non-Malawian fieldworkers, and provide the former with an idiom of critique that not only preserves local knowledge as their domain but also reclaims the authority, wisdom, and locality their age and experience afford them. In a sense, fieldworkers framed checking as a practice rooted in tacit knowledge, even as we note that this and other forms of local knowledge emerge rather from a portfolio of skills and bits of information acquired through exposure to research projects (Prince 2014).

ECONOMIES OF TRUST IN RESEARCH WORK CULTURES

Researchers, especially those new to working in Malawi, recognized the importance of assembling a fieldwork team composed of professional, trustworthy, and competent fieldworkers. They, and the fieldworkers themselves, saw a direct correlation between a professional, committed team and high-quality data. Foreign researchers drew on knowledge from peers in their research networks who were working in Malawi. Dr. Smith, an American principal investigator for RAM, recalled her original naive fieldwork plan: she had planned to go to the University of Malawi and hire research assistants there. However, in discussions with other researchers, she came to understand how important it would be to have experienced fieldworkers on her team. Eventually, the stamp of approval from a fellow foreign researcher in her network was enough to convince her to hire John as her supervisor and delegate to him the authority to determine the composition of the field teams.

In recruiting and retaining fieldwork teams, researchers emphasized that they sought out people they could trust. This resonates with scholarly framings of the relationship between interpersonal trust and the production of good knowledge. Steven Shapin (1994) shows, for example, how the codes and conventions of gentlemanly conduct in seventeenth-century England also determined which people (and by extension, which knowledge claims) were credible, reliable, or trustworthy (see also McCook 1996). Trust, however, is not something inherent to an individual; rather, it is built over time and within unfolding social relations. Although Dr. Smith trusted John enough to allocate him significant (hiring) power in prefieldwork planning, he would also have to continue to earn her trust for the duration of fieldwork. Trust between researchers and fieldworkers was established within a distinct research culture as it mapped onto an underlying social field. The cultural norms of research by which trust is built up are rooted in a certain interested disinterest on the part of both researchers and fieldworkers. This interested disinterest upholds the shared misrecognition of large economic and educational gaps between researchers and supervisors (Redfield 2012; Geissler 2013b).

Research work culture encompasses norms for social interaction, expectations of sharing (of everything from blankets to food to workload to billiards games in a local drinking joint to music files to stories), and guidelines for behavior. Interactions and impressions that transpire outside of the bounded workday inform not only how fieldworkers interact with one another, but also how much or how little foreign researchers come to trust individual supervisors or interviewers. Trust informed researchers' evaluations of the data collected by a certain supervisor's team of interviewers, how much independence a specific fieldwork team was granted, whether a researcher allowed an interviewer to borrow his computer, or whether a graduate student loaned a supervisor 100 kwacha (at the time) for dinner. Because trust must be continually and consistently performed and negotiated, becoming trustworthy—effectively recruiting a new person into one's network—is a full-time job. Whether distant from the eyes of their bosses or sitting next to them at dinner, they maintained an interest in being deemed good fieldworkers.

Disagreements or conflicts between supervisors and researchers were rare, even if behind-the-scenes talk sometimes indicated friction. Both parties were uninterested in conflict that could threaten their mutually beneficial relationship to one another: to oversimplify, researchers wished to collect data as efficiently as possible, and supervisors wished to run an operation that was stress free and earn a salary. Relationships between fieldworkers and researchers were effective not only in producing knowledge but in proving useful to individuals even amid antagonism (Schumaker 2001, 249). Dr. Smith (RAM) explained:

> When you're working with a big project like this one, you can't have all the control. People have told me, you know other researchers, that they think I don't supervise fieldworkers enough. They say, "Your supervisor is a free agent!" And, well, it's true. My supervisor is not here every minute, even on days when we are doing data entry. Like yesterday afternoon he was off in the car scouting [scheduling interviews for the next day with local leaders]. And I know when he's out that he's taking care of his own personal business, but the thing is, overall, he is available to us twelve hours a day. He gets his job done.[21]

She knows her supervisor often conducts his own business or errands on the clock, even though he does not explicitly inform her of this. Her assumptions are borne out by my own experience in the field, where some supervisors engaged in brief business meetings, dropped off or picked up family members from nearby spots, stopped to meet friends, visited the market, or picked up a laptop from a computer repair store. However, this does not break the trust between them—trust is a give and take. The researcher surrenders some time and money in exchange for assurance that the job will get done. Indeed, the supervisor explained that he preferred working for RAM over others because, he said, "They [RAM's researchers] are not constantly looking over my shoulder." In this way, a mutual disinterest in conflict or confrontation that might have created bad feelings and negatively influenced fieldwork ensures that both parties achieved their interests.

In addition to being trustworthy, fieldworkers were expected to possess local knowledge useful to outside researchers. In discussions with supervisors about why the research project may have hired them over other possible individuals, they consistently mentioned trust and their possession of local knowledge as major factors. I quote one supervisor, speaking at length, to illustrate the kinds of knowledge that the local experts themselves think researchers are seeking:

> Most of the time . . . when people from outside come here to do their research, the main advice they ask from us is [about] the processes they have to pass through for them to do their research in a proper way. So maybe you go to a site: which people should we meet first so that our job should go smoothly? So we tell them, "These are the authorities we have to meet first so that things go well." Aside from that, like, cultures in local areas . . . we have to explain, to say, okay, we are in this area, and this is what we are expected to do in this area, and we should behave like this. . . . For example, the Yaos mostly don't drink because they are Muslim and on Fridays they go to mosque so we tell the researchers to do interviews in non-Yao areas on Fridays so we don't disturb them in mosque. . . . We may even have to tell these kinds of things to interviewers, as well. Like one time an interviewer offended a Yao man who had been cooking us lunch by bringing in one of his [the interviewer's] mice for lunch. The Chewas do prefer to [enjoy] eat mice, but the Yaos . . . it's taboo for them, you know?

This supervisor's comments indicate that fieldworkers have become familiar with the expectations, demands, and needs of foreign researchers. Through sequential interactions with growing numbers of projects and research- ers, they come to possess an increasingly convincing, packaged, and com- moditized form of local knowledge, scripted to match the anticipations of foreign researchers. Notably, the examples of local knowledge stated here deal with logistics or with cultural caricatures of ethnic or religious groups (e.g., Chewas like eating mice). They exemplify the unstable, shifting, and constructed nature of local knowledge as it fits into and is shaped by a mar- ketplace; fieldworkers broker their embodied human capital—stores of in- formation, habits, and practices—to researchers who wish to enlist it so as to produce valuable data.

Though research projects take for granted their need for local knowledge, the content and meanings of the category itself often go unremarked. In many projects and contexts, foreign researchers solicited local or cultural knowl- edge from their Malawian supervisors or interviewers. They asked, for exam- ple, about the specific differences between types of traditional healers in the rural areas (see above), about the details of initiation ceremonies, about the availability of antiretroviral medications (ARVs) at local hospitals, about local perceptions of female condoms, or about widow inheritance or other cultural practices.[22] Researchers often assumed the responses given by experts to be experiential, authentically local, or, in Dr. Smith's words, "from the horse's mouth."[23]

Researchers generally overestimated the amount of logistical local knowl- edge possessed by their employees. It was in the interest of fieldworkers to appear familiar with the research area in question, even if it was terra incog- nita. Once in the vans for the day, distant from the eyes of the researchers, the team's peripatetic meanderings betrayed their nonknowledge of certain regions or villages. The fieldworkers maintained flexibility and nonchalance, cobbling together directions from young children or women on their way to the borehole (often giving them rides in exchange for directions to a chief's house, for example), hiring a local scout (often the son of a village head- man), and/or asking door to door to learn the location of a certain village, household, or headman. Many times, teams were lost amid dense grasses or stuck on the wrong side of a bridge felled by mudslides in the rainy season. However, so long as the team made sufficient progress that day, fieldworkers maintained their credibility.

In the case of both cultural and logistical information, it is notable that fieldworkers often explicitly attributed their own local knowledge to their past work on research projects. In a conversation about whether young girls in rural areas fall in with sugar daddies who give them money or gifts in exchange for sex, for example, a supervisor prefaced his response with, "When I was with the adolescent intervention pilot study, we found that . . ." The research studies these fieldworkers have participated in, then, enjoy a new citational life distant from the world of Google Scholar. Local knowledge was not ready-made, but fashioned and packaged via mobility and exposure to the national landscape through research project employment. In this sense, local knowledge reflects the economic and epistemological context in which it attains value. Whereas discussions around data among researchers often center on the impact of fieldworkers on data (they have the capacity to ruin or improve data), we note that data also very much impact fieldworkers as they engage with them.

Fieldworkers cultivate an ability to display the very kinds of expertise and competence that researchers seek out as they clock time working with research projects, and researchers recognize the value that continuity and cultivated expertise add to their data. American fieldwork manager Patrick told his audience at a training session, "The more time you spend with us, the more valuable you are to us." He asked that fieldworkers sign a contract in which they promised to stay with the project for the duration of data collection. Later, he explained to me that it had been difficult to find interviewers this field season because the project was competing with the national census, which paid much better for similar work.[24] The value of sticking with a project for the duration of fieldwork and over the course of many years is weighed pragmatically by fieldworkers. Each project job is a platform for expanding social connections and increasing the probability of future financial gain. John, RAM supervisor, explained why he had "deserted" a project that originally hired him many years earlier to work for another one: "They didn't bid high enough for me!" Andrews, too, elaborated on the dynamics of the marketplace of expertise: "Research is getting much more expensive. . . . Even I am getting more expensive myself. Now I can negotiate, say things like, "They [another project] are giving me this and that." Working for the same employers year after year also allowed supervisors more room to negotiate for raises and better living conditions in the field. Clocking more time in research worlds and learning the ins and outs of the marketplace of expertise enabled fieldworkers to more effectively broker local knowledge to possible employers, to increase their negotiating power, to access resources, and to earn more trust from their international counterparts.

Living Project to Project: Itinerant Knowledge Work

FLEXIBLE ACCUMULATION IN THE CONTACT ZONE

Although project employees frequently voiced complaints about grueling work schedules, they were better off than most of their peers because they had a temporary but guaranteed salary. Even if financial remuneration for work on research projects was low, the research project offered diversified social connections and social capital, defined by Pierre Bourdieu (1986, 248) as "an aggregate of the actual or potential resources which are linked to possession of a durable network of more or less institutionalized relationships of mutual acquaintance or recognition." International research projects are crossroads of social and informational capital that can often be converted into economic capital, as others have documented for an array of global health projects in Africa. Transfers and exchanges of this sort occur every day during fieldwork. A research project is a contact zone, a place where diverse actors meet and engage in transactions and relations that are mutually transforming, even as they play out in asymmetrical relations of power (Pratt 1991). Pratt's concept helps us to look beyond both data themselves and the temporary institutions in which they are produced; in this section, I show how alternative forms of value are produced as side effects of research itself, often redirecting fieldworkers' imaginations, hopes, and anxieties.

Fieldworkers accumulated many kinds of capital during fieldwork; indeed, even as they wished they could stop living project to project, they recognized the potentials inherent in proximity to a transnational research collaboration. First, valuable material objects regularly changed hands between foreign and Malawian project staff members. At first glance, the transfer of secondhand objects from foreign to local staff at the close of fieldwork periods might seem insignificant. However, such objects were often reinvented or revalued as they passed hands, not only from the staff member to a local counterpart but from the counterpart to family or friends in the future. Clothing or running shoes were sometimes kept for personal use but also served as highly valued gifts to kin living in rural areas, who often expect monetary or in-kind gifts from wealthier relatives. Despite the ephemeral nature of research work and relatively low salaries, it was nevertheless assumed by kin of project staff that they would share the wealth the staff member accumulated through employment. Both middle-class and poor Malawians outfit themselves in kaunjika (secondhand clothes for sale at rural bomas and city markets), an important stylistic and practical resource in a country where international clothing outlets are not present. The secondhand clothing, backpacks, or coats given to project staff members were usually of better quality and newer than that available at weekly markets. Other gifts were much more highly valued. Very frequently, friends to American staff would find themselves with a mint-condition cell phone at the conclusion of fieldwork, an item that could be used personally or sold for a large sum. American staff members were compelled to give things away at the close of fieldwork and frequently referenced the poverty and difficulty of finding electronics in Malawi as motivations for, in some cases, bestowing an iPod, digital camera, old laptop, or USB key (flash drive) on a research colleague. Such gifts were likely to be kept and not sold, due to the high status they would give to their owner at a time when access to technology and connectivity was coveted.

Though the material utility of such objects is apparent, it should also be noted that they often played a key role in the ability of individuals to market themselves to future projects. Namely, researchers prefer to hire research staff members who are "well versed in English and understand what we as Americans are looking for."[25] Often, the Americans who are charged with the task of hiring fieldworkers are relatively young (either graduate students or recent PhDs) and, therefore, likely to find common ground with a young Malawian. As often as American research team members shared their music with Malawian counterparts, they also exhibited a hunger for Malawian or Zambian music they could share with friends back home. Flash drives became a future-oriented object for their owners. The owners of these drives could use them to store résumés or cover letters to potential employers and access these documents quickly at Internet cafes (in 2007–2008, smartphone or wireless access to the Internet were minimally available to elites in Malawi). Flash drives often enjoyed wide circulation among groups of close friends; upon inserting one into your computer you were likely to, first, contract a virus and, second, to observe files named for multiple people. In more than a few cases, project staff members would give or sell laptop computers at affordable prices to Malawian staff members. Obviously, this object's potential for enhancing future career and social prospects is very significant. It should be noted that familiarity with and a clear ability to use technology significantly enhances one's chances of being hired at a higher level on a research project, especially in 2007–2008 when smartphones and laptops had yet to achieve mass circulation in Malawi. Working as a supervisor or interviewer, for example, requires an ability to work with digital recorders (to record interviews with research subjects), iPods (used by some projects as transcription devices), cameras (to photograph research subjects), GPS technology (for mapping sample sites), and laptops (if one is on the data entry team or a typist of interviews).

Joining a research community was also an opportunity to acquire social capital. First, the friendships that formed between foreign and Malawian research staff members became a resource to be tapped into later, when the former returned to Malawi for another round of fieldwork or to start up another project. American research staff told me that before returning to Malawi for "another fieldwork season," they would e-mail or SMS friends in Malawi to inquire whether there was anything they needed. Most research staff members suggested that being a courier for gifts was "the least they could do" since their friends in Malawi had very little access to the commodities and technology Americans took for granted. Furthermore, project staff would often furnish loans or monetary gifts (via one of the many Western Union outlets in Malawi) to help their Malawian colleagues "[go] on in school" or "[start] a business"; loans were disbursed in person or with the help of e-mail, Skype, and Western Union after foreign project staff members returned home. Thus, an open line of communication to a friend across the ocean became another node of support in already existing networks of kin and acquaintances. One supervisor who worked on numerous research projects told me, "Many of us tend to each have our own azungu," a person from abroad who was most intimate with him or her.[26] (I am, I gather, a number of Malawians' "own azungu.") Especially in cases of emergency or tragedy, such nodes could be easily activated.

Social capital was often converted into financial capital through recommendations for employees passed from people who had spent time in Malawi and people who were anticipating arrival in Malawi; a longtime supervisor explained, "These researchers employ people they know, who they have worked with.... They know someone they are familiar with already will do a good job."[27] In more tragic cases, too, the friendship networks born in the space of the research project were immensely important to Malawians. In mid-2009, members of GSIP received news that a Malawian supervisor had passed away; news from LSAM via a Listserv reported that an elderly woman who had worked as a cook for the project had endured a forcible break-in at the project's housing compound. Most recently (2016), a former MAYP supervisor experienced severe financial hardship. In these cases and others, digital connections mobilized financial and other resources from Americans and Europeans affiliated with the projects directly to the family of the deceased and the affected individuals, respectively. Americans and Europeans who have worked on survey projects in Malawi have also raised money via e-mail, GoFundMe, and so on for colleagues in Malawi experiencing financial hardship. Of course, individual relationships often include transfer of funds to support businesses, educational plans, or children's schooling fees as well. In this way, transnational social networks forged within projects have unpredictable value in the future (Jackson 2012).

Working in the field, distant from the eyes and ears of foreign research staff, sometimes permits local experts to accumulate resources by siphoning them from the project. Various forms of siphoning such as conducting personal business on project time (as described above) remained hidden and did not necessarily threaten researchers' authority or project protocols; were the fieldworkers to make these actions explicit, however, they would lose credibility and trust. In some cases, research project supervisors used their own cars for some work-related tasks, necessitating reimbursement for fuel used on project time. Fieldworkers could often take advantage of the nonknowledge of their bosses of, for example, the price of fuel to fill their gas tank for the next week (if they used their own car for project business). Another benefit commonly siphoned from projects was mobile phone airtime. Projects provided airtime cards to fieldwork supervisors so that they could check in with their interviewers about their progress or locate them if they were lost. In the field, supervisors almost never phoned interviewers (airtime depletes very quickly if it is used for phone calls); if absolutely necessary, they would send an SMS, which cost significantly fewer kwacha. Supervisors used their siphoned airtime for personal calls to friends, lovers, or family and viewed these *maunits* (airtime units) as a perk of the job. If supervisors knew that the boss providing them with the airtime had little knowledge of how long units last, they might try to negotiate for more by claiming they had depleted their units making phone calls in the field that day. In some cases, project staff who stayed in the office failed to realize that many of the rural fieldwork sites lacked reliable cell phone coverage in 2007–2008, making both phoning and SMS messaging difficult or impossible.

John, an experienced fieldworker, managed to draw on and activate social capital with great acumen. When we first met in 2005, he was working as an interviewer for LSAM; by 2008, he was the head supervisor for RAM.[28] Since 2005, he had married, had a child, started a minibus business, completed a master's degree abroad, and traveled widely. He dressed well, often wearing a tie and dress shoes to work on days when we stayed in the field office. In the years following 2005, he visited numerous international cities, often staying with researchers or graduate students affiliated with the research projects he had worked for. In addition to his role as a head supervisor, John also ran a business in a suburb of Blantyre, Malawi's commercial capital. John is exemplary (though not representative by any means) of the imagined social mobility this chapter depicts. With each serial job for research projects, he gained increments of credibility, status, expertise, and authority that subsequently permitted him to expect and negotiate for more money, resources, trips, and benefits. Early in his project-to-project career, his personal laptop computer and mobile phone were acquired through his work with research projects. At times between 2005 and 2008, John capitalized on the distance between himself and his employers to take on work from more than one research project simultaneously, a feat made easier because one employer attempted to oversee John's work from abroad via Skype.[29]

In 2008, projects began to put in place contracts stating that an employee may only work for a single project at a time. In June 2008, the recruitment and training for LSAM happened to overlap in time and space with the recruitment and training for National Statistical Office census enumerators. The statistics office posted a list of local people who had won positions as enumerators on the bulletin board at the front of the building where LSAM was holding its training sessions. A supervisor noticed the name of one of the project interviewers on this list; although this interviewer had already been selected as an enumerator for the census a week earlier, he had attended two days of LSAM's training. This "eating from both sides" was deemed underhanded, and the interviewer was not paid for the trainings he attended.[30]

Although some Malawians working for research projects were duplicitous with their employers, it makes sense to view all such tactics to maximize social position and financial gain in the context of the flexible labor pool they occupied. Again and again, research supervisors told me that being flexible is essential in this kind of work. The descriptor "flexible" was fitting for many reasons, not least of which involved the efforts of these individuals to diversify their social and financial capital networks. Their strategies were diverse, but work on a research project became a platform for forging profitable relations and practices. One twenty-nine-year-old male who worked as a research supervisor for ten years explained that he grows tobacco by reinvesting the money he earns doing research to do farming. From these earnings, he employs six men who monitor and harvest the tobacco each year. In 2007, he supplemented his income by selling thousands of kilograms of tobacco. This supplementary livelihood strategy is an example of his flexibility; he can go to his home in northern Malawi three times a year to check on the tobacco and still earn money as a research supervisor. Today, he is well employed— still in the research world—as the research manager for a consulting firm that helps foreign researchers set up and carry out data collection in Malawi. He has traveled frequently abroad and is a coauthor on several academic articles.

For some individuals, then, knowledge work has become a contemporary form of migrant labor that enhances rural accumulation in a village home; "mobility is . . . a lifestyle in which improvements in the village are pursued through a stay in town," where "town" stands in for the field (Englund 2002, 139). We might even suggest that the thin mattresses and simple accommodation in rest houses rented by research projects have become a contemporary corollary to the workers' living quarters associated with mining camps in South Africa and Southern Rhodesia.

ON BEING STUCK IN PLACE

Fieldworkers were perpetually poised to learn of better opportunities, higher pay, and rumors of new projects coming to Malawi. Research world gossip networks were efficacious in spreading invaluable information: who was working for which project, how much a project was paying, and the paths and trajectories of in-country azungu. The going rates for one project versus another were important forms of knowledge for interested would-be interviewers and supervisors. Gossip gleaned from known social network members was the main channel of such information. However, it is important to note that even opportunities to move upward within the research world were tempered by close analysis of the social and economic benefits; John, for example, was invited by a group of Americans to be one of the Malawian trustees of a new organization but declined this offer when he discovered that a Malawian law prohibits trustees of such organizations from working for the same organization.

Fieldworkers rely on a larger structure they have little knowledge of or access to. For example, in late 2007, a large research project received word that their proposal had not passed ethical review and therefore could not be immediately implemented. Anticipating approval, the project had already begun training its staff, including nurses who would act as VCT counselors for the project. When the researchers received the news, they passed it on to a cadre of well-qualified nurses who had expected months of steady employment but were left suddenly unemployed. Similarly, fieldworkers who were part of ready-made field teams contracted out to research projects often complained that their salaries were not paid on time by the consulting firm or center they worked for: "They will just call us and say, 'You'll get the money in two weeks.' And, well, we have no choice but to wait for it."

Because most of the interviewers and supervisors were typically in their twenties or early thirties at the time of this fieldwork, they harbored career aspirations; males and females alike complained about the instability of this kind of research work, where they were forced to live project to project. They described how they became stuck in the work of research: "This kind of work doesn't propel me forward at all. I've just been getting some money but I am starting to think I need to make a next step. I am just . . . stuck." Victor, a long-time supervisor on research projects, and his wife, Margaret, a data entry clerk working for numerous projects, wanted to study for an MBA and a master's in development studies, respectively, he said, "so that we can stop this working constantly for other people and just have our own organization." Victor tried to diversify his income by investing in a minibus using money he had made working on research projects. He was thrilled at this prospect, and his business plan exhibited much foresight in its desire to market the minibus to all the projects he worked with (projects paid about 8,000 kwacha [$57–65 at the time] per day to rent a minibus and driver to conduct fieldwork). However, his plan came to a tragic end when he "went in" with a colleague who promised to buy the bus while in South Africa for a business trip. Victor fronted as much of the price of the minibus as he could afford and waited eagerly for the bus to arrive. When it did, his friend handed him back the sum Victor had fronted and proclaimed that he had decided to do it alone. Victor accepted the news ambivalently: "I'm sad but he just had more capital than me. He has worked longer than I have in research, and he had the financial means to double-cross me."

Fieldworkers tended to internalize feelings of failure if they "were just staying, sitting idly" while "others were working." Many supervisors were graduates of the University of Malawi and were embarrassed if they failed to secure employment for even a short period of time. Nonetheless, research jobs were scarce, which meant college-educated young people stayed for some portion of the year in the village (or the town) they were from. Whereas foreign project staff members assumed that fieldworkers were happy to go home at the end of a long and exhausting fieldwork contract, they dreaded returning home where they would no longer be earning money. Esau, a supervisor with LSAM, said, "You know, in the old days it was very easy for anyone who went to college to find a job because graduates were so scarce and there were lots of new companies coming in [to Malawi]. But now there are just so many of us and jobs want five years of experience and, well, if I don't know someone, I won't get a job anyway." Following his work with projects in 2007–2008, Esau did eventually find stable, if relatively low-paying, work as a school-teacher in a lakeshore district.

Certainly, since 2008, a number of fieldworkers—primarily supervisors and those with a college education—have enjoyed success: enrolled in graduate programs, found work with NGOs or other international organizations, taken positions in government bodies such as the National AIDS Commission, became entrepreneurs, or found work in survey administration or as consultants. In particular, LSAM has made significant investments in a core group of its longtime supervisors: they have found well-paying work in research worlds, obtained graduate degrees, traveled to present papers on which they are coauthors at foreign conferences, and so on. Yet it was well known at the time that the likelihood of moving up in the world of research was small. Nonetheless, even as they felt stuck in place by living project to project, fieldwork jobs stoked hopes and generated new imaginings of alternative futures and careers. Living project to project simultaneously provides opportunities for and blocks to social mobility. A person's position in the social field of a research project correlates with chances of achieving financial or career success. Though rhetoric and public talk on the part of project members celebrates the equality of all team participants, status distinctions and hierarchies within the project are often preserved and maintained through talk and practices. Chisomo, an LSAM supervisor, described how interviewers (who had only finished secondary school) saw their superiors and notes the spatial hierarchies implicit in their accommodations in the field: "[They] tend to think we think we are too good for them. You know, we went to college and had this shared experience and they didn't. And also, you can see on the project how this pans out; while we [supervisors] get the nicer chalets [at the rest house where fieldwork was based] as accommodation, they complain about how they are there in the public, crappier rooms."

In my rough map of the rest house where LSAM was based in mid-2008 (figure 2.2), the spatial distribution of project staff members is evident. Namely, the "nicer chalets" are self-contained (with bathroom) and set off to the side of the main building beneath shade trees. They are quieter, cleaner, and more expensive per night than the "public, crappier rooms." These rooms were darker, cramped, and generally less clean, and their occupants had to share bathrooms they often complained were not well kept. Additionally, the interior rooms, if not fully occupied by fieldworkers, were sometimes rented by the general public (often truck drivers who were rumored to bring sex workers into their rooms at night), creating a sense that the project members in these rooms were no different than everyday guests who could afford only this cheap accommodation. While supervisors largely stayed in the same caliber accommodation as foreign project staff members (chalets), the fieldworkers, data entry clerks, and drivers were relegated to the interior rooms. Despite rhetoric of collaboration and equality that dominated research work

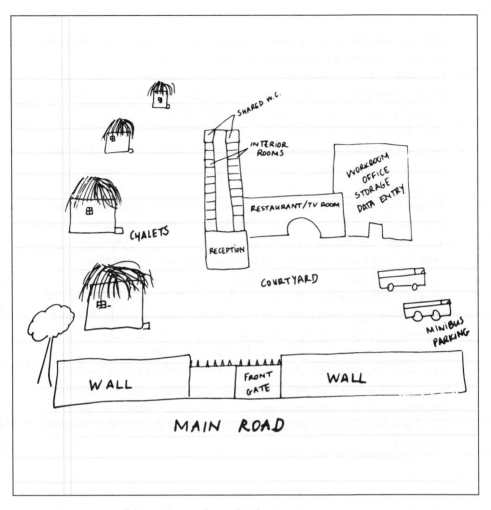

FIGURE 2.2. Author's rendering of LSAM headquarters, 2008.

cultures, the spatialization of inequalities at the Mpaweni is a metaphor for the boundary work that upholds status distinctions and hierarchies between project staff members, made explicit in American field supervisor Patrick's suggestion, "I think the level of room should reflect the hierarchy and status of the person."[31]

When supervisors went out for drinks or billiards in the evenings, they would often restrict invitations to other supervisors or foreign graduate students and framed the exclusion of interviewers as professional (e.g., "We cannot drink with those who work for us"). Only interviewers who had finished college were hired by MAYP and RAM, so interviewers and supervisors socialized more freely during nonwork hours. Nonetheless, in conversations among themselves, supervisors often expressed pity for interviewers who became jobless when a project moved from one site to another. Indeed, a number of supervisors viewed their role not only as a professional one but saw themselves as mentors who aimed to train their charges, as well, in good work ethic. I observed, for example, a conversation between LSAM supervisor Andrews and a novice interviewer—whom he referred to later as *kamwana* (childish, not grown up)—who was struggling to follow the instructions for data collectors in the field. Andrews told him that he knew the interviewer was capable of doing the work and suggested, "In life it means nothing to have potential if no one knows [you have] it." Later, Andrews told me he thought it was important that interviewers gained skills besides simply doing fieldwork working on projects like LSAM.[32] They considered firing interviewers one of the most difficult parts of their job and often asked foreign project staff members to do it for them. Because they had less contact with those who had hiring and firing power on research projects, interviewers were least likely to move up in a project. Thus, although knowledge work could lead to upward mobility or increased capital for fieldworkers, interviewers and supervisors led a precarious existence characterized by differential levels of ambivalent stagnancy based on their role in the project and specific social connections and intimacies. In the process of making valuable data, fieldworkers also fashioned new kinds of value and aspirations: the fates of data and their creators are linked.

Conclusion

This chapter has shown how brokering and translation on the part of hundreds of fieldworkers are central ingredients in data collection and add value to data. The commodification of data for consumption by researchers and policy makers has likewise commodified the kinds of expertise and knowhow central to its collection. Local knowledge, often taken for granted, is performed and constructed in the space of social relations, and such performances betray the different, competing interests of the variety of persons who encounter one another in the contact zone of fieldwork. As Lekgoathi (2009) illustrates in his study of the construction of apartheid-era knowledge about the Transvaal Ndebele, African researchers and informants play a central role in making African societies accessible (logistically and culturally) to outsiders. Northern researchers reinterpret Malawian ideas, traditions, customs, behaviors, and contexts through the prism of their training in a certain discipline and their scripted impressions of Malawi—most influentially, however, they complement these perceptions with the local knowledge they so highly value (Watkins and Swidler 2012). Yet becoming a good fieldworker does not entail mastering a body of stable local knowledge or being native to a geographic or cultural place, but rather learning and embodying new ways of seeing that rely on and reproduce difference and distance between knowers and known, science and culture, and office and field. Data collection is an endeavor that is shaped by and shapes the subjectivities, aspirations, and dreams of those who collect it. In this sense, the rhetoric of cooking data might also be read as an idiom mobilized by overworked fieldworkers to level critiques against their employers and negotiate the low morale that might result from being stuck in place (Gerrets 2015a).

Maintaining focus on the relations and practices that make up fieldwork, chapter 3 centers the encounters and transactions between fieldworkers and interviewees in the process of data collection. Specifically, it considers how a kind of standardized reciprocity—where respondents are given a bar of soap as token of thanks for information they surrender—becomes a site of negotiation and debate about the value of health data for different actors in research worlds.

THREE

CLEAN DATA, MESSY GIFTS

Soap-for-Information
Transactions in the Field

Ndema, an LSAM interviewer wearing his project T-shirt and name badge, with a clipboard and two bars of soap, leaves the minibus to locate the respondent he is meant to interview. When he arrives at his assigned household, he shouts, "Hodi!" (May I enter?) and Mary, his respondent, emerges. They engage in polite conversation and introductions before sitting down on a mat on Mary's verandah to begin the survey. Ndema summarizes the long consent form for Mary, who claims she can read the rest, and she signs her name on the form. For the next 1.5 hours, Ndema asks questions and Mary provides answers that he records on the questionnaire's twenty-five pages. As the research encounter concludes, Ndema thanks Mary for her time, handing her two bars of soap; she quickly folds them into the chitenje tied around her waist.

In this composite sketch of a typical research encounter in the field, Ndema, a fieldworker who lives in Mary's district, embodies the kinds of mannerisms and practices he has been taught in the prefieldwork training sessions discussed in chapter 2: he is respectful, professionally dressed, gracious, and careful in administering the survey tool. Yet as a bridge between his community and survey projects, he modifies standards and guidelines for administering questionnaires to adapt to unfolding conditions in the field (Kingori 2013; Madiega et al. 2013; Reynolds et al. 2013; Sambakunsi et al. 2015). Finding the informed consent form too long, he summarizes it instead of reading it verbatim, for example. Ndema and Mary's interaction foregrounds the stranger intimacy of the research encounter, a site where private information and gifts are exchanged.

From June to August 2008, thousands of rural Malawians like Mary were given a gift of two bars of soap (*sopo*)—red Lifebuoy and yellow Sunlight—in exchange for their responses to LSAM's questionnaire. Recipients held diverse opinions about this gift. Ruth, a woman living in Balaka District who has been in LSAM's sample for many years, expressed ambivalence: "Whatever the [researcher] gives me, I will receive. A gift is never small [*mphatso sichepa*]." Individuals who fell outside LSAM's random sample were envious of those who received gifts, however small. Yet though they accepted this gift gratefully, many survey participants did consider it too small to properly express appreciation for the time they invested in answering questions. Members of Malawi's research ethics board and researchers, meanwhile, viewed soap as a gift fitting to the Malawian context and, importantly, one that would not coerce survey participation or dirty their data. Depending on perspective, soap can become welcome compensation, too small a gift, a symbol of jealousy at uneven distribution of benefits, a way to build solidarity, a commodity with explicit exchange value, or a promise of a better future.

Having so far explored how health data are shaped by and shape actors and practices in survey design, fieldworker training, and fieldwork phases of research, I now focus specifically on transactions that undergird the administration of household-level surveys in the field. Researchers consider soap an appropriate research gift because it not only serves as a small token of thanks but also does not threaten to contaminate their data. A larger or more meaningful gift could be construed as remuneration and elevate the risk that respondents will lie (provide bad data) in order to receive payment, for example. The logic of giving a small gift for research participation emerges from human subjects research ethical standards rooted in an ideal-type agentive subject who participates altruistically in research and thus provides pure, untainted (truthful) information. Yet, in Malawi, as elsewhere in the global South, expectations that people should participate in research altruistically or for the public good are in tension with research fatigue, a legacy of exploitation and unfulfilled promises at the hands of global projects, and therapeutic misconception, in which research participants mistakenly attribute therapeutic intent to research procedures (Benatar 1998; Aiga 2007; Stewart and Sewankambo 2010). Centering encounters between the fieldworkers described in chapter 2 and their research subjects, this chapter reveals the contested value of data in survey research worlds and exposes how clean data rely on messy transactions—obscured by the benevolent figure of the ethical gift—to materialize. Close analysis of the soap gift foregrounds how assembling good (clean) data relies not just on the practices and planning of the researchers and fieldworkers we have met so far, but on relations and transactions between projects—represented by fieldworkers on the front lines— and their research subjects. This chapter conceives of research subjects and researchers not as fixed or preexisting actors but as emergent workable forms that, like data themselves, are assembled in research worlds.

In what follows, I first draw on interviews with foreign and Malawian demographers and members of Malawi's institutional review board (IRB) to show how soap embodies ethical standards for research with human subjects in Malawi, emphasizing how its material characteristics make it a clean and easy gift in the field. Drawing on interviews I conducted with participants in LSAM and MAYP surveys, I then analyze the claims and contestations that recipients of the soap gift raised about soap-for-information exchanges amid research fatigue. Showing how they come to view soap and research benefits as rights they are entitled to, as wages for the labor of research participation, and as a symbol of their exploitation by projects, I reveal that naming soap an ethical gift relies on a bounded definition of research that abstracts it from its particular time and place. Efforts to arbitrate whether soap or other items are ethical gifts do not attend to the fact that soap-for-information transactions inevitably convert objectified categories of persons (researcher and research participant) into personified actors whose intentions, personhood, and stakes are distributed across the research / real world divide (and the individual/society divide) that ethics presumes (Strathern 1988). Rather than the cog in the assembly-line machinery of research that demographers imagine soap to be, then, this ethical gift unravels normative ethics and highlights how collecting high-quality data is less a clean assembly-line process than a messy and unpredictable life course.

Soap, Standards, and Ethics

By the 1990s, blood samples and information were seen by global ethics organizations as embedded in power relations and subject to constraints of ethical disclosure, consent, and sensitivity to context. In the context of global health research in Africa, where poor research subjects enroll in studies led by wealthy foreign institutions, projects like the ones described in this book are subject to tight oversight, monitoring, and rigorous review processes. All projects (including the author's ethnographic one) discussed in this book submitted proposals to both their home universities' IRBs and to a Malawian IRB for review. These boards judge proposals on the basis of universal ethical principles— justice, beneficence, and respect for persons—encoded in key documents (see NCPHSBBR 1979; CIOMS 2002; WHO 2011). Local IRBs—composed of Malawian bioethicists, researchers, and scholars—are charged with arbitrating whether material benefits for research participation are appropriate in light of a "community's gift exchange and other traditions" (CIOMS 2002, 31). Recourse to culture, as in whether a gift is culturally appropriate, obscures material inequalities between researchers and the researched, and relies on the assumption that a place like Malawi is internally homogenous and steeped in "traditions" (Carrier 2003). As Folayan and Allman (2011, 100) point out, whereas researchers earn money, status, and accolades for their work, research participants are expected to understand their role as voluntary, altruistic, and toward the collective good. Research ethics—anchored in the image of an individual agentively consenting to research participation—mandate that participants volunteer in the absence of incentives or coercion to do so.

The Council for International Organizations of Medical Science (CIOMS) provides guidance on informed consent and recruitment, specifically "inducement to participate in research": "Subjects may be reimbursed for lost earnings, travel costs, and other expenses incurred in taking part in a study. . . . Payments . . . should not be unacceptable recompense. . . . *Payments or rewards that undermine a person's capacity to exercise free choice invalidate consent.* . . . Payments in money or in kind to research subjects should not be so large as to persuade them to take undue risks or volunteer against their better judgment" (2002, 31, emphasis added).

From the perspective of demographers who designed surveys and oversaw their implementation in the field and the Malawian ethics board members who reviewed their research proposals, soap fulfilled these criteria. Ubiquitous and with small monetary value, soap does not threaten to induce participation nor to invalidate consent, the gold standard of human subjects research.[1] Soap is an accomplice in informed consent's ruse: to equate research subject and researcher, stripping them of social and economic trappings within a bounded, contractual moment devoid of specificity. Soap is enlisted into a document-based ritual of verification that produces researchers and the researched as objectified, impersonal, and homogeneous categories at the heart of our imaginings of ethics (Kelly 2003, 192; Petryna 2005; Jacob and Riles 2007; Brives 2013; Kingori 2013; Bell 2014; Hoeyer and Hogle 2014). A respondent's signature or thumbprint on the signature line of the consent form stands in as evidence of a project's ethical relation to a research subject and converts the information he or she provides the fieldworker into data under the ownership of the project. Notably, the informed consent ritual produces the kind of workable subject it requires: the idealized autonomous, agentive individual that is consent's grounding. In being premised on freedom and autonomy, this ritual emphasizes the autonomy of "the researched" and performs the sleight of hand of obscuring or "unknowing" profound material differences between the project and its participants (Geissler 2013b, 18). The overwhelming symbolic value of the consent form lies in its ability to mitigate prior injustice and mute deep inequities of interpretation around research transactions by creating partial and temporary alignment of competing narratives in the name of an imagined common good (Reddy 2007; Simpson 2016, 330). Soap and consent forms are standards, backed by the authority of IRBs, that make data collection possible under regimes of ethical governance (Timmermans 2015, 79).

Following Turnerian (1969) ritual progression, the informed consent ritual takes place outside the flow of normal life: fieldworkers such as Ndema were encouraged to find a quiet place to protect the privacy of the respondent and preserve confidentiality of responses. Incidentally, this emphasis on privacy or separation was sometimes interpreted as secrecy and generated suspicions on the part of relatives of a respondent: in February 2008, the parents of an MAYP respondent said they felt uncomfortable with an interviewer taking their daughter off to a quiet spot under a tree to talk about private family matters, for example.[2] Together, soap and informed consent forms are central standards without which data collection would be impossible under global health's regimes of ethical governance. For research respondents, meanwhile, the consent form and soap are material indexes of a past relation and touchstones for imagining future possible relations.

In 2007–2008, the standard gift for participating in LSAM's or MAYP's survey was two bars of soap; researchers on these and other projects explained that they often communicated with one another to prevent gift inflation.[3] Malawian fieldworkers working on project-to-project contracts, too, preferred gifts to be equivalent across projects, so they would not have to explain to research participants why one project gave better gifts than another. A small commodity with consistent shape and monetary value, soap is a standard gift.[4] However, even as researchers and ethics boards standardized compensation in line with ethical principles, their rationales were diverse. Dr. Payson, the American demographer heading up MAYP's data collection, recalled feedback received from the Malawian IRB about the language she used to discuss compensation: "In the U.S. you always have to talk about reimbursement on a consent form, and they [ethics board] didn't want me to talk about reimbursement. . . . It wasn't the issue of coercion—it was more the issue of making people in the future less likely to participate in research if they're not going to be paid."[5] While reimbursement connotes monetary payment, a gift is given freely. In a conversation about research gifting in Malawi, a former Malawian ethics board member expressed to me his dismay that research participants viewed soap "in terms of money" even after "we [the ethics board] worked so hard to make [the exchange] into a gift exchange."[6] The effort to keep soap clean of dirty money's taint comes into friction, however, with the meanings assigned to soap in Malawi. Soap is often framed as something a male lover or husband, for example, is obliged to give his female partner. "He didn't even give me soap!" stands in as moral critique of a man's inability to provide for his partner, a form of material dependence in the context of sexual intimacy that Mark Hunter (2010) terms "provider love" (Swidler and Watkins 2007; Mojola 2014). In Uganda, meanwhile, family planning volunteers placed soap at the center of claims they made on the program they worked for: "[We] do not even have money to buy soaps" (Flaherty and Kipp 2004, 53–54). A request for soap can thus euphemistically refer to broader fundamental needs meant to be fulfilled by relatives, lovers, employers, or other patrons.

Like soap mobilized as critique of an intimate partner, so too is the soap mentioned on consent forms moralized; however, its bureaucratization as research gift endeavors to delete local contingencies of exchange and to produce a kind of forgetting whereby a one-off bureaucratic gift carries no past or future meaning, confounding Mauss's ([1922] 1967) interpretation of the gift as enduring social glue.[7] This effort to standardize and bureaucratize reciprocity, however, is complicated by respondents' investment in the past and future means by which they engage with research projects and other institutions that provide forms of care amid precarity. In some cases, rural Malawians kept yellowing piles of consent forms in their homes, a material palimpsest of research participation and a "figurative residue" of research encounters (Graboyes 2015, 203). Participants' complaints about soap documented below are about more than just soap: they point to projects' failure to provide them a means to acquire "soap" for themselves and critique the impersonal relations inherent to global health worlds where they give more than they get.

Soap as Clean and Easy Gift

In addition to deeming soap appropriate recompense in line with ethical guidelines, researchers framed it as an easy, convenient gift. In reflecting on other possible gifts (some of which had been given in the past), they rationalized that soap was cleanest: easy to transport and carry, noncoercive, and unlikely to affect data quality. First, soap's small size and cellophane packaging made it an attractive gift. Giving bags of sugar, for example, wasted money and time since bags could burst on bumpy van rides, and they weighed down fieldworkers walking long distances in the sun. Whereas rectangular cardboard boxes filled with bar soap could be easily stacked along the walls of the field office, cumbersome bulk bags full of individual one-kilogram bags of Illovo brand sugar took up more storage space. Another shortcoming of sugar gifts, according to Malawian fieldworkers, was sugar's potential to interfere in bodily processes. They recalled respondents who, in the past, fell ill after ingesting sugar or cooking oil and blamed the project that had given them these "poisonous" items. Similarly, fieldworkers refused to gift their empty water bottles (*botolo*) to children who coveted them, explaining that if a child fell ill after filling one, relations between villagers and project might be soured.[8]

While research respondents commonly stated they wished to receive money (*ndalama*) for participation, researchers and Malawian fieldworkers generally believed that giving money would promote a culture of dependency or handouts, perhaps expressing salaried fieldworkers' anxieties around poorer relatives' incessant requests for money. Amid long-standing debates about how to properly compensate research participants (Dickert and Grady 1999), money is generally deemed unacceptable compensation in its presumed potential to coerce participation in impoverished settings like Malawi, even as its withholding paternalistically mutes research participants' claims that they know best what they need (Geissler 2013b, 18, 23–24). A clean and neutral gift, soap seems to avoid the pitfalls of ndalama by ensuring information remains free of charge and that participation is not coerced, but agentively chosen or voluntary. Yet some suggest that information should not be free of charge but properly remunerated as a form of wage labor, and others call upon projects to not only collect data but also redistribute resources (Ndebele, Mfutso-Bengo, and Mduluza 2008; Folayan and Allman 2011; Cooper and Waldby 2014). Emanuel (2004) meanwhile argues that there is no justifiable ethical concern about high incentives for research participation that is not excessively risky, confounding the dominant narrative that money is necessarily coercive. Ethical guidelines around gifting practice—and the aversion to payment, in particular—align with researchers' generalized impressions that information or bodily samples that have been paid for are contaminated (Titmuss [1970] 1997). Altruism or purity of intentions, in this model, is a necessary precondition for clean data.

Second to money, research participants mentioned they wished to receive secondhand clothing (kaunjika) for answering survey questions. (Some respondents mentioned they would appreciate blankets as a gift instead of soap, a need likely brought to the fore during the chilly winter months when LSAM was collecting data.) In response to stated preferences for kaunjika over sopo ("I already know what you [fieldworker] have in there [your bag] and it's just soap. I don't want that for [a few] kwacha [per bar]—bring us a bag of kaunjika and we can . . . [pick] what we like!"), foreign researchers' and Malawian fieldworkers' main concern was that if people "pick . . . what they like," a gift is not standardized. Soap's shape, size, utility, and price—the very things that make it an alienable commodity—construct it as a suitable gift in research worlds. Its status as clean gift obtains not only from its hygienic uses, but from its position in a bureaucratized world where gifts do not aspire to produce but aim to foreclose messy social entanglements that may result from their exchange (Anderson 2008). Marcel Mauss ([1922] 1967) showed us that gifts function because of the hidden "interested" forethought invested in them under tacit temporal constraints: the triple obligation of giving, receiving, and returning gifts cements social bonds and produces a sense of obligation between transactors. In research worlds, however, soap functions despite the standardized, impersonal, and time-insensitive conditions under which it is dispensed. Soap enters a system of relations as a gift and reflects standards of that system (Star and Lampland 2008). Yet, much to research participants' chagrin, soap—and by proxy research—does not transform their lives or communities, nor does it engender meaningful obligation on the part of projects.

Giving soap to research participants recalls the gift of soap brought to Africa via colonial hygiene projects that envisioned modern, consumerist subjects (McClintock 1995; Burke 1996). Imperial soap production exacerbated status distinctions and smuggled in governing projects under the sign of health and hygiene. In late 1920s and early 1930s correspondence between soap producers and Nyasaland's government, about the merits of import duty on soap, writers attributed "increasing demand for soap among people who [previously] knew little about soap" partially to the return of migrants from South Africa and Rhodesia who "swaggered" about in the villages and set an example of cleanliness for "village boys." District commissioners instructed villagers in the "direct bearing soap has on their hygiene and general advancement," and noted the "lack of [cleanliness among natives] in [Nyasaland]." The comptroller of customs, in attempting to prove that locally manufactured soap was inferior to imported soap, observed that local soap was often given away freely as *banyira* (a small top-up or gift that accompanies a purchase in the market) (CAA S1/1382/29; CAA S2/14/32).

The centrality of soap—as a symbol of health, racialized modernity, and cleanliness—to both colonial-era improvement projects and present-day projects opens a space for considering how this tiny object is laden with overlapping meanings and legacies. The gift of soap in research worlds dramatizes the difference between researchers and the researched along intersecting axes of race, economic status, and health: soap seems to be a gift that works especially well across such gradients. Though everyone uses soap, Malawian fieldworkers' sentiments, such as "[Villagers] are grateful for the soap and really need it," emphasize differences in financial and social status between project employees and research subjects (see Englund 2006, 70–98, for an analysis of cultural dispositions of elitism that reinforce boundaries between Malawian activists and the grassroots). When RAM gave bars of soap to wealthier, urban-dwelling churchgoers in June 2008 in return for their participation in interviews, they were offended and refused this gift intended for the poor. Some suggested RAM donate the soap instead to their home church for use in health kits that home-based care volunteers used to administer to the rural poor.[9]

Consumption and use of soap in Malawi has long been an index of personhood, has played an important role in the development of self and other, and has by now come to acquire meanings beyond an imperial civilizing tool (Durham 2005). In fact, soap as research gift—given by projects to some individuals but not others—reflects the logics underlying the rise of humanitarian design amid diminished faith in nation-states, entwining market and ethical logics. Like the increasing number of well-intentioned devices produced by social entrepreneurs to improve lives in the global South, soap responds to immediate individual, rather than collective or social, needs and offers a direct conduit for expressing care, even as it produces forms of value for its givers

(Redfield 2016, 175). Notably, however, the 2011 rollout of a national sanitation campaign that placed "handwashing with soap" at its core illustrates that soap remains an enduring prop in the state's production of clean citizens and modernity (West 2016, 80–85). Malawian families identify soap as a fundamental need; their desire for this basic object aligns nicely with researchers' desire to give a gift that is cleaner and healthier than bottles of Coca-Cola or sugar. Comparisons between soap gifts and sugar gifts (with preference for the latter) commonly arose in conversations with Malawians living in project sample areas. Many people in Balaka District, for example, recalled that LSAM had, in the past, given sugar as a gift; some had heard rumors that they discontinued the sugar because research participants had accused them of lacing it with contraceptives. One woman reported that the consent form she signed had listed that she was to receive a gift of soap and sugar, but she had only received the former. She explained that the word "sugar" had been blacked out with a pen. After some investigation, I determined that the teams printed a form from a previous survey year and so, instead of wasting paper, blacked out "sugar" and administered them. Research participants' nostalgic recollections of a bygone sweeter gift—and the paper trail it left behind in archived consent forms—point to how legacies of giving and taking inform present-day moral economies of exchange.

Notable, as well, is the way in which standardizing reciprocity—and the material gift exchanged—balances ethical commitments to giving something in return for information with anxieties that gifts or incentives might dirty or contaminate data by altering the responses of those in the sample (making them more or less accurate or complete), or by stoking expectations that create friction between projects and respondents—potentially increasing frequency of refusals, for example. Even if receiving a gift raises respondents' motivation, it may prompt them to lie: to provide answers more pleasing to the interviewer who gifts it to them or that make respondents appear more deserving of future gifts from the interviewer (Stecklov, Weinreb, and Carletto 2015). Generally, there is evidence that gifts increase data quality by exerting a positive effect on retention, strengthening the external validity of surveys (Weinreb, Madhavan, and Stern 1998; Bignami-Van Assche, Reniers, and Weinreb 2003), though most of these studies are confined to contexts outside the "least developed countries" where even the smallest of gifts may exert influence on respondents (Knoll et al. 2012; Singer and Ye 2013). Gifting has by no means been validated as a best practice and may have effects on the quality of the responses collected (Stecklov, Weinreb, and Carletto 2015, 15; adams et al. n.d.). In short, gifting is simultaneously a way of standardizing ethical investments—doing the right thing when collecting data in impoverished contexts—and producing messy expectations, relations, and unevenness. Soap, validated as an ethical gift, carries the potential to either contaminate data or make them better and cleaner.

Soap's material form—small, packaged, lightweight, cheap—ensures it meets the needs of Malawian ethics boards, foreign researchers, Malawian fieldworkers, and research participants. As it travels, soap accumulates multiple and competing meanings yet remains recognizable as a rhetorical gift by all parties; its efficacy lies in its fluidity (deLaet and Mol 2000). By maintaining the integrity of diverse actors' interests, soap enlists them as allies to research (Star and Griesemer 1989, 389). In its flexible standardization, soap resembles the modular humanitarian kits developed by Médecins sans Frontières for frontline crisis responders (Redfield 2008). Soap and humanitarian kits work because they possess material characteristics that enable them to literally fit into and streamline larger research or humanitarian infrastructures, even as their physical forms are imbued with dense meanings by those who encounter them. Consider other instances from the ethnographic record where objects' material properties reflect or limit their social lives and relations they cohere. Annette Weiner (1976, 7), in her work on Trobriand women's banana leaf bundles, foregrounds how bundles' materiality—qualities like new, old, clean, dirty—registers differences and hierarchies between persons who exchange them. Like soap, bundles are not signed, not exchanged between two specific partners, and divisible into units that achieve relative equivalence, about one cent Australian. Sharon Hutchinson (1992, 299), meanwhile, notes that until the 1960s, Nuer refused to accept paper currency for cattle because paper notes were ill suited to the hot, wet, and windy climate, or were eaten by white ants. The material forms of soap, humanitarian kits, and banana leaf bundles are central, rather than incidental, to the social relations they cohere. Paper currency and sugar, for the Nuer and Malawian fieldworkers, respectively, failed as gifts not because of their value or meanings, but because of their mundane material characteristics.

Complaints about Soap: Unraveling Ethics, Revaluing Data

The justification for research in impoverished settings relies on a presumption that it will improve the collective good or bring abstract future benefits to participants, but participants, as we will see, often expect their lives in the present to be transformed (Titmuss [1970] 1997, 281; Reynolds et al. 2013). While anthropologists document how research transactions of blood, information, and benefits activate multiple gift economies that come into friction, soap, even as it is assigned competing meanings, works because its transaction is legitimated as ethical by both participants and researchers (Lairumbi et al. 2012; Sambakunsi et al. 2015). Yet naming soap ethical does not preclude critical engagements with the ensuing production of value and knowledge from information collected. In what follows, I consider the heterogeneity of meanings cathected onto the soap gift to reveal that naming soap as ethical relies on a bounded definition of research that abstracts it from its particular time and place. Even as soap appears to facilitate the collection of data and keep the gift relationship clean, it produces new kinds of subject positions, forms of value, and expectations in its transaction. Transactions in research worlds produce not only data but new kinds of social bonds (and social ruptures) and, thus, new kinds of social persons (Kelly 2015; Meinert 2015).

SOAP (AND RESEARCH) AS RIGHTS

For some survey respondents, soap was a symbol of injustice and a metaphor for failures of state and nonstate administration of aid, resources, and gifts. The distribution of the seemingly innocuous soap gift sometimes engendered suspicions and distrust in sampled areas. Although soap is a standardized gift (in that all who participate receive equally), it is interpreted as an unjust gift because some people are left out. The lopsided social terrain of lucky insiders and unlucky outsiders created by random sampling grafts onto a landscape pockmarked by other instances of uneven distribution. People living in sample areas drew parallels between random sampling and exclusions produced by the government's annual distribution of limited fertilizer coupons to the poor, widely perceived to be inefficient, corrupt, and unfair. One participant in LSAM's survey mobilized an aphorism to critique the pitfalls of randomization: "[Chimanga] chimalora opanda mano!" ("Maize always goes to those who don't have teeth," that is, good things are wasted if given to the wrong people), while another wondered why LSAM "skipped some houses."[10]

Survey respondents for LSAM and MAYP pointed out that some who received soap were the wrong people: drunkards, village fools, or others who did not deserve to participate and would do a bad job as respondents. Critiques of the mode of reciprocation necessitated by random sampling—where only participants are given a gift—resonate with Paige West's (2006, 47) observation of the bind faced by a Papua New Guinean biodiversity conservation project whose gestures to pay back individuals and communities for their labor and cooperation with gifts such as school fees or jobs were criticized for rewarding some individuals more than others or for failing to give gifts befitting the project's ample resources. In Malawi, a locally fitting gift—soap—meets formal ethical standards for any single research encounter but does not address expectations that a project should not skip houses, nor does it respond to critiques that individuals and communities are entitled to more than just soap.

Survey participants explicitly coded research and soap as rights good citizens were entitled to, using both the English and Chewa terms (*ufulu wachibadwidwe*, freedoms one is born with) when talking about these entitlements. Some of my informants, for example, suggested it was their human right to receive health care or medicines if a project found them suffering. Like fertilizer coupons distributed by the state, soap prompts reflection on the political relationship of citizens to institutions in their midst (Bornstein 2012; Samsky 2012). Soap triggers its recipients to consider the value of information they surrender, and complaints voice needs that might be fulfilled by one among the many projects Malawians often lump together (Prince 2012). In terming soap a human right, participants upend normative ethics based in liberal human rights and individualist personhood to resituate rights as material and, often, collective entitlements (Englund 2006). Though it may not generate the *hau* (spirit of the gift) that Mauss ([1922] 1967) observed between Maori transactors who thus continued a cycle of giving and receiving between them, soap makes the mismatch between interpretations of the value of research a problem for negotiation, even as it seeks to make them commensurate as mere misunderstandings.

Refusals to participate in surveys were symptoms of respondents' dissatisfaction with past research encounters. When I visited the household of a middle-aged man called Dominick who refused to participate in LSAM's survey, he was initially reluctant to speak with me, coding me as a representative of another project. When I explained that I wanted to hear his reflections on research in the format of a conversation and not a survey, he elaborated on his refusal to answer LSAM's questions: "I won't answer those silly [survey questions]; people already came here [a few months back] and some of my friends chose some bottle caps with kwacha [money] on them and, me, I chose a cap and it had nothing on it. If they are coming here to fool us again, just tell them don't even come!"[11] In 2004, LSAM began HIV testing respondents in its panel survey sample. Because those tested would need to report to portable tent test result centers two to four months after their initial test to receive the results, LSAM implemented an experiment to determine how small monetary incentives might affect respondents' likelihood of coming to the test centers. The experimental design featured respondents drawing bottle caps marked with amounts ranging from 0 to 300 Malawi kwacha ($0–3, at the time) from a bag or hat and receiving a voucher to be redeemed upon pickup of results (Thornton 2008; Obare et al. 2009). In 2006, this incentives program was not implemented because of the advent and feasibility of rapid testing, which meant respondents received their results immediately. However, that year LSAM initiated another incentives program, this time an HIV-prevention experiment. A portion of individuals who received an HIV test in 2006 (whether the test was positive or negative) were enrolled in an incentives study whereby they participated in a similar bottle cap lottery that promised them the monetary amount depicted if they maintained their HIV status for the next year. In 2007, LSAM distributed the incentives, which ranged from 0 to 4,000 kwacha ($0–32 at the time), based on which bottle cap a respondent had chosen back in 2006. Despite efforts to educate participants about experimental design, villagers interpreted random distribution of incentives (via a lottery system of choosing a bottle cap with a monetary amount on it from a hat) as unjust. Dominick, for example, felt fooled because he had not received what he felt entitled to, and feeling wronged motivated his decision to abstain from the 2008 survey, even though it did not include incentives in its design.

Refusal to participate in research is likewise refusal to accept a gift (soap), yet these refusals (so long as not too numerous to reduce sample size significantly) may legitimate research's ethical claims by proving that potential subjects have agency to choose not to participate. Rather than viewing Dominick as a Maussian "moral person," LSAM encounters him as a depersonalized and categorical research participant whose refusal to accept the soap gift does not injure the researcher; rather, his refusal, in a sense, reproduces a research community or, at least, does not undo it (McGranahan 2016, 322). His refusal is not socially but numerically coded, easily digested by statistics that measure sample retention. Though the survey associated with his name does not carry data, his refusal does not threaten data quality but perhaps enhances it from the perspective of an ethics rooted in an agent's ability to refuse. Dominick's critique that he did not receive the money he felt entitled to, and the rationale underlying his refusal to accept a gift of soap in 2008 goes unaddressed by research ethics that rely on those in the sample receiving soap and others outside the sample receiving nothing. Despite researchers' efforts to clearly explain study design and dispel misconceptions of therapeutic effects, Dominick cast them as a homogenous and undifferentiated group of people who sought to fool him and others like him. Moreover, while demographers often blame interviewers—their appearance and mannerisms, for example—for refusals or nonresponse by respondents (Lynn 2008), Dominick indicated that it was his interaction with a corporate entity (the project) rather than any one individual that mediated his refusal (Reynolds et al. 2013). Further, Malawians often make little distinction between the many projects in their midst. As Miller, Zulu, and Watkins (2001, 171) point out, LSAM respondents in early waves of the survey perceived that fieldworkers were associated with the national family planning program, despite their explicit introduction as affiliates of LSAM (see also Graboyes 2015, 34–36).

SOAP AS PAYMENT AND RESEARCH AS WORK

While some researchers suggested that survey participation could be a way for participants to break up an otherwise uninteresting day, participants often viewed research participation as a job, raising complaints about the value of soap in a discourse of labor, even as they continued to call it a gift. Many respondents complained that they saw "no profit" in research participation. A female LSAM participant suggested, "I expect more than soap because it is not equivalent to the job I do as a respondent. . . . It's a very big job; [interviewers] can ask you so many questions on so many topics and sometimes you just reach a point where you run out of answers and just look at the interviewer."[12] She is not paid for her time but volunteers it, ostensibly to benefit her larger community, in line with Lochlann Jain's (2013, 119) observation that randomized controlled trials "absorb . . . the individual into a potential yearned-for advantage . . . further institutionalizing [a] fantasy of hope for the next generation of [research] subjects." Yet even as research participants seem interchangeable from the perspective of projects fixated on sample size rather than individuals (Biruk 2012), people in sample areas indicated that research participants can do a good or bad job. In explicitly framing participation as working (*kugwira ntchito*), research subjects make political claims on projects tied up in a distributive economy of care and social welfare (Ferguson 2015). Soap, coded as an antonym of monetary payment, is resignified as a commodity whose exchange value is inadequate remuneration for good work.

Andrews, fieldwork supervisor, suggested research participants increasingly see research as a job:

> In Malawi . . . we have these rules that in research you [cannot] give people money. But, you know, things are changing. Times are changing. . . . Nowadays for you to get anything you need, you need money. If somebody comes to your house and then tells you let's sit down [and] we should chat, that means you have lost that time. That could have been productive time, but yet you spent that time chatting with some-

body. So . . . people . . . are really starting to value their time. [When] someone gives them something, they can look at it and value it and say, okay, from that job I've got this.[13]

He notes that participants carefully calibrate time and labor and contests the legitimacy of research rules, prescriptive ethics that name money as an inappropriate gift for what he sees as a job (Folayan and Allman 2011).[14] Sitting and answering survey questions is a drain on time and energy: in early August 2008, Henry, an interviewer, arrived at a sample household to find his assigned respondent. Relatives went to fetch him from where he was working in the fields nearby. He and Henry initiated the interview, but when Henry went to verify the names provided for his parents-in-law with his wife, he found upon returning that "[his] respondent had abandoned [him]" or run away after losing interest in the long-form survey. Fieldworkers, in general, voiced concerns that projects they worked for relied on gifts not to build but to evade social obligations, consistent with Kingori (2013) and Madiega et al.'s (2013) findings that field staff of medical research projects in Kenya were wary of obligations that impoverished research subjects imposed on them as representatives of a wealthy foreign project. Another LSAM supervisor reflected on the large number of refusals the previous day:

> It was better in 2004, when [LSAM] came here . . . but we camped in the villages. There, right there in that field [pointing to a big open field near the tea room]. If people had questions they could come ask us, and we managed to eat and drink with them [the villagers who made up the research sample]. We also brought money to them by hiring local guards for the campsite, cooks, or buying goats and other foods from them. For long-term projects like this one, that is a must. Not this simple coming and going.[15]

In his view, proper exchange entails more than one-off gifts. He deems contributions to the local economy and spontaneous social interactions that arise when projects are sited among the people, as opposed to nearby rest houses, as demystifying LSAM's objectives and creating amity between strangers. In his account, a gift of soap symbolizes not reciprocal social bonds between projects and participants, but rather the coming and going typically associated with market-based transactions. His comments echo the emphasis on moral responsibility beyond formal ethical practice endorsed by fieldworkers and other intermediaries across contexts (Kingori 2013; Sambakunsi et al. 2015). Further, they illustrate how a gift can be ethical when evaluated from a perspective within a research world but unethical when evaluated in light of historical memory and experience in a particular time and place. While this verifies the gap between prescriptive and situated ethics (or field ethics) identified by anthropologists and others (Molyneux and Geissler 2008; Graboyes 2015), it more importantly shows how soap's status as a culturally appropriate gift simultaneously makes it ethical and brings into question the social value of research for those who wish their payment was more befitting of the labor they contribute to data.

Research participants employed the metaphor of hunger to accuse Malawian fieldworkers of "eating [their] money": "They come here and instead of fetching food for the children, we sit here wasting time *kucheza* [talking]. . . . They go home and eat good food, rice, meat. . . . They leave me hungry and make money as they do so."[16] This accusation finds intertextual meaning in a history of "eating money" as a critique leveled against elites, scammers, relatives, governments, or "big men" who fatten themselves on the spoils of the poor or gain wealth corruptly (Bayart 1993; Geschiere 1997; Hasty 2005; Smith 2008; Dahl 2014).

Participating in an interview means surrendering productive time. While talking, a respondent is unable to, for example, obtain food for her child (though women often shelled maize or cooked during interviews). One respondent suggested that if he went in search of piece work instead of sitting for an interview, he would have been able to buy bars of soap himself. Fieldworkers often sought out men absent from their households in trading centers or fields where they worked. While respondents answer questions for up to three hours, time is money, or its equivalent in food, and longer-form surveys may exacerbate participants' frustrations with lost time (Aiga 2007). As participants experience a net loss, they see interviewers "getting fat" from the information (and salary) they collect. Some even accused LSAM interviewers of "eating our money" explicitly, invoking again the 2006 HIV-prevention incentives experiment: "[The interviewers] take the bottle caps with zeros on them and put them on top [of the pile in the bag] . . . so we pick them and the people in T-shirts [LSAM interviewers in project T-shirts] eat our money." Indeed, it was common for respondents to furnish interviewers with small gifts during survey administration in line with local hospitality norms: sugarcane to gnaw on, groundnuts, fruits, or even *nsima* and relish at mealtimes. Such gifts were given without ethical compulsion (but rather in the spirit of hospitality), in contrast to the soap that flowed the other way. The soap gift aimed to fast-forward a social relationship that did not exist before the interviewer arrived at the household by making him seem trustworthy or kind (Weinreb 2006), but framed this relationship as ethical, rather than social or economic. For research participants, projects were not only eating their time and leaving them hungry but creating a new hunger for a better future they would likely never taste.

Fieldworkers, meanwhile, struggle to reconcile their desire to forge meaningful relationships with respondents with pressures to meet interview quotas each day and with guidelines imposed on their behaviors in the field by researchers. Like the community health workers Swartz (2013) documents in South Africa, fieldworkers balanced their empathy for impoverished research subjects with their pragmatic investment in completing tasks crucial to their own economic survival. Thornton (2008) notes that in a pilot of the LSAM HIV-testing incentives project in 2004, nurses gave out higher incentives than they were supposed to, feeling sympathetic to poor villagers, dirtying the theoretical distribution of randomized incentives; nurses were instructed that continued employment was contingent upon following the randomization standards. Patricia Kingori (2013) likewise observes how data collectors in Kenya sometimes modified standards to favor their own personal ethical values and motivations as they witnessed the suffering of the research subjects they encountered, and Geissler (2013b, 19) shows how clinical trial staff in Kenya gave private gifts to poor research subjects, viewing them as kin or friendship relations.

The metaphor of eating also surfaced in accusations that research projects were "sucking" (a form of eating) research participants' blood (*kupopa magazi*). These stories fit into a larger transhistorical genre that demonizes dangerous others (colonial officials, researchers, politicians, physicians) who steal or accumulate bodily material or information for mysterious ends (Musambachime 1988; White 2000; Geissler 2005; Fairhead, Leach, and Small 2006; Anderson 2008; Kaler 2009; Kelly et al. 2010). While the bloodsucker stories circulated around survey projects, for the most part they only minimally affected daily data collection, though fieldworkers often had to convince reluctant respondents that the stories were not true before they would agree to participate. Notably, however, GSIP—which included a cash incentives component—fieldworkers were "literally chased from villages" in a district where they were piloting the survey in October 2007 when the project's SUV was pelted with stones by villagers who claimed the vehicle carried bloodsuckers. This project subsequently relocated to a different site. In a neighboring district, the district health officer reported to me that government health surveillance assistants newly assigned to a rural post were chased by villagers who vandalized the clinic overnight and threatened them with violence, illustrating that it is not just foreign projects that are cast as outsiders by the rumors. In fact, the scariest thing about the bloodsuckers is that they might blend in or disguise themselves as something or someone benevolent.

Around the time when bloodsucker rumors were circulating, local newspapers featured numerous headlines that sensationalized the rumors, such as "Bloodsuckers Terrorize Chiradzulu!" (e.g., Mmana 2007; Muwamba 2007; Malikwa 2007). Media coverage serves, at least since the early 2000s, as a makeshift archive of flare-ups of bloodsucking rumors. In December 2002, for example, then president Bakili Muluzi made public statements to disassociate his government from stories that it was sucking people's blood in exchange for maize donations from foreign governments (e.g., Munthali 2002; Tendani 2002 McFerran 2003). In October 2007, meanwhile, the Malawi government declared that anyone spreading such rumors would be arrested, and many of those who feared the bloodsuckers interpreted this edict as evidence that the state was not interested in providing for their security, or might even benefit from their insecurity. Similarly, many months later, rural Malawians living in or near LSAM sample villages sometimes accused their chief of allowing the *opopa magazi* to access their blood in exchange for "a few kwacha" given to him or her by survey projects. A colleague at the University of Malawi observed that bloodsucker stories were not "like maize or the rains," which come every year; "You never know when they will surface," he suggested. Reflecting on the rumors, a traditional authority (similar to a chief) in Zomba District traced them to "politics," explaining, "This area is a UDF [political party] stronghold; [other political parties] put the magazi in people's heads here to hold back development so that when people chase the projects from here they move to other places, ones which are supportive of the ruling party."[17] Importantly, he linked projects to development and acknowledged that projects were unevenly distributed across the local landscape; it was perhaps the randomness of this distribution that raised questions about just distribution of benefits. Later in the conversation, he suggested that although people are eager for research and development projects to help them, they also do not believe it is possible to get something for nothing and assume that anything they are given might need to be paid for. Similar sentiments surfaced amid the Community Based Rural Land Development Project, a resettlement scheme initiated in 2005, whereby people who were relocated to distant districts and given inputs to develop and farm new land were fearful of having their blood sucked or being held in corrals to fatten them up to take their blood.[18]

In interviews I conducted with a random subsample of respondents who had participated in LSAM's 2008 survey, some suggested that survey projects were sending their "blood" abroad to get money or to "do business," or admitted they did not know what happened to the answers they provided to surveys. Though previous studies of vampire stories have largely focused on "blood stealing" by medical institutions, stories in Malawi also placed survey responses at the center of their accusations. In fact, it is important to note that many research participants framed taking an HIV test and receiving knowledge of their status as a major *benefit* of research participation, challenging dominant assumptions that Africans are superstitious about blood. Like intimate liquids, responses that locals give belong to them. Tiwonge, a survey participant, framed the information she surrendered to LSAM in bodily terms: "Research is important. The findings can help improve our lives. But I ask . . . why are they [researchers] stealing my voice?"[19] In reflecting on the conversion of her responses ("voice") into findings, she embodies a postcolonial history and collective memory characterized by theft of voices, bodily tissues, land, and labor by research projects, the state, and the Employment Bureau of Africa, the recruiting organ in Malawi of the South African Chamber of Mines. She indicates that her voice, in its translation to data on a page, is not fully alienated but stolen. The soap gift is not equivalent to the voice she gives. For Tiwonge, soap may be ethical, but it is not enough.

The kinds of suspicions and mistrust evoked by the circulation of opopa magazi rumors find historical corollary in correspondence and discussions surrounding colonial health surveys in Nyasaland, where a major concern of colonial officials and researchers was gaining the trust of their research subjects, whom they speculated would refuse to give "samples of blood [and] dejecta" for fear they would be used for bewitching and sorcery (M2/14/1 1935). Vaccination teams in the mid-twentieth century, too, noted that when they arrived in the villages, children would run into the bush to avoid being inspected or vaccinated, and officials involved with a stool survey to determine the prevalence of parasites in Zomba District faced resistance that prompted them to begin examining stool specimens in the open and disposing of them by "public burial," not unlike LSAM's practice many years later of disposing of HIV test kits in a respondent's pit latrine to alleviate suspicions (S1/986 (A11)/25 1952). Though refusals were relatively uncommon in the surveys I spent time with, on occasion a respondent would hide in her latrine or tell her child to tell the fieldworker she was not home. As is discussed in more detail in chapter 4, respondents also sometimes faked their identities—posing as someone else—in order to access a gift they were not entitled to by virtue of being outside the sample.

Unraveling Ethics?

In its claim to foreclose future obligations between a project and members of its research sample, in its classification as "appropriate recompense" rather than coercive incentive, in its presumed noneffect on the quality of data collected, in its connotation as healthy, and in its standardization and convenience, soap is deemed an ethical gift. However, when viewed from the perspective of the field, soap becomes a contested—hardly clean—object laden with competing meanings and claims that reflect and cohere the interests and positions of actors across different scales of the research world. The claims on and meanings attached to soap discussed in this chapter do not become data, as they fall outside that which survey projects seek to measure and document (Geissler 2013b, 21).

Demographers' epistemic investment in clean, high-quality data is borne out not only in meticulous attention to survey design (as we saw in chapter 1) and in intensive trainings to harmonize fieldworkers' behaviors and practices, but also in ensuring that ethical standards are adhered to during data collection, as this chapter has shown. The informed consent ritual—and the exchange of soap—are visible manifestations of human subjects research ethics that privilege autonomy and agency as consent's grounding. As data collection proceeds, transactions of soap for information produce the workable subjects of researcher and research subject. While the thicket of contested meanings and claims that adhere to soap come out in the wash, so to speak, when data are transferred to databases, scrubbed, and become statistical evidence, it is clear that the transactions of soap on the ground produce hopes, expectations, and conflicts that endure long after a single project has left the field.

Receiving soap means being a member of a community (or sample) that imagines ongoing research participation as linked to future entitlements or benefits well beyond soap. Jerven (2013, 72), writing on the case of the 2006 census in Nigeria, tracks a shift from a colonial-era fear of being counted to a postcolonial "race to be included" in enumerating exercises. In this case, the interest in being counted was so strong that people in Nigeria's southern region accused enumerators of counting animals—in addition to people—in the north to further political agendas. In 2001, LSAM drew its sample incorrectly, leading fieldworkers to conduct duplicate interviews before researchers realized their mistake: very few respondents told the fieldworkers they had already been interviewed, likely in order to receive more soap (Bignami-Van Assche 2003). Ferguson (2015, 85) suggests that the poor may today see in forms of enumeration and surveillance forms of incorporation, support, and recognition that are otherwise unavailable. While survey projects travel local landscapes lightly and thinly—they do not build hospitals or provide medicines, for example—they nonetheless create economies of speculative hope around future entitlements or incorporation. A good-enough gift, soap is an empty signifier onto which people project multiple stakes and meanings regarding their intersecting futures as researchers, fieldworkers, and research participants.

Deciding what to give research participants in exchange for information or blood samples is an ethical dilemma that must be addressed in order for data collection to proceed smoothly. Because the fruits of participation in research projects may be realized far into the future, demographers worry that respondents might refuse to answer questions, particularly in overresearched areas. As Riedmann (1993, 56–57) shows in her historical analysis of fertility surveys carried out in 1970s Nigeria, some subjects requested *naira* (Nigeria's currency) before answering questions, in much the same register as survey respondents in 2007–2008 Malawi. Similar concerns likewise troubled Nyasaland colonial official staging development schemes that required unpaid labor (M2/4/2 1931; NSZ 1/5/1 1938), and researchers implementing the Nyasaland Nutrition Survey (1938–1943) pondered whether "tangible rewards" would gain the "confidence of the people" and improve participation (Berry and Petty 1992, 20).

Likewise, a 1938 meeting of district commissioners featured discussion of how to balance "the commercial view point that bulk[ed] ever large in the native's mind" with what they saw as the erosion of "the communal system of village life." It was with great reluctance that the British Colonial Office began to contemplate compensation for those who participated in community development schemes, and community development enthusiasts continued to see individualism and competition—exacerbated by payment for work they thought should be voluntary—as threats to African societies (NSZ 1/5/1 1938; Vaughan 1982). In 1930, a series of letters from missionaries working in Nyasaland to the director of medical and sanitation services argued that Africans participating in medical training programs should be paid; one missionary based at Livingstonia Mission urged the government to subsidize missions to pay native hospital assistants, who, he said, "after being trained, tend to find their way to neighboring territories where they are engaged with pay, unlike here" (M2/4/2 1931). The long history of the politics around monetary transactions in research and development worlds indicates a delicate balance between giving too little and giving too much, and illustrates enduring racialized assumptions inherent in fears around "giving Africans money," around fostering dependency, and around eroding self-sufficiency (Ferguson 2015).

As others have shown, gifts can be wrenched from their embeddedness in social solidarities in shifting economic landscapes (Andaya 2009). This chapter has illustrated how the ethical gift of soap given to survey participants produces rather than reconciles expectations. Intended to avoid undue inducement to participation, soap comes to be seen as insufficient payment even as it maintains its status as a gift. According to the logics of an ethics rooted in the principles of liberal human rights—autonomy to decide without coercion whether or not to participate in research—soap is an ethical, even an ideal gift: Malawian research participants did not contest its status as such. But, as we have seen, they nonetheless raise many grievances about the gift: soap and research benefits are material entitlements or rights that are improperly distributed; research participation is unpaid labor; and research projects are bloodsuckers.

Such grievances are often mitigated by researchers' insistence that they are misunderstandings and by the forward march of projects whose focus is on collecting more and more data in the most efficient manner possible (Crane 2013; Meinert and Whyte 2014). As Graboyes (2015, 203) astutely points out, many research sites (or fields) across Africa are "static backdrop[s] for new researchers to experience the same difficulties [as past researchers] and explain them with the same tired tropes: uneducated Africans and well-intentioned researchers rebuffed for no good reason." A close examination of the particular transactions that produce data illustrates, however, that contrary to dominant opinion, research participants' critiques and grievances do not arise from therapeutic misconception—where subjects misunderstand that all aspects of research will benefit them directly. Rather than misunderstanding research, research participants situate projects they encounter within historical experiences and legacies of the extraction of data and other resources, pointing out that the benefits that researchers accrue in the process of making their responses into data are far greater than those they receive. They call on projects not only to give more but also to account for their extractions of data toward ends often misaligned with local priorities (Muula and Mfutso-Bengo 2007; Dionne 2012). Such critiques recall Malawian peasants' resistance to antierosion conservation measures (widely referred to as *malimidwe*) imposed by the colonial government that required them to expend free labor—for example, building ridges in gardens—toward ends they deemed not in their best interest. While the colonial government cast rural residents as resistant to conservation, Mulwafu (2011, 151–153) shows that this resistance stemmed from legitimate frustrations with new conservation laws that not only asked them to work for free but also stripped them of traditional rights of ownership and control over land, which in their view was being stolen from them in the name of conservation.

Projects such as LSAM and MAYP aim to avoid thick local involvement—indeed, becoming too generous might muck up data—by giving an ethical but distancing gift, but participants seek substantive engagement across difference. A bicycle taxi driver operating in MAYP sample villages, for example, said, "So many projects are coming here and not giving us anything and breaking their promises, unfulfilled promises. It's time for them to stop asking us so many questions and start doing something for us."[20] An elderly LSAM research subject told me she thought researchers collected surveys to "make sure everything works all right, and if it doesn't, after *amasankha bwinobwino* [they analyze/count the answers well] they come back to us *kuti tigwirizane nawo* [to bridge the gap]."[21] For her and many others, the soap gift symbolizes the injustice of projects that not only take more than they give, but also fail to come back. Yet research participants continue to deposit information in a data bank that might yield returns in the future, even if researchers' coming and going makes this a risky investment. In their stance of refusal and critique, they insist on the possible over the probable (McGranahan 2016, 323).

At first glance, the soap-for-information exchange in Malawi seems to highlight tensions between Malawian and foreign cultural codes of giving, calling forth the distinction between commodity and gift exchanges that has preoccupied anthropologists in the wake of *The Gift* (Mauss [1922] 1967). Rural Malawian research participants, we might suggest, simply view gifts differently than researchers: they see soap-for-information transactions as personal and generative of social obligations. Researchers, coming from a commodity-based society, on the other hand, view the same exchanges as expedient, impersonal, and not producing future interdependence. This reading, however, not only Orientalizes rural Malawi as a gift society but presumes that researchers and the researched inhabit different worlds characterized by competing interests and bounded cultural norms, flattening the hybrid subjects and objects of survey research worlds (Carrier 2003). Further, reading Malawian resistance to research in this manner fails to attend to the ways in which flows of research, benefits, and gifts are mediated by social, moral, and economic practices produced in the encounter between forces glossed as local and global

(Masquelier 2012). Soap is recognized as a gift not across worlds, but because it is a central ingredient in cohering a new one (that nonetheless mobilizes fragments from old ones): a research world. Exchanges do not occur between preformed persons but rather highlight how new kinds of persons and new future trajectories are produced and imagined through transactions that activate "sciences' pasts and futures" simultaneously (Tousignant 2013, 730; see also Strathern 1988; Wendland 2012).

If we presume that research worlds and the subjects who inhabit them are produced by transactions, our investments in normative ethics—which aim to govern preexisting subjects rather than respond to the expectations and relations that arise in the course of data collection—are unraveled. Even as projects successfully minimize harm by carefully obtaining informed consent, protecting confidentiality, avoiding deceptive practices, and inviting participants to refuse participation, respondents still feel wronged. Writing from the position of an ethnographer of global health, Nyambedha (2008, 775) proposes that we define "harm" more capaciously to include raising research subjects' expectations or hopes without addressing them. Such a proposal invites us, especially when read through the lens of Deborah Thomas's (2011) "reparations as a framework for thinking," to consider how the transaction of an ethical gift activates memories of unfulfilling and unjust research encounters in the past, and prompts imaginings of alternative, better futures. In line with anthropologists' calls to move away from culture-centric critiques of ethics to center structural inequalities that constrain their operations, reparations as a framework for thinking invites a radical reconceptualization of ethics' categories and assumptions. Ethics necessitate the imagination of racialized subjects who are both more in need of protection and more disposable than those who do the imagining; they also presume preformed subjects, obscuring how it is through research transactions that people (and data) are made and unmade. This framework might help us more closely attend to continuities between histories of expropriation at the hands of colonial science and present-day modes of bio- and informational capital extraction in order to build an ethical framework responsive not merely to narrow project-based parameters but also to the histories and political economy in which projects as a whole are situated. Peterson et al. (2015) show how research institutions in Malawi likewise take a diachronic approach to ethics, documenting how proposals for HIV preexposure prophylaxis (PrEP) clinical trials were deemed unethical by Malawian ethics boards not because of worries over trial practices, but because the protocol did not explicitly deal with questions about future research agendas, future drug access, and so on. While these trial proposals adhered closely to normative ethical standards, they failed to address potential adverse effects that may exceed those most visible to researchers (Crane 2010a). On-the-ground protocols in place were deemed ethical, while the expectations and imagined futures the research would generate at the individual and national level were not.

A narrow focus on meeting or exceeding formal rules and ethical standards obscures the historically informed meanings that participants assign to research transactions (Biruk 2017). Neither, however, does a situated, contextually attentive analysis of ethics address the concerns of Malawian participants documented in this chapter. As Wendland (2008) points out, normative ethics presumes that research is a distinct entity governable by rules and codes that rely on its autonomy from larger spheres of life. Yet, for research participants, as this chapter has shown, research is a realm of negotiation over proper distribution (a rightful share) of past, present, and future benefits, of which soap is just one (Ferguson 2015).

In Africa, the accumulated knowledge of researchers was extracted from captive donors without payment or ethical governance, often in the service of empire and capitalism (Titmuss 1970 [1997], 284; Tilley 2016). Ethics, as a corrective to that history, is a realm internal to—not autonomous from— political economy: it is the enabling regulatory condition for the market in research participation as work (Cooper and Waldby 2014, 14). This chapter has troubled the underlying premise of research activities: that information should be freely given. It is the volunteerism of impoverished Malawians that enables the collection and circulation of high-quality data. Yet ethics viewed from the bottom up seems mostly to work to ensure that projects can accomplish their ends—collecting good data as efficiently as possible—without being held accountable for how research transactions shape the very communities and individuals they aim to document or study. Clean data can only materialize within and through messy social relations and transactions: people, ethics, and data are made and remade as research activities are carried out in a particular place and time. The hybrid subjects and ethics produced along the way invoke and imagine pasts, presents, and futures through the transaction of soap and information. Crucially, however, these memories and aspirations are rooted in a critique of the material inadequacy of a present that attempts to settle rather than meaningfully redress claims its recipients make on its givers.

Coda: The Anthropologist and Soap

> Today I received the list of my respondents from Dr. Jones. She provided
> me with 20 people drawn randomly from six enumeration areas, all of
> whom were in the larger MAYP sample. The list contains the enumera-
> tion area number, household identification number, and name of each
> of the twenty respondents I will speak to. I checked in with Dr. Jones
> and Dr. Payson about giving respondents gifts, and although they sug-
> gested that either soda, cookies, or soap would work, we collaboratively
> decided that the best thing would be to use the same gifts distributed
> during "regular" interviews so as to not cause uneven expectations or
> affect the general data in the future.[22]

In my role as an ethnographer of projects, I not only participated in everyday fieldwork activities but also conducted my own interviews with projects'
survey respondents, which my research assistants jokingly termed "research
on research" interviews, even coining an acronym, ROR, to describe them. In
the field notes above, I record the pre-ROR interview preparations and com-
munications I conducted with MAYP's principal investigators via email. Both
were happy to allow me to conduct ROR interviews and to collect qualitative
data alongside MAYP fieldwork but provided me with a random sample of
respondents to ensure that my research activities had minimal impact (future
or present) on the survey data they were likewise collecting. (The anthropologist, too, has the potential to contaminate or dirty data.) The list I was
provided with was my guidebook and map for the next few weeks. With my
research assistant, I found myself seeing like a demographer, even as the data
I was collecting were qualitative rather than quantitative. Instead of engaging in more traditional anthropological fieldwork interviewing respondents
known to me or from a single village where I had spent a lot of time, I was a
kind of parasite on MAYP (and later on LSAM, when I conducted ROR interviews a few months later), visiting the households of—poaching—a random
sample of their respondents. I found myself relying on the same means as
project fieldworkers had in the prior weeks to find the households: scouts,
maps, and word-of-mouth directions. Because MAYP's teams had already left
the district, however, I could no longer rely on project minibuses or SUVS
to carry me to the households: my research assistant and I spent long hours
walking or riding in bicycle taxis or rickety public minibuses in an effort to
find my assigned respondents. While the content of my questions and form
of the interview encounter differed from those my respondents had engaged

with MAYP fieldworkers, the performance was similar. While fieldworkers asked mostly close-ended questions and recorded answers in pencil on survey pages, I asked mostly open-ended questions and recorded the conversational interviews on a recording device. Yet my encounters with subjects relied on the same kind of stranger intimacy documented in this chapter.

Complicit in the sampling logics of MAYP and LSAM, I also ended up rewarding respondents in the same way that MAYP and LSAM did, at the request of the demographers who granted me access to members of their sample. I relied on the soap as a gesture of goodwill, an ethical act, and a corollary to the bureaucratized ethics symbolized by the consent forms I too administered. My ROR interviews with both MAYP and LSAM respondents differentiated me from the fieldworkers because I was not administering a survey and sought stories not numbers, but the mode of my engagement with respondents mirrored that of projects: I talked with people in a (mostly) one-off way, relied on soap as an imperfect but workable gift, and used the technology of random sampling to source respondents. Ironically, my interviews served—among other things—as a space for respondents to voice complaints about soap even as I would gift it to them following our conversations. In this way, even as this chapter stages an important critique of the extractive logics of survey research from the perspective of its target populations, the ethnographic data it enlists have complicated social lives that are not outside of, but constitutive of, survey research worlds and the anthropologist studying them. Whether data are qualitative or quantitative, their finished forms (statistics and ethnographic accounts, respectively) rarely reflect the messy transactions that both made them possible and, as we saw in this chapter, threatened to contaminate them.

Like chapters 1 and 2, this chapter has ethnographically probed top-down standards and imaginaries undergirding the collection of good data that take form in the office by highlighting the messy side effects they produce in the field. I do not aim to arbitrate what might be the best gift to give respondents in surveys (or even whether a gift should be given at all). Instead, I hope the competing claims I excavate in this chapter help nuance our understanding of human subjects research ethics that underlie health research and intervention in sub-Saharan Africa and beyond. Even if soap works as a good-enough gift as adjudicated by all parties to survey research, its transaction nonetheless opens a space in which the value of data for different parties can be contested and debated. Informed consent forms and soap (as research gift) are the alibi of clean data, but a narrow focus on the recipe for human subjects research ethics obscures the messy and competing meanings and valuations that actors in survey research worlds assign to soap and data themselves. Continuing this chapter's focus on research encounters between fieldworkers and survey participants, chapter 4 explores how standards governing the collection of clean, accurate, and reliable data—conjured in the office—are, first, imparted to fieldworkers during intensive trainings, and, second, embodied by fieldworkers as they collect data in the field.

FOUR

MATERIALIZING
CLEAN DATA IN THE FIELD

It is early morning in mid-February 2008, and the MAYP SUV forges its way awkwardly through grasses taller than its roof, becoming mired every few kilometers in mud. Each time its wheels spin in the muck, we exit the vehicle to help dislodge it. Before fieldwork begins for the day, we are thoroughly covered in mud. Anticipating a long day with many impediments to smooth data collection, the eight of us (a driver, a supervisor, five interviewers, and myself) packed a small cooler with bottles of water, yogurt, and Mahewu (a grainy maize drink that is a favored field lunch). We also carry a loaf of bread, knowing it will be difficult to find chips stands or tearooms in the remote enumeration area (EA) that is the site of today's fieldwork.[1] The EA is located in Thuma Forest Reserve, an area of rugged topography in central Malawi about twenty kilometers from the main road connecting the capital, Lilongwe, to the lakeside town of Salima. Each of the five interviewers will visit three households by the end of the day to collect survey data for MAYP. Spirits are a bit low on the heels of a frustrating few days of fieldwork dogged by flooded bridges, impassable roadways, long walks in water-saturated shoes,

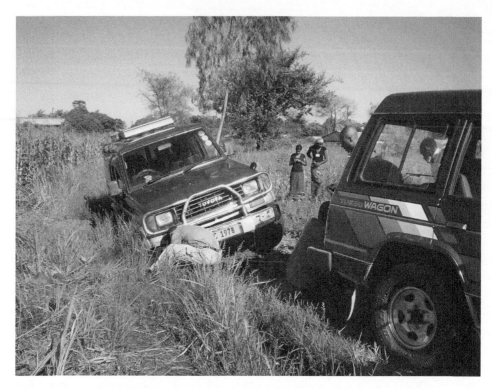

FIGURE 4.1. An SUV belonging to MAYP stuck in the mud, 2008. Photo by the author.

and the slow progress common to fieldwork during Malawi's rainy season. Pushing the SUV and slipping in the mud, fieldworkers recall other rainy season fieldwork mishaps, laughing about the time they hired canoes from local people and navigated through "crocodile-infested waters" to visit sample households unreachable by a washed-out road (see figure 4.1).

As we slowly make our way toward the EA, Chifundo, the team supervisor, opens a thick brown folder with the EA's number written on it in black marker and distributes to each interviewer a collection of items: three questionnaires, consent forms, crude maps of the area drawn by teams in previous years, headshot photos of assigned respondents (referred to as "snaps"), bars of soap for gifts, and yellow handheld GPS devices to be programmed with household coordinates. We scrutinize the maps to plan a time-efficient strategy of attack, and the SUV stops frequently to allow interviewers to disembark one by one, sometimes still a few kilometers' walk from their assigned households. Most interviewers carry umbrellas to cope with intermittent downpours. Chifundo points to a baobab tree that rises above grasses that stretch as far as the eye can see, indicating that the SUV will wait at this landmark to collect all the interviewers at the end of the day. One interviewer returns to the tree shortly after being dropped off, unable to locate his assigned household. Chifundo sets off in search of the local chief to inquire about its location, meeting two men in army fatigues who patrol the reserve for poachers.

As interviewers finish their assigned interviews, they return one by one, covered in mud, to the SUV to submit their completed questionnaires to Chifundo and myself for checking, play bao with the curious young children who congregate near the SUV, sleep, or listen to music. By the end of the day, thirteen of fifteen damp questionnaires are successfully filled in. The team groans in frustration: we will have to return to the bush again in the coming days to find and interview the two respondents who were not at home today (a man who was out buying maize and a woman who was at the district hospital delivering a baby), consuming time and fuel in the process. Chifundo takes this news ambivalently: "These are the challenges we face *kukapita field* [going off to the field]!"

. . .

This scene, re-created from my field notes, foregrounds the logistical challenges faced by fieldwork teams, especially on rainy days when data are being collected in remote areas like Thuma. The SUV caught in the mud is a fitting metaphor for the messy impediments projects like MAYP encounter everyday in their quest to collect clean data. While the ideal vision of researchers conjures efficient interviewers visiting all sample households and recording accurate data as neat pencil marks on questionnaires, fieldwork teams find themselves navigating many unexpected obstacles in the field. Distant from the eyes and ears of the demographers and economists who design the surveys and outfit teams with maps, clipboards, and other accoutrements meant to streamline data collection, fieldworkers embody—if imperfectly—the epistemological investments of their employers. Fieldwork places a set of demands on perception, subjectivity, and performances that help materialize data. Nonetheless, tensions between the abstract standards that govern data collection and the material circumstances of the field engender creative tactics on the part of fieldworkers who seek to manage, if not eradicate, uncertainty and errors in the data they collect.

As will become clear in this chapter, collecting clean, high-quality data entails learning to "see like a research project" (Biruk 2012). Not unlike James Scott's (1998) state, survey projects in Malawi utilize tools and technologies to better see their subjects: maps, questionnaires, photos, GPS devices, and sampling, for example. These tools collect and organize heterogeneous information that is converted into valuable numbers and are central props in structuring ways of seeing, gestures, and other forms of body work exhibited by fieldworkers (Boyer 2005, 259–260; Vertesi 2012). As a supervisor told a new crop of LSAM data collectors during a prefieldwork training session, "*You are the project.*"

In what follows, I trace how researchers' scientific investments in pure, clean data—symbolically represented in surveys that act as a recipe for data collection—are made and unmade by practices and processes on the ground. Through close analysis of the embodied techniques and technologies employed by fieldworkers during data collection, I illustrate how frictions between epistemological metrics for data and the particularities of everyday fieldwork produce—and come to validate—the numerical evidence we use to understand the AIDS epidemic in Malawi. I focus, in particular, on the cultural translation of survey concepts such as probability, the techniques and technologies used by fieldworkers to uncover the truth of rural Malawian social realities, and researchers' intensive efforts to harmonize encounters between fieldworkers and research participants. The chapter pays careful attention to how evidence is fashioned through technologies and relations that add value to numbers and codes recorded on a page, even as those processes also threaten to undo that value by cooking them, in the eyes of project designers.

In highlighting the production of data's value within the social relations and processes that make up the fieldwork phase of research, I bring to light the provisional and contextual nature of the value and uses of quantitative evidence that we usually encounter in a form detached from its contexts of production (Guyer et al. 2010; Lampland 2010; Ballestero 2012; Erikson 2012; Sangaramoorthy and Benton 2012; Day, Lury, and Wakeford 2014). Chapter 2 shows how fieldworkers perform and cultivate a marketable kind of local expertise aligned with researchers' expectations and described how data collection relies on the production of a spatiotemporal difference and distance between the field and the office. This chapter likewise centers fieldworkers' role in assembling data, but presents a fine-grained analysis of the nature of their interactions with data themselves; it considers how their bodies, affects, and practices in the field and the data they collect are coproduced. We will see that the embodiment of standards for clean data by fieldworkers is a central part of the coordination of data collection across thousands of research encounters.

As elaborated in chapter 1, the material form of the survey questionnaire, with its text waiting to be read aloud to respondents, boxes waiting to be checked, and empty space waiting to be filled in by data collectors, is a template for the collection of good data in the field. The questionnaire plays a key role in the inscription processes of survey fieldwork by acting as a script for interviewers who are meant to translate the heterogeneous realities they document into usable units of data as they record them on the page (Callon 1986; Latour 1987). By shared demographic standards, data are expected to be clean: accurate and reliable, efficient and timely, and collected from sufficiently large, pure, and representative samples. The visions of researchers produce and rely upon conventions and tools that are organized, but not governed or controlled, by any one actor, and both enable and limit the movements and perspectives of those who populate research infrastructure (Knorr-Cetina 1999, 11). A survey project's fieldworkers need not visit every household in a given village to administer surveys, but only those included in the project's predetermined sample, for example. Researchers' investment in the sample as reservoir of data trickles down to fieldworkers whose everyday movements and interactions become conduits through which abstract disciplinary values and designs are translated into the field. The questionnaires they administer are boundary objects, a means of translating between intersecting social worlds (the village, the research project, the office, and policy), and various social groups (villagers, interviewers, data entry clerks, researchers) (Star and Griesemer 1989).

From start (survey design) to finish (eventual publication of articles based on survey data), the assembly line envisioned by researchers confronts threats, many of which arise during data collection in the field: mistranslation, lying respondents, respondents who refuse to participate, respondents who have migrated or are out of town, interviewer effects, poor weather conditions, inaccurate data entry, and lost data. High-quality, clean data attain value from their relative scarcity: not all projects can equally invest the resources, time, and energy needed to effectively manage uncertainty, as defined by a set of demographic epistemological norms. Fieldwork is expensive: fieldworker salaries, per diems, lodging costs, fuel, and constant car repair are some of the expenses evident in the opening scene of this chapter.

Scholars, institutes, and policy makers seek out data whose brand they trust and are familiar with; numbers and statistics carry the aura of the research project that produced and packaged them. Andrews, a longtime fieldwork supervisor with LSAM, reflected on the difference in brand between data collected by the June 2008 Malawi National Census and the data being collected by LSAM at the same time: "Those guys [National Statistical Office, NSO] are just hiring whoever because they need so many people to enumerate.

This is bad—their data will have problems. You can just look back to 1998 [year of the last census] to see how many problems come up with the data, all from hiring people [fieldworkers] without experience!" Andrews's endorsement of the LSAM brand devalues NSO data as flawed or dirty. High-quality, clean data are a vestige of a distant local reality faithfully and authentically captured by experienced and trustworthy fieldworkers and arbitrated at all steps along the way by checks and audits (Lyberg and Biemer 2008, 421).

Taking demographers' epistemic investment in high-quality, clean data as an entry point, this chapter argues that seeing like a research project necessitates standardization of habits, scripts, practices, and social interactions across thousands of social encounters in the field. It also shows how the unfolding practices and instruments of fieldwork shape the very objects they are meant to count and track (Haraway 1989, 171–172; Mol 2002; Asdal 2008; Lorway and Khan 2014). As Kapil Raj (2007, 226) suggests, the stabilization and collection of immutable units of information by fieldworkers associated with the nineteenth-century Indo-British exploration of Central Asia was rooted in the mutable nature of men themselves, and the knowledge and skills they embodied. Jamie Lorimer (2008, 391), too, highlights how surveyors for the U.K. Corncrake Census learned to reorganize their bodies and senses to better see, hear, and count corncrakes, a species of migratory bird. Yet because the standardizing values of enumerative projects are materialized in fieldworkers' bodily techniques (Mauss 1973), they also enfold uncertainty, which manifests in numbers that are profoundly provisional, even as they are immensely valuable as expedient placeholders for realities (Lampland 2009; Verran 2013). Standards of data collection make stability and fixity in numerical representation possible, despite—or perhaps because of—their customization by fieldworkers in the field.

Clean Data, Messy Field

The completed questionnaire must be NEAT, CLEAR, READABLE, ACCURATE, UNBEND [sic], AND CREASE OR OIL FREE.... The questionnaires you are using are very sensitive to any manhandling. They should be kept unsoiled.
—2008 Population and Housing Census Enumerator's Manual (NSO, Zomba, Malawi)

The mandate for clean, unsoiled questionnaires is taken from manuals distributed to enumerators for the Malawi National Census in 2008; it invokes the tension between clean and dirty data that likewise preoccupied LSAM, GSIP, and MAYP in 2007–2008. The imperative delivered from NSO to a cohort of enumerators demonstrates an explicit aversion to bent, creased, oily, and messily written questionnaires in their material, paper form, but, more importantly, it draws a link between the questionnaires' physical forms and the quality of the data they will produce. During the 2008 census exercises, in fact, enumerators complained that they needed raincoats and other materials to protect census documents from winter rains and warned the NSO that if they were not properly equipped, data would be lost (Phiri 2008). Similarly, the district commissioner of Kota Kota (present-day Nkhotakota) in 1939 was concerned that census sheets distributed to village headmen to track basic demographics in their villages were—in the absence of a binder or container in which to collate them—so "dirty, dog eared and torn" as to be completely illegible (CAA 1939). Unsoiled questionnaires are the initial step in producing clean data, and maintaining the purity of the survey's white paper in the face of dust, rain, and greasy fingerprints is a fitting metaphor for the labor that goes into making clean data. In this section, I illustrate how clean data— usually considered to be an after-the-fact product of statistically based data cleaning or scrubbing procedures in the office—are an epistemic commitment that places demands on fieldworkers' perceptions, practices, and bodies in the field. Data and their collectors are made and remade by one another as data are assembled.

In order for them to achieve value for audiences who seek to use them, data must be accurate and reliable. Accuracy dictates that data must be as true a representation of reality, an individual, or a social phenomenon as possible. Reliability mandates that data and findings resulting from them must be replicable—obtainable in the same form again and again. Data cleaning is typically a method of dealing with data problems that occur: it can be glossed as the screening, diagnosis, and treatment of suspected errors in compiled data. Finding such errors requires familiarity with all phases of data flow, as errors can arise from bad initial planning, inadequate piloting (of surveys and people), and so on (van den Broeck et al. 2005). Common sources of error include missing data, input errors by data entry clerks, fabricated or invented data, coding errors, and interviewer or measurement error.[2] Though data cleansing or scrubbing techniques are usually applied to data that are already housed in databases, my informants emphasized the importance, as well, of keeping data clean during fieldwork.

Dirty data, from fieldworkers' perspectives on the ground, implied spelling mistakes or wrong numerical codes, forged or cooked data, incorrect data associated with a question, incomplete or sloppily entered data, missing data, or duplicate data. Field teams were well aware of their role in the larger process of making clean, valuable data. If an interviewer neglected to ask a question of a respondent, for example, the blank space on the survey page became a stumbling block later on for the data entry team member who must enter that blank space into the database as "missing data." (During a training session for LSAM, a supervisor, Esau, informed a new crop of interviewers, "The absolute worst crime you can commit is 'missing data.'") Collecting data that are accurate and reliable entails meticulous attention to both linguistic and cultural dimensions of translation and to harmonizing and surveilling the behaviors of interviewers and data entry teams in prefieldwork training sessions and the field.

THE PROMISE AND PERILS OF BEANS: VERNACULAR PROBABILITIES

In chapter 1, I discuss that a major objective of prefieldwork survey design sessions and meetings between foreign and Malawian researchers is to translate hundreds of survey questions from English into local languages—Chewa, Yao, and Tumbuka—and to anticipate how such questions might be confusing to either respondents or interviewers. In addition to linguistic translation, survey design and fine-tuning necessitated attention to what might be termed accurate cultural translation. The twenty-five-page survey used by LSAM consisted of nineteen sections ranging from "Group Membership and Social Capital" to "AIDS," to "Marriage," to "Economic Situation," and so on. One of these sections, titled "Expectations Questions," assessed respondents' subjective expectations of future outcomes such as HIV infection, economic shocks, or illness. Researchers suggest that understanding such expectations is crucial to designing and evaluating policies in health, education, and so on (Attanasio 2009; Delavande, Giné, and McKenzie 2011).

This section of the LSAM survey was identified as a problem by interviewers and supervisors, making it an ideal site for exploring the potential and pitfalls of translating potentially complex concepts (here, probability) into simplified forms for a target audience with low literacy. In an attempt to ensure clarity of meaning of probability for its low-literacy sample of rural Malawians, LSAM implemented an exercise using beans that came to be known as *nyembanyemba* (beans, reduplicated) among fieldwork teams and research participants. Respondents were asked to place a certain number of beans in a dish to estimate how likely it was that they would, for instance, experience a food shortage or contract HIV/AIDS (one bean if it was unlikely to happen, ten beans if it was certain to happen; see figure 4.2). As an interactive elicitation technique, researchers consider the beans to be visual, intuitive, and fairly engaging for respondents and, importantly, view it as a translative

X2 Pick the number of beans that reflects how likely you think it is that...	# of beans in plate
a) You will have to rely on family members for financial assistance in the next 12 months	[____]
b) You are infected with HIV/AIDS now	[____]
FOR MARRIED RESPONDENTS **(INTERVIEWER: if respondent is not married → X2f)**	
c) Your spouse is infected with HIV/AIDS now	[____]
FOR UNMARRIED RESPONDENTS	
d) Your romantic partner is infected with HIV/AIDS now (INTERVIEWER: if no romantic partner, write 99 and → X2h)	[____]
e) You will be married one year from now	[____]

FOR BOTH MARRIED AND UNMARRIED RESPONDENTS	
X3 Consider a healthy woman in your village who currently does not have HIV. Pick the number of beans that reflects how likely you think it is that she will become infected with HIV...	# of beans in plate
a) During a single intercourse without a condom with someone who has HIV/AIDS	[____]
b) Within the next 12 months (with normal sexual behavior)	[____]
c) Within the next 12 months if she is married to someone who is infected with HIV/AIDS	[____]
d) Within the next 12 months if she has several sexual partners in addition to her spouse	[____]
e) What about if this woman we just spoke about [in X3d] uses a condom with all extra-marital partners? How many beans would you leave on the plate?	[____]

FIGURE 4.2. The beans exercise from the LSAM questionnaire, 2008.

technology that promises to increase quality and value of data collected from an imagined villager (Delavande and Kohler 2007; Delavande, Giné, and McKenzie 2011).

Respondents' and fieldworkers' responses to the beans were largely negative. Research participants tended to view the beans as infantilizing (a common reaction was, "If you want to play, go over there with the children!"), and the beans were an important site of friction between actors across different levels of the project.[3] Fieldwork supervisors negotiated carefully between top-down efforts to standardize implementation of this activity, their own skepticism about the beans, and the incessant complaints from fieldworkers that the beans exercise was silly, time consuming, and boring for respondents. Supervisors chastised interviewers for being lazy and encouraged them: "Improve your attitudes—the bad morale among your villagers [research participants] is coming from you! These guys [respondents] observe us. They can tell you think nyembanyemba is *chabe* [worthless] and this allows them to protest [against it]." They also occasionally spied on interviewers as they interviewed respondents to ensure they were not cheating the project by failing to do nyembanyemba and just filling in numbers at random (the most flagrant form of cooking data) in the boxes provided in the beans section. However, at nightly meetings with American researchers, the supervisors suggested that the beans exercise was a "misfit with Malawian culture" and difficult for Malawians to understand. They also suggested that respondents grew bored with the instrument and observed that they "tended to pick the number you give as example" when demonstrating the exercise. For example, he explained, if you taught the respondent about the beans using five beans as a halfway point between a high chance of rain today and no chance of rain today, respondents tended to continue to pick five throughout the remainder of the exercise.

A culturally relevant tool from the perspective of the researchers was, in local estimation, a failure in the Malawian cultural context.[4] At a technical level, fieldworkers complained that respondents often suggested they couldn't know what would happen in the future or suggested that only God could know such things. We note that nyembanyemba, a script for the capture of individual datums that would later become evidence of the probabilistic orientations of rural Malawians, became a site of struggle where data were malleable entities, perhaps more representative of negotiated research encounters than the rural reality they sought to represent.

My field notes recorded at households where nyembanyemba was implemented highlight some of the issues that arose when this tool was translated into the field and make clear that numbers recorded in the boxes in the beans section of the survey are contingent and still unsettled renderings of the realities they seek to enumerate. In June 2008, Tapika, a twenty-four-year-old female LSAM interviewer, interviewed a thirty-five-year-old man, Josiah, in a village in central Malawi. After he showed us the tobacco balers he purchased to collect fees from his fellow villagers who used it, the pair (and I) sat behind his house on a mat he set out on the ground, and the survey interview proceeded smoothly until we reached the beans exercise (Section 15). Although Josiah was initially a bit baffled by the instructions ("I really should do this? [Move the beans around.] Can't I just answer the questions?"), he was a relatively willing participant.[5] Halfway through the long section, however, he grew tired of the beans and began to mention numbers without manipulating the beans and the dish in front of him. At this point, Tapika grew visibly frustrated and proceeded to pick up the number of beans Josiah said each time and place them in the dish, as if to indicate that Josiah must continue to use the beans. Josiah grew increasingly annoyed, and the defeated Tapika completed Section 15 without the beans.

In this encounter, Josiah made known his own reasonableness by making an effort to go along with the beans exercise he initially found unappealing. His later lack of interest, however, marked his effort to disengage from a social dynamic in which an interviewer asserted her status by requiring him to play with the beans. Tapika, as a younger woman interviewing an older man, negotiated the relationship carefully and likely felt compelled to perform the scripts and standardized implementation of the beans she had learned in training sessions, not least for the benefit of the anthropologist in her presence. Tapika's desire to be identified as a good fieldworker trying to convince a difficult research subject to participate correctly in this activity performs her absorption of the project's vision to collect accurate and precise data (Madiega et al. 2013, 23). Yet Tapika's effort to translate nyembanyemba in a standard and normed fashion intersected with the contours of her unfolding social encounter with Josiah. The promise of nyembanyemba to collect high-quality, more accurate information about rural Malawians' subjective expectations was in ongoing tension with the difficulties interviewers faced in implementing the exercise precisely, that is, in a standard and consistent manner across respondents. A culturally relevant tool, then, is encumbered by the coconstruction of culture itself. In touching, manipulating, and debating the beans—a material technology validated by demographers across many research contexts—a close reading of Tapika and Josiah's encounter exposes accurate data as inherently cooked: the numbers scrawled on the survey page and subsequently aggregated with those supplied by other respondents to other interviewers are not stand-ins for reality but rather provisional and improvised artifacts of a social negotiation.

Tapika and Josiah's interaction with the beans recalls the well-known metaphor of bean counting or the bean counter, a phrase that refers typically to a person who is excessively concerned with accounts or figures, often to the detriment of other aspects outside the figures and numbers. The act of counting beans, tiny tokens with minimal to no value, also carries the negative connotation of misplaced focus, a metonym perhaps for global health experts' uncritical investment in numbers as the sole or most important measure of efficacy and success (Adams 2016a; Erikson 2016). Tapika takes up LSAM's mandate to count the beans, but the frictions that arise between her and Josiah during the research encounter reveal the absurdity of the activity and foreground how bean counting, rather than accessing true probabilities held in Josiah's head as it seeks to, is reduced to child's play in his and other participants' eyes. Yet, Tapika—the reluctant bean counter in this scenario—makes every effort to ensure each bean is counted for the sake of the quality of LSAM's data.

Bean counting has not always carried its familiar negative connotation. Bean ballots were common to colonial New England elections, for example, when people voted with "Indian beanes" or black and white peas for their desired candidate (a practice likely imported from England), and bean counters were people of demonstrated integrity ("The General Laws and Liberties" 1672; Bishop 1893; Gross 1898; Leonard 1954). In ancient Greece, "pebbles" of "small, thumb and finger size" were the quintessential symbol of Athenian democracy. Beans were used whenever there was recourse to counted votes and in law courts when voting for the plaintiff or defendant (Netz 2002, 337; Everson 1996). In one Athenian practice, the beans themselves elected candidates via a randomization device called a *kleroterion* that had two columns with individual vertically stacked slots. Plaques with candidates' names were arranged and dropped into the slots on one side. Into the other column were dropped balls, some black and some white. As the counting machine dropped out a name and a ball in parallel, white would indicate the person had been chosen, and black would disqualify him from election. The "beans," then, acted independently of human agency to control the results of important elections, minimizing the possibility of human corruption tainting a democratic system (Netz 2002, 337). The nyembanyemba exercise, even as it aspires to collect the cleanest and most accurate data related to a respondent's felt probabilities (thus positioning the fieldworker as bean counter), is not unlike the kleroterion; in practice, the beans exercise often seemed to resemble a divination session, throwing the bones, or casting lots more than a scientifically validated tool for collecting better data.

PROBING FOR THE TRUTH

Another important dimension to collecting accurate data entails ferreting out lies or false information provided by respondents, and ensuring that no blank space is left on a survey page. The main technique employed to achieve these objectives is probing, or *maprobing* as interviewers and supervisors termed it. Probing, or fishing for more information than a respondent initially provides in response to a question, is a key skill for good interviewers to cultivate. During project training sessions, fieldworkers were taught how to avoid being cheated by respondents who might lie or feign nonknowledge for various reasons.[6] Richard, a supervisor, cautioned the interviewers on his team: "Watch out for contradictions, or things that seem illogical, like, 'I'm twenty-one and I have six children.'" Such warnings encouraged interviewers to be vigilant seekers of the truth.

In particular, LSAM emphasized the importance of probing to ensure accurate responses to sections of the survey focused on assessing the economic shocks (Section 5) experienced by a household in the past five years (death, illness, poor crop yields, loss of income, natural disaster), listing individuals a household might seek help from in the event of future shocks (Section 6, "Potential Transfers Roster"), and listing the actual individuals a household received assistance from in the past two years (Section 7, "Actual Transfers Roster"). Patrick, the American LSAM fieldwork manager, told interviewers, "We want to see economic shocks [recorded on your surveys in Section 5] because research shows they happen. Don't leave this section blank. Probe!" Later, in reference to Section 7, where respondents were asked to list the names of up to ten individuals who actually provided them with financial assistance in the past two years, Patrick again emphasized the importance of probing: "If they say they haven't gotten help from anyone in two years, you know they are lying. You are Malawian." Similarly, he discouraged interviewers from using Code 24 ("did nothing") in response to the question, "Munachita chiyani pofuna kuthana ndi vutoli?" (What did you do to overcome this shock [problem]?): "You *know* 'doing nothing' is not what happened!" A good interviewer, he suggested, should use this code very sparingly and only after serious probing failed to uncover the answer. "It's better to have something there than nothing," he said. In the advice presented here, we note that uncovering lies presumes a kind of local expertise and local origins ("You are Malawian"), consistent with the constructions of local knowledge elaborated in chapter 2. The supervisors, in this case, traffic in advice that furthers the epistemic investments of projects themselves: collecting accurate data by ensuring a completed survey contains no blank space or false information (see West [2016, 92], who documents the same among health surveillance assistants in rural Malawi).

Probing was also framed as an effective mnemonic device to improve recall of information, particularly that related to age of respondent or relatives. Mba (2014, 14) notes that age falsification by the respondent, ignorance of age, or cooking of age data by enumerators have long been major contributors to poor data quality on age across censuses and demographic surveys in sub-Saharan Africa.[7] Interviewers were taught how to deal with respondents who claim they are unable to recall their (or their child's) year or month of birth. To zero in on a date to fill into the survey, an interviewer could pose a variety of probing questions, such as whether they were born around independence (1964), whether their child was born during a harvest month, whether it was cold outside (June–August), and so on. However, even amid such probing efforts, evaluations of age-related data drawn from multiple African national censuses indicate that both male and female respondents preferentially report ages ending in zero or five, throwing into question the truth captured by such techniques (Mba 2014, 23).

In training sessions, probing was cast as a key technology for collecting true information. Before commencing real interviews, trainees were expected to try their hand at survey administration during pilot surveys, which had the dual purpose of piloting the surveys to catch mistakes in the content or linguistic translation, and of piloting the interviewers themselves to determine whether they were able to individually reproduce the collective standards for data held by the project. This liminal period between the completion of training sessions and the commencement of full field research was a time of significant anxiety—a rite of passage—for potential fieldworkers, who understood themselves to be under close scrutiny by supervisors and project leaders. Fieldworkers aimed to masterfully perform the skills and techniques they were taught a few days before, and to return with a neat, complete survey in a reasonable time frame. During the liminal period before potential fieldworkers transitioned into full-fledged employees, they sought to showcase their competence in the interest of earning a job for the next few weeks or months.

On one occasion, an LSAM fieldworker sought to pilot the survey at a household where the respondent refused to answer two sections of questions, and was forced to return to the minibus with an incomplete survey. He insisted to the supervisor that he probed tenaciously but was thwarted by the respondent's staunch refusal to answer his questions. So worried was he about losing his job that he pleaded with his supervisor to accompany him back to the household so he could prove that the blank space on the survey was the fault of the respondent, and not a symptom of his poor interviewing skills. Interviewers' economic interest in earning a daily wage for the duration of a fieldwork season motivated them to internalize and attempt to embody the expectations and standards for data collection to the best of their ability.

Importantly, the rhetoric of probing and lying respondents positions the research project as endowed with the ability to see or make visible the truth, betraying a primary investment in collecting data that are representative of an imagined authentic rural social reality, a reality that is always already prefigured by the questions that capture it. Research encounters were also imagined as mimicking or reproducing a real-life conversation; supervisors often emphasized to their interviewers that probing is a way to show a respondent "you are really listening, and not just recording information down on a paper." But seeing like a research project circumscribed the nature of this chat. Interviewers soon discovered that some responses provided by respondents did not easily fit into the options, codes, or boxes provided by the tangible survey in front of them. After piloting, interviewers for MAYP pointed out that some of the survey questions did not allow for commonly given responses. For example, one question asked which district in Malawi the respondent and family had originated from. Since a common response was "Zambia"—a neighboring country—fieldworkers complained about the built-in limitations of the survey (MAYP later added a note: "Record country if not born in Malawi").

On a household roster for MAYP, interviewers were asked to insert the appropriate code next to each listed name to indicate relationship to the respondent. Interviewers argued that the code "1: Husband/wife" did not sufficiently capture the relational category "cowife." Though they coded this response as either "1" or "12" ("other relative"), they suggested that it surfaced so frequently as a response that it deserved its own code.[8] Similarly, LSAM interviewers suggested to their supervisors that a code be added for the third of a four-part question about the number of sexual partners the respondent's best female married friend had in the past year (see figure 4.3). When asked a question about how they knew how many sexual partners their friend had, many respondents responded idiomatically, something like, "She was caught red-handed." When fieldworkers suggested this be added as a code for the question, LSAM researchers generally agreed that the questions should be

S19c Mukudziwa bwanji kuti anagonanapo ndi amuna amenewa? *How do you know she had sex with these partners?*	She told me..1 Saw her coming & going....................2 Rumours/other people told me..............3

FIGURE 4.3. Question S19c from the LSAM questionnaire, 2008.

amended to improve accuracy. However, as Patrick, the American demographer managing fieldwork at the time, explained to the supervisors who brought him these suggestions, "We can't add a code without messing up things in terms of the past, data we have already collected. We must keep the phrasing and translation of the questions consistent, even if they aren't the most accurate. It's too late. . . . In order to measure change, we have to ask things in the same exact way. We have to have the same codes every wave even if they're not correct. So, just fit those responses [i.e., those mentioned above] into the existing categories."

Seeing like a research project, in this regard, necessarily implies a certain conservatism of vision. Patrick's suggestion that altering codes or phraseology of questions in the present would "mess up things in . . . the past" indexes a tension between accuracy (collecting the most true answers) and reliability (collecting such answers in the same way year after year). In his words, we note that, rather than collecting the most complete picture of rural social realities, research projects collect data that are always already, and self-consciously so, incomplete and incorporative of errors. Interviewers' embodied decisions and negotiations in the field reconcile the gap between sometimes dueling epistemic investments (accuracy and reliability) and place the onus of clean data on interviewers. The probing skills so valued by researchers are key to collecting the truest data, but, in Malinowski's ([1922] 1984, 192) classic words, these data may not be "full-flavoured" but "squeezed out of reluctant informants as a trickle of talk." In reflecting on the effects of probing on data collected by fieldworkers on projects in five sub-Saharan African countries, Randall et al. (2013, 780) echo Malinowski: the interviewer "extract[s] data from the respondent" and may "make respondents say things they had not thought about or possibly do not want to say." As is evident in the case of LSAM's questions about household shocks and probabilities, respondents fulfill their role in research by simply providing a plausible answer, as arbitrated by the fieldworker they encounter.

	SUPERVISOR	LOGGED BY	CHECKED BY	ENTERED BY
INITIALS	_____	_____	_____	_____
DATE	_____	_____	_____	_____

FIGURE 4.4. The life course of data (taken from LSAM questionnaire first page, 2008).

PERSONALIZING DATA: CALLBACKS AND CHECKING

The plausibility of respondents' answers, however, is meticulously measured and technically mediated at many points along data's life course. Figure 4.4, taken from the front page of the LSAM survey, shows the path that data take as they are manufactured, and whose hands they pass through as they are converted from raw information (survey responses) to valuable data (statistics derived from a database of good numbers). When an interviewer returns to the field supervisor with a completed survey, the supervisor checks the questionnaire to ensure there are no immediately obvious inconsistencies between responses and no missing information or blank spaces. If the supervisor discovers missing information, the interviewer is sent back to the household to collect it. Once the survey questionnaire is deemed complete, the supervisor initials and dates it. It is carried back to the field office in the minibus and deposited in a "to be logged" box, where it waits to be logged by a data entry team member. Next, it is checked again by a data clerk; if inconsistencies are discovered, it is sent back to the field the next day to be corrected by the initial interviewer via a callback. Finally, when a survey is deemed complete, consistent, and credible, it is entered into the database by a data clerk. At this point, the survey has passed through many hands, indicated by the differently colored pen marks and initials on the front page. After being logged and entered, surveys are scanned and archived in boxes labeled with village numbers.

The product of all this labor—clean data—is valuable precisely because it passes through so many hands. The initials scrawled on the front page not only signal the phases through which data pass but also point to the logic and mechanisms of seeing like a research project. No one person arbitrates the quality of data; instead, a number of individuals whose habits and ways of seeing have been harmonized (to various degrees) all claim ownership over data at one point in time. In the snapshot of data's life course in figure 4.4, we see how the different cogs that constitute the machinery of the research project are supposed to work together. Even if data in their final form—statistics or numbers derived from a database—may appear to be abstract and unanchored from their origins at a rural household, data are personalized at every stage, even in their raw forms. Notably, however, the persons who handle data along their life course are typically "the most poorly paid and least well qualified link[s]" in the data production process even as they, in reality, might have the most influence on the value of data collected (Randall et al. 2013, 784).

This personalization works as a push and pull mechanism to ensure standardization and collection of high-quality data through self-surveilling checks and balances. In the process of fieldwork, the callback acts to clean data as they pass between an interviewer and supervisor. Supervisors who discovered inconsistencies in the pages of a recently collected survey would summon the interviewer to question the inconsistency. If there was no viable explanation, the interviewer was sent back out to the field to revisit the same respondent to find out the truth. Callbacks were loathed by interviewers, who put in extra effort during a first research encounter with a respondent to avoid having to revisit a household. Having too many callbacks marked an interviewer as incompetent or lazy and put one's job in jeopardy.[9]

Esau, an LSAM supervisor, discovered an inconsistency in the way an interviewer called Edward on his team had recorded information about the number of children his respondent had in his first and second marriages. Esau suggested Edward find the respondent and ask the question again to be certain he got the numbers correct. Edward protested and, since it was dusk, it was decided he would go collect the information the next morning. A few hours after fieldwork began the next morning, Edward returned with his survey; he had neatly crossed out the number given for children in a second marriage and replaced it with the correct response. However, upon receiving the callback survey, Esau accused Edward of cooking the number, implying he had made it up. On our way out of the village at dusk that day, Esau ordered the minivan to stop near the trading center where the respondent in question was based. He inquired directly with the respondent whether Edward had revisited him that morning, and the respondent indicated he had not. Edward sat in the back of the van, shamefaced and quiet as Esau chastised him in front of his team members. As we disembarked at the field office half an hour later, he exclaimed, out of earshot of Esau, "*Eeee . . .* they [supervisors] don't know how difficult it is to make someone sit for hours asking them questions, and then to go back again yelling 'Hodi!' [standard Chichewa greeting used to request entrance or announce arrival at someone's compound or home] a second time. . . . You become a laughingstock."

The negotiated friction between Edward and Esau indicates that data's travels are circuitous and do not follow a straight path. Lying—most obviously framed as a common practice among rural respondents—manifests also as a deviation from standardized habits and practices entrained into fieldworkers as Maussian techniques of the body (Mauss 1973). Even as lying appears in the final data as gaps, error, or messiness, it operates tactically in the field as it does in everyday social life (Salamone 1977; Bleek 1987).[10] Peterson (2002, 388), for example, in an examination of colonial census data collected in French postwar southern Mali, suggests that respondents were motivated to declare the religion they thought was the safest vis-à-vis outsiders and the state, which led to a false significant increase in Muslims counted. Recall, as well, how in chapter 3 we saw how people impersonate individuals in the sample to receive the soap gift projects distributed to their respondents.

LEARNING TO WRITE (AGAIN): HARMONIZING INTERVIEWERS AND MUTING INTERVIEWER EFFECTS

Working in the field is determined by the field itself. . . . You can't plan from the office the things that will come up out there. —Chifuniro, LSAM supervisor

Chifuniro's advice to a new crop of interviewers points again to the discursive spatiotemporal boundary drawn between the clean and orderly office and the messy and unpredictable field. While one can plan for and attempt to predict the impediments and challenges to be faced during data collection, it is nonetheless an endeavor determined by the field itself. In this way, prefieldwork training sessions for interviewers seek to, as far as possible, mitigate what demographers term interviewer effects, or measurement error due to interviewers' characteristics or practices in the field. Training sessions are crucial moments of standard setting, where the project seeks to establish uniformity in fieldworkers' comportments and practices by introducing a set of agreed-upon rules for data collection (Bowker and Star 1999; Timmermans and Epstein 2010).

Of course, it is difficult to control for effects that an interviewer's age, gender, or ethnicity might have on a respondent's answers in a given encounter.[11] Nonetheless, projects employed tools to attempt to document and measure such effects. The last page of LSAM's survey was an interviewer's questionnaire, which directed the interviewer to answer eight questions "soon after the interview." These questions were meant to capture (1) potential role-independent interviewer effects (e.g., social identity) on the course of the research encounter or the data it produces; and (2) potential measurement error due to lying respondents. First, interviewers were asked to rank the respondent's physical attractiveness relative to other persons of about the same age and sex on a scale of 1 (much more attractive than average) to 5 (much less attractive than average). These questions were attempts to access the effects of social characteristics on respondents' answers. These data were then collated with data collected from project supervisors, who were asked during fieldwork trainings to rate the attractiveness of all the interviewers on the same 1–5 scale.

The interviewer's questionnaire also served as a system of checks and balances on prior responses to the same questions asked during the course of the survey. For example, interviewers answered the question: "Does the respondent's house have a pit latrine?" (yes, 1; no, 0). In bold capital letters, a note to the interviewers compelled them to check for themselves to determine the answer (in trainings, interviewers were encouraged to request to use the toilet at some point during the interview to subtly ascertain whether or not a latrine was present).[12] This (like trap or red herring questions embedded in questionnaires, as well) was meant to check whether the respondent had answered the same question posed back on page 2 accurately, or had lied, which might call the truth of other responses into question also, a built-in means of determining potential measurement error at the level of a respondent (Kasprzyk 2005, 172–173). The interviewer questionnaire collected a set of mimetic metadata that implicitly indexed patterns of response variation and added value to the data collected (Vemuri 1994). The auxiliary data collected in a survey that help describe the data collection process are commonly referred to as "paradata" in demographic parlance, and reveal researchers' massive investment in monitoring data quality.

In training sessions, research projects focus on minimizing measurement error due to role-restricted interviewer effects or differential response patterns that might result from interviewers' different interviewing styles, their differential adherence to guidelines or survey scripts, and so on (Sudman and Bradburn 1974; Stecklov and Weinreb 2010). Relational politics between interviewer and interviewee, too, can affect data collected: Loveman (2007, 91–96) analyzes data from the 1910 and 1920 rounds of the Puerto Rican census to show how interviewers brought assumptions to bear in their classificatory decisions around the race of their respondents, with a "whitening" effect on the census data. Interviewers' primary labor during fieldwork is recording responses with pencil on the pages of questionnaire after questionnaire, long the dominant mode of data collection in developing countries and known as paper-and-pencil personal interview. In recent years, survey projects have begun implementing tablet- or smartphone-assisted personal interviewing, but at the time of this research, interviewers used paper questionnaires. Before pencil goes to paper, however, interviewers relearn how to write. In addition to writing neatly, interviewers must ensure they leave no blank spaces, follow the script and instructions of the survey meticulously, and accurately translate raw information into the appropriate codes.

The training sessions discussed in chapter 2 were the primary site in which projects sought to harmonize the behaviors and writing practices of project interviewers. Clean surveys necessitate that all interviewers record information (or lack of it) in the same fashion. Learning to write (again) was a long process that entailed going through the survey questions one by one and painstakingly providing specific instructions on how to properly record information. On the first page of the survey, where interviewers were meant to record accurate information about the respondent, including age, birthplace, father's name, and so on, no codes were provided; rather, the interviewer had to neatly write out given answers. As we moved through the survey pages in a training session, we often paused to reach consensus about how to record information consistently: "We should now agree that instead of leaving a blank space on the first page, we must write in a dash instead," with the trainer drawing a dash on the flip chart at the front of the room.[13] The directive was followed by a question that functioned to index consensus and progress throughout the training sessions: "Eti? Onse pamodzi?" (Is it so? Are we all together here?) The fieldworkers' ritualized response ("Eeee! [Yes!]") cements the solidarity and collectivist orientation—centered on the research project's-eye view that is the imperative of these trainings (Vertesi 2012, 405).

Training sessions also familiarized interviewers with skip patterns in the survey. Skip patterns—highlighted by instructions for the interviewer embedded in the survey itself—chart a course for interviewers as they proceed from question to question and page to page of the survey in the field. Two skip patterns, indicated by >> (see figure 4.5), direct the interviewer to proceed, in the first case from question 10 to question 12 and, in the second case, from question 11 to question 13. In addition to observing the skip, interviewers were expected to treat the blank space produced by a skip in consistent and harmonized manner. While some projects encouraged interviewers to mark a skipped question with a dash, others taught interviewers to leave a blank space.

For the numerous interviewers and supervisors who worked on many different research projects, these idiosyncratic preferences were difficult to master, and their relevance to the quality of data collected often opaque. Supervisors often absolved themselves of responsibility for these guiding rules, using the term "azungu" (Chichewa term for foreigner) to emphasize the fact that such directives came from above and were out of their hands: "The

10.	11.	12.	13.
Do you have electricity working in your dwelling?	Is your electricity from ESCOM, a generator, solar panels, or some other source?	Although you do not have electricity here, is there electricity within 100 meters of this dwelling, whether from ESCOM, a generator, a solar panel, or some other source?	Is there a <u>landline telephone</u> in working condition in the dwelling?
1= Yes 2= No (>>12)	1= ESCOM 2= Generator 3= Solar panel 4= Other, specify (>>13)	1= Yes 2= No	1= Yes 2= No

FIGURE 4.5. A skip pattern embedded in the LSAM questionnaire.

azungu do not want you to write any leading zeros, so do not do it" or "The azungu want us to use the code 'Other' as sparingly as possible, so avoid it." Despite the emphasis on observing skips and the ample attention paid to writing practices in the trainings, they became a source of much frustration for interviewers during survey administration in the field. During fieldwork pilots, many interviewers felt discouraged by all the red ink on the pages of their completed surveys, indicating their supervisors' many corrections. The red marks identified errors of content (e.g., inconsistencies between responses or responses that were not likely true) or errors of form (e.g., where interviewers had failed to observe skip patterns, used the wrong marks to signal a missing response, neglected to ask a question, or written sloppily).

Often, techniques to ensure accuracy and techniques to ensure harmonization and efficiency came into friction. As discussed at length above, probing is a valuable skill for interviewers to cultivate and helps ensure that interviews flow more naturally and take the shape of real conversation rather than sterile survey encounter. During training sessions, interviewers were encouraged to think of the questionnaire as a form of chatting (*kucheza*); however, this often threatened the quality of data collected by increasing the influence of interviewer effects on data. In early June 2008, Ishmael, an LSAM interviewer, explained that he most enjoyed administering the vignettes section of the questionnaire. "I have fun with them because I like to tell the story in my own way," he suggested. The vignettes, inserted into the survey by a sociology graduate student, were meant to measure a respondent's perception of agency as played out in fictional stories constructed to have local relevance and solicit data of value to researchers (see figure 4.6).

V5	Rose is married to a man who moved around with [had sexual relations with] a girlfriend for many years while they were married. When she found out, she told him to stop seeing the girlfriend or she would divorce him. He stopped. How easy is it for Rose to protect herself from getting infected with HIV/AIDS?	Very easy Easy Difficult Very difficult Don't know	1 2 3 4 88
V6	Beatrice caught her husband "red-handed" having sex with another woman. She took her case to the ankhoswe [traditional marriage counselors/advisers] and said she wanted a divorce because she was afraid of getting HIV/AIDS and she was no longer able to trust her husband. The chief granted her the divorce and she didn't have to pay any money. Beatrice went through with the divorce despite her husband's protests, and she returned to her parent's home. How easy was it for Beatrice to protect herself from getting infected with kachilombo [HIV]?	Very easy Easy Difficult Very difficult Don't know	1 2 3 4 88

FIGURE 4.6. Two vignettes from LSAM questionnaire.

Though Ishmael was widely known to be a well-performing interviewer, his supervisor reminded him that it was essential he read the vignettes exactly as they appear on the survey page, to ensure that all respondents hear the vignettes in the same way (and thus to mitigate measurement error resulting from role-restricted interviewer effects). This advice betrays the project's interest in collecting timely data; interviewers were left to negotiate a small space between administering a questionnaire like a chat and collecting complete data as quickly as possible.

On one visit, I accompanied Janet, a twenty-six-year-old female interviewer, to her meeting with a thirty-nine-year-old woman called Namoyo. When we arrived, Namoyo and her mother were shelling maize on the *khonde* (verandah). Before getting down to business, the four of us sat quietly together, each working at the maize. Maintaining our place on the khonde and continuing to shell maize, we began the questionnaire. Now and then, children, goats, and chickens darted across a walking path nearby, disrupting the flow of the survey. Janet introduced the survey as an informal chat: "Naphiri [my Chewa name] and I are just here to have a chat with you!" In both English and Chichewa, kucheza (to chat) implies conversing in an informal, nonlinear, undirected, and non–temporally bounded manner—free-forming a conversation. But as soon as Janet brought out the questionnaire and her pen, it became evident that this particular chat would closely follow the order of the questions written on the survey pages.

The first portion of the chat involved Janet verbally eliciting and carefully filling in the household roster (for a sample roster, see appendix). This roster was a table with fifteen columns and ten rows. After asking Namoyo to list each member of her household, Janet wrote the names one by one into the blank rows. Once all the names were recorded on the sheet, she asked a series of questions about each household member: "How old is X? What is X's relationship to you? Is X's mother alive? In what year did X move here? What is the highest level of schooling X went to? Is X married? Is X ill?" Many of the answers provided by Namoyo had to be coded by Janet with a relevant number. In cases where she did not recall the codes, Janet paused the chat while she leafed through an accessory packet of questionnaire codes in order to find the proper one. A month earlier, Janet had attended a training in which project interviewers had been taught to maintain good penmanship and be careful and consistent in filling out project surveys. As Namoyo delivered her responses to the survey questions, Janet took care to record the responses neatly; she even used a ruler as a straight line beneath the letters she wrote. The chat was marked by long periods of silence as Janet monitored her own penmanship to ensure she was seen as a good interviewer, not only by me but by the researchers and data entry clerks who would see the marked-up questionnaire later in its life course.

Despite the recipe provided by the survey from beginning to end, survey chats were certainly not linear. The encounter between Namoyo and Janet confounds survey researchers' claim that modules or sections of the survey should match the order in which the interview is to be conducted so as to mirror natural ordering (Glewwe 2005a, 41; Dillman 2008). Namoyo could not recall the names of her parents-in-law when initially asked by Janet; later in the survey, however, she suddenly remembered them, interrupting the flow of the interview session and prompting Janet to flip back a few pages to enter the information. Like the rhythmic shelling of maize, the survey's chronology served as a mere backdrop against which our interaction meandered. The interview encounter was a negotiated space of flows and stoppages of data symptomatic of the interests of the interviewer and interviewee, respectively. As was the case in most of the interviews I observed, the interview between Janet and Namoyo was marked by interlocutors' mutual testing of the waters.

Early on, Namoyo commonly responded to questions with "I don't know," or by providing other noncommittal answers. When Janet asked her about the amount of money she loaned to others in the past year, she claimed "none." Janet looked at her dubiously, laughed, and probed, "Not even five kwacha [about 4 cents USD at the time]?" Namoyo laughed, and then agreed that she had indeed loaned friends, neighbors, and family members money in the past year. Later, Janet had to return to this box on the survey again when it turned out that Namoyo could remember the amounts she donated to individuals she listed by name. Similarly, she claimed she could not remember the ages of her own children. When Janet pressed her, she could.

Finally, over the course of a series of questions that covered wealth indices, Namoyo grew frustrated and visibly annoyed at having to provide verbal responses to questions that she felt were self-evident to Janet. As a good interviewer who had been taught never to miss a question, Janet enunciated each question: Does your household own a TV? Solar panels? Does your household have a metal roof? Namoyo laughed in the face of such questions: Janet could easily see that she possessed none of these items—she was poor! Yet when Namoyo laughed, Janet still pressed her to verbalize her actual response: "No."[14] Often, respondents' ambivalence about participating in a survey aligned with the interviewers' own ambivalence about the agenda of the project that employed them (May 2008). Janet's affective orientation to Namoyo's sighs of frustration showed that these questions were not her own; she made it clear that she was merely a mouthpiece for LSAM. Namoyo, picking up on Janet's apparent disinterest, made repeated stabs at taking control of the interview encounter by being selective about which questions she answered, by providing inconclusive or vague responses, or by feigning nonknowledge before finding an answer. These efforts tested the contours of the interview as a social space: How invested was Janet in securing answers to each of the questions? How much could Namoyo reveal? Was Janet able to detect when Namoyo provided bad information?

In the space of the formal survey, Namoyo relished the chance to talk to Janet and me; as outsiders, we were a valuable and novel source of information. Namoyo asked us how things were in other districts to which we had traveled with LSAM, whether we had any children, and so on. Again, the linear form of the survey meandered when it was inserted into the social relations and space of the interview encounter. The standards and guidelines for collection of good numbers that interviewers learned in training sessions translated into the field in unpredictable ways through the instrument of the fieldworker (Mauss 1973). The imperative to write neatly appeared in the field as awkward silences, with goats bleating in the background and informal conversation filling the gaps. The mandate to ask every question became the site of a negotiation, with both interviewer and interviewee trying to gain a foothold to express and secure her interests. The command to leave no blanks on the survey prompted push-and-pull exchanges between Janet and Namoyo, with the former probing for pieces of information and the latter recalcitrant about providing it. The chronological time presumed by the numbered pages of a survey and the project's emphasis on efficiency and timeliness were enacted by Janet's careful administration of the survey but came into friction with both her desire to be a good interviewer (which often involved slowing down to record data well) and her circuitous and slow time encounter with Namoyo.

OPTIC TECHNOLOGIES: POLICING AND PATROLLING THE SAMPLE

Producing high-quality data presupposes meticulous sampling strategies. It is impossible for projects to interview all Malawians, but in order to attain high-quality numbers, a sample must include a large enough number of households to support the eventual claims made from the data. Beyond ensuring that the absolute number of sampled households is sufficient to ensure that data will be of high quality according to epistemic investments in statistical power, projects must also protect sample purity; the sample must capture not only ten individuals living in sample households, but the correct ten individuals.[15] In demographic terms, this entails interviewing the same individual year after year. Panel survey projects must minimize threats to sample representativeness that may arise from how a sample is chosen and followed over time, participation rates in a survey, and the procedures of data collection.

Like researchers, fieldworkers were well aware of the importance of both sample size and sample purity, which manifested in their everyday embodied practices as concerted efforts to locate and successfully interview all individuals in the sample. Over time, they came to see the sample as a cohesive whole, even as they interacted with its individual members on a daily basis. For example, in discussing the importance of properly introducing research project objectives to local traditional authorities such as chiefs, supervisors told their fieldworkers, "We must respect the sample at all times." Seeing like a state (or a research project) entails deploying a set of techniques and tools designed to guide people's conduct as individual units of a population (sample). Much like Foucault's ([1978] 2007, 137) metaphorical shepherd cares for his flock, research teams, too, care for the research sample from birth to death over longitudinal time. The sample is an organizational and, as will become clear, a political unit. Whereas a top-down view of the sample might suggest that its individual members are interchangeable, a bottom-up view indicates quite the opposite: producing high-quality data relies on the systematic collection of freely given information from thousands of individuals, each enmeshed in complicated social networks, each with a unique geographic location, and each with his or her own agenda.

Recalling James Scott's (1998) elaboration of the efforts of eighteenth- and nineteenth-century German scientific forestry to manage and order the ecological messiness of forests, we note the important role that tools and technologies such as maps, devices to measure tree size, and surveys played in allowing the state to narrow its focus or vision to see only what it wanted to see: the revenue from timber extracted annually. Survey research in the age of global health employs techniques not unlike those taken up by the state in census or other national projects. Technologies of enumeration make visible slices of reality that are of interest or valuable to a particular situated gaze.

Survey researchers are well aware of the detrimental effects of attrition—failure to find or reinterview individuals who were surveyed in earlier waves or visits to the field—on the quality of their data. Attrition leads to a decreased sample size that reduces power in statistical analyses and is a major factor in poor data quality in sub-Saharan Africa (Alderman et al. 2001; Bignami-Van Assche et al. 2003). Mobility of respondents, failure to find respondents, and respondent refusals are major threats to data quality. Epistemic investments in sample purity and sample size translate on the ground into various techniques and tools that help a project efficiently and effectively see a sample. Emulating the unfolding relations of the field, I provide two ethnographic vignettes to bring to life how the sample is bounded and how data's purity is maintained by the improvised and unscripted practices of fieldworkers.

Even as research teams come to see the sample as a single entity, it is a living, breathing organism whose shape-shifting nature perpetually threatens to exceed or escape the gaze of the research project. To combat sample attrition, field teams are outfitted with an arsenal of instruments meant to allow them to see and keep the sample pure on a daily basis. The movements, meanderings, and interests of respondents, however, challenge these optic tools.

Nonetheless, these instruments allow the project to patrol the borders of the sample sufficiently to produce numbers that are good enough, if not perfect.

> The large table in the common room of the MAYP field office is littered with hundreds of envelopes. These are the tool kits of the fieldworkers who will collect data tomorrow from villages within fifty kilometers of the office. Each contains a set of tools necessary to locate and interview a single respondent; indeed, the contents of each packet stand in for and create a sort of enumerable person. Within each folder is a color photograph of an adolescent male or female. I remove one and see a boy, age seventeen, in a blue T-shirt standing against a backdrop of bricks likely to be his home. He squints into the sun and holds a white paper across his chest that reads 102_Madumbo_34. This placard indicates for the interviewer assigned this boy the enumeration area, traditional authority, and household number (e.g., EA_TA_HH). A small white sticker below the photo lists the name, sex, schooling status (in or out of school), and nickname of this respondent. Aside from the survey itself, the envelope also contains a map, hand drawn by the fieldworker who visited the same respondent last year. The maps include landmarks ranging from trees to shops to football pitches [soccer fields] and churches, represented in the unique hand of interviewers. These maps—which capture reality from the perspective of an observer on the ground—contrast with the large official maps kept in the field office and are complemented by the GPS coordinates of the household, included on the same page as the map. The teams were provided with bright-yellow, heavy-duty GPS devices, though they were rarely used in practice.[16]

This excerpt from my field notes highlights the arsenal of optic tools utilized by projects to bound and see realities of interest: photographs, enumerative labels, GPS devices, and hand-drawn maps. In fact, each envelope stands in as a proxy for a real person, valuable to the project as a coherent unit of data. Here, we see how much the project already knows about its subjects, and come to understand the labor and technologies invested in finding and successfully surveying each of these individuals.

The technologies for locating respondents are numerous, but nonetheless respondents employed tactics, either deliberately or by virtue of being absent, to escape or evade the project. A respondent could be out: working in the *dimba* [wetland garden] or trading center, on a trip to South Africa, in the city, at the hospital, completely relocated to another residence outside the

Respid: _____   **Name:** _____

Nickname:

Gender: male

Age: 39

Marital status:

Head Compound:

Childname:

Anthro registration? (Y or N) | y |

Outcome of Visit 1: | 1 | *CB*   **Outcome of Visit 2:** | | **Outcome of Visit 3:** | |

Date of Visit 1: 30/07/08   **Date of Visit 2:** _____   **Date of Visit 3:** _____

1=Completed, 2=Refused, 3=Hospitalization, 4=Dead, 5=Not Known, 6=Temporarily Absent, 7=Moved, 8=Other

Comments from visit: *interviewed* _____

Number of spouses: 1

Spouse ids:	Spouse Name:	Still Married?
20 ▪▪	▬▬▬▬▬▬	☑
		☐
		☐
		☐
		☐

FIGURE 4.7. Log form for recording interview outcome, LSAM.

spatial bounds of the sample, or, in some cases, passed away since the previous interview. When an interviewer arrives at a household and hears "Alibe! [He/she is not here]," the interviewer proceeds to record the reason on a log form with eight possibilities, depicted in figure 4.7.

Each outcome entails a series of next steps that illustrate how finding respondents—even those who have disappeared—is a cat-and-mouse game. For example, if it was determined that a respondent was deceased, the interviewer proceeded to administer a mortality questionnaire, also called a "verbal autopsy" by the research project teams.[17] The verbal autopsy entailed interviewing a family member or other person close to the deceased to, as closely as possible, ascertain and document the cause of death of the respondent. Even in death, then, respondents did not escape the gaze of the project; their movement out of the sample needed to be documented to preserve the integrity of the sample. Each respondent designates, from the view of demographers, interchangeable lives and deaths that somehow belong to the research project (Stevenson 2014, 27). Death may be beyond the reach of biopolitical power, but it is not outside the view of statistics: "Power has no control over death, but it can control mortality" (Foucault 2003, 248).

In many cases, a respondent was temporarily away, and an appointment could be set for the following day for a return visit by the interviewer. If

> **Characteristics of the Core Respondent**
>
> a. Has the core respondent moved permanently or temporarily? [___] 1= Permanently
> 2= Temporarily
> b. Where does [...] currently live?
> c. District (or country): _____ TA: _____
> d. Village/town: _____
> e. Area type [___]
> 1= Major urban   2= Boma   3= Rural
> f. Head of compound: _____
> g. Name of household head: _____
> h. What is the nearest market or trading center? _____
> i. Is there a landmark close by to where [...] stays? (such as a school, junction, etc.)
> _____
> j. Approximately how far is this location from here? (indicate the main means of transport
> as well as the approximate time, and/or distance)_____
> k. What is {...}'s marital status? [___]
> 1= Single →Q3e   2= Married
> l. Name of spouse:_____
> m. Why did [...] move?
> 1= To work or look for work   5= Following new spouse
> 2=To look for land   6= Don't know
> 3= School   7= Other, specify_____
> 4= Following parents
> n. What was the approximate date of [...]'s move out? (note: should be after ~June/July
> 2007)
>   Month: [___|___]
>   Year: [___|___|___|___]

FIGURE 4.8. Tracking form for absent respondents, MAYP.

interviewers were told a person was in the fields or at the trading center, they would walk or take a bicycle taxi to search for the respondent, and perhaps interview him while he was ironworking, farming, or selling mobile phone airtime units. Some respondents were away more permanently due, for example, to relocation or migrant labor. During tobacco season, many men sought casual labor planting and harvesting, and would live away from home for a number of weeks or months; a person might also be away closer to home engaged in *ganyu* labor.[18] In figure 4.7, we note that this particular respondent was "interviewed" (a successful outcome). In many other cases, however, respondents had relocated to South Africa since the previous survey wave ("6=temporarily absent"). Indeed, migration is the main reason for sample loss or attrition in Malawi (Anglewicz et al. 2009). In such cases, the project would complete a tracking form (see a portion of MAYP's version of a tracking form in figure 4.8), collecting as much information as possible about the whereabouts of the individual: who he is staying with and which neighborhood he is living in, for example.

At the close of fieldwork, teams would use these forms to track respondents, using piecemeal information collected from relatives and friends to find them. For example, at the close of MAYP fieldwork, seventy-five respondents needed tracking, among these, twenty-two in the study district of Salima, nineteen in Lilongwe District, and three in Dowa District, covering over 11,000 square kilometers.[19] "We will find them—don't worry," Hastings, a MAYP supervisor, exclaimed when fieldworkers questioned the utility of collecting this information, showing the extent to which the project was willing to go to preserve the sample. Finally, although interviewers were encouraged to work hard to avoid refusals, some participants, as we saw in chapter 3—though in LSAM's case, remarkably few—did refuse to participate (Kranzer et al. 2008; Reniers and Eaton 2009; Obare 2010). This, too, had to be documented on the form, and interviewers were asked to record some notes on the reason behind this refusal. Similarly, respondents who were too ill to be interviewed—or in some cases too drunk on *kachasu* (a variety of locally distilled liquor popular in rural areas)—were coded as refusing.

The arsenal of tools meant to track respondents who were away worked to effectively reduce attrition in the sample; however, even finding respondents who were present was not easy. Namely, before beginning an interview, fieldworkers had to verify that the respondent was who he claimed to be. As supervisor Andrews explained, "These guys have been in our sample *kalekale* [since a long time ago]. We know them! But we have to make sure we get the right person." Maps hand drawn by fieldworkers in past years often worked to help interviewers find the households they were assigned (see figure 4.9 for a sample hand-drawn map). Sketches of miniaturized trees, churches, vegetable stands, paths, and soccer fields helped fieldworkers find their way through terra incognita, though, of course, trees or kiosks could change from year to year. Each crop of interviewers was instructed to correct or improve the maps as needed and often drew over, crossed out, and refined the maps to make them more accurate in the present. In this way, these maps from below became accumulative condensations of archived project knowledge, collaboratively created, transmitted from one generation of fieldworkers to another, and owned not by an individual but a project.

Teams often relied on word-of-mouth directions, and, in especially rural or difficult-to-navigate EAs, teams would often hire a scout. This person, assumed to be a reservoir of local knowledge about the social landscape and

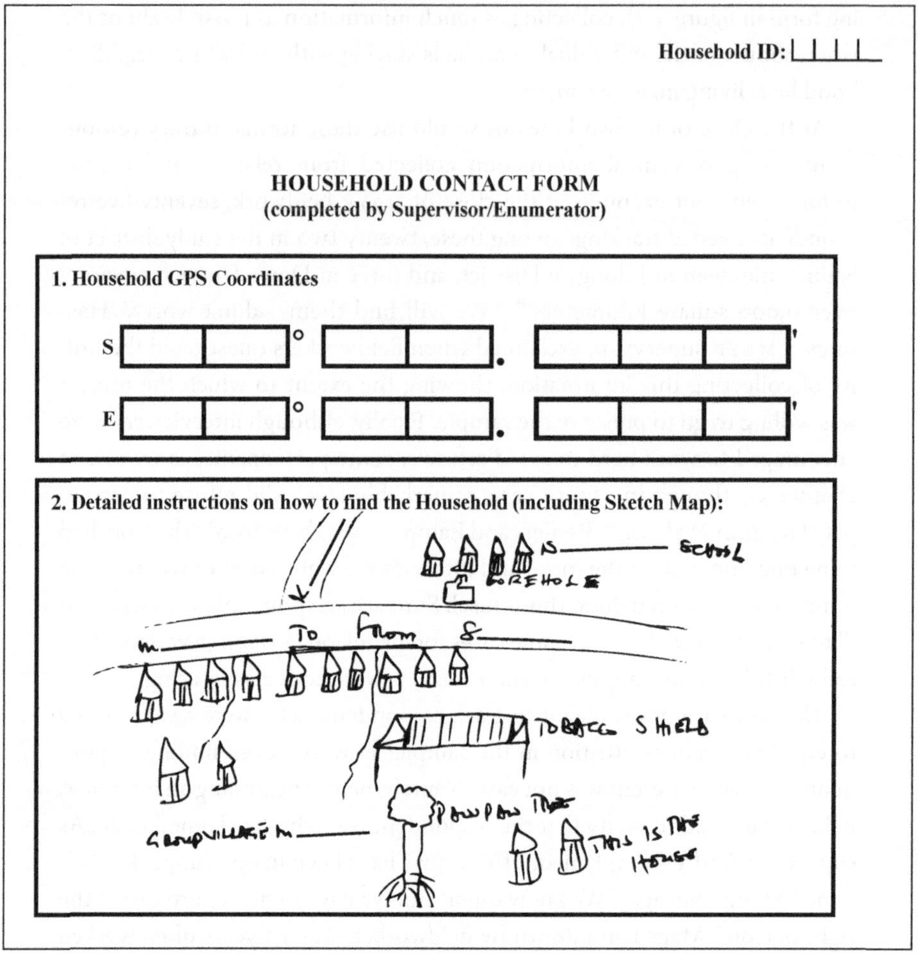

HOUSEHOLD CONTACT FORM
(completed by Supervisor/Enumerator)

1. Household GPS Coordinates

S ▢ ° ▢ . ▢ '

E ▢ ° ▢ . ▢ '

2. Detailed instructions on how to find the Household (including Sketch Map):

FIGURE 4.9. A map hand drawn by MAYP fieldworker (anonymous).

composition of villages in the sample, was paid a daily rate of 500 kwacha (about $3.50 USD at the time) and was often asked to locate and book appointments with respondents ahead of time to save time and ensure respondents were present when teams arrived. Scouts were often appointed by the chief of a certain area, who frequently recommended a son or other relative for the job.[20] Scouts took significant pride in their few days of employment and emphasized their status by carrying a clipboard that listed the names of respondents to be interviewed. Teams also relied on more informal channels of finding respondents, inquiring about the whereabouts of individuals by showing photos to bicycle taxis or giving women carrying buckets of water from the borehole a ride in exchange for information about the locations of sample households. In general, the array of tools available for seeing a household—that is, making it visible against a background of village life—were very effective. On only a few occasions were respondents not trackable at all.

In coming face to face with a respondent, however, an interviewer had to verify that this individual was who he or she claimed to be. The supervisors' advice to their fieldworkers that "respondents are always trying to trick [research teams]" was sometimes borne out by interactions in the field. Names did not always work as a unique fingerprint, since relatives can share the same names or similar names. When someone claimed to be the sought-after respondent, interviewers often held up the pixelated photo next to the person's face to scrutinize the match. Often, they noted a tree or house in the background of the photo and asked the respondent, "Where is this tree?" or "Are these the bricks that appear behind you in the photo?" In some cases the numerical code of a household was scrawled in white chalk on the house itself, a visible marker that the household was in the sample. Next, the interviewers cross-checked the names, age, and nickname.

Nonetheless, a number of hiccups arose. Fieldwork teams encountered imposters, or people who would pretend to be the respondent and proceed to answer the questions. On some days, LSAM supervisors grew frustrated with the prevalence of what they called "imposter syndrome" and blamed it largely on the "hunger for kwachas" the incentives project that passed through previously had created. People posed as members of the sample because they assumed being in the sample meant receiving money or other possible benefits now or in the future. Though imposter stories became the stuff of fieldwork folklore after the fact, in the moment, imposters were a drain on time, resources, and patience. For example, Collins, a MAYP interviewer, spent one morning searching for Moses Banda, a respondent in the sample. It was well known in the sample villages that MAYP was expanding its sample that year to include spouses of respondents. When we turned up at Moses's household—according to the map in the envelope—we were greeted by Mercy, a woman who claimed to be Moses's wife. She assured us that Moses was out but would return shortly; in the meantime, in line with the sampling strategy to add spouses to the sample this year, Collins decided to interview his wife. However, about two hours later—while Mercy and Collins were still immersed in the interview—Moses arrived, and it soon became clear that Mercy was not Moses's wife, but the wife of his brother who lived in Lilongwe. Collins stopped the interview immediately, visibly frustrated at being tricked by Mercy.

The supervisors debated whether Mercy should receive the bars of soap or not, ultimately deciding to give her the gift in exchange for her time, even if the information would never become data. Mercy, motivated here by her own interest in acquiring the soap she knew would be forthcoming, pretended to be someone she was not, throwing a temporary wrench into the works of the project and threatening the integrity and purity of the sample as an interloper. As we saw in chapter 3, soap sometimes motivated respondents to pose as someone else; in a few cases a legitimate respondent did not want to answer questions and suggested a friend or relative stand in for him or her to receive the soap the respondent was entitled to. On the ground, the sample was a political and politicized unit. An optically bounded, neat and tidy entity as viewed from above morphed into a messy, shape-shifting political community on the ground, rife with spillovers and leakages (Adams and Kasanoff 2004, 344).

In the case of LSAM, the longest-running survey project I worked with, people in sample areas were very aware of who was in and who was out of the sample. Even as some people expressed frustration with the meager soap gift, there was a sense that being in the sample was better than not being in the sample, and it held a certain promise of benefits to come in the future (Prince and Otieno 2014, 940). Often, people saw the conspicuous mini-buses passing through the villages and flagged us down, asking if we could ask them questions as well. The teams often promised they would see them soon, but without knowing whether these particular individuals were in the sample or not.

Certainly, the sample was the narrow lens through which both the project and its fieldworkers bounded the social reality of interest to them. In the same way that fieldworkers are taught to conceive of the field as separate from, distant from, and different from the office, the sample has to be treated in a certain way in order to ensure the collection of pieces of information in a standardized and orderly manner. Even before teams gain access to the sample, they must first engage in formal meetings with district commissioners, traditional authorities, district health officers, and local police to alert them to the teams' presence in the district for the coming weeks. The epistemic commitment to sample purity produces the sample as a thing autonomous and disconnected from the world surrounding it, an entity whose borders should be patrolled. Yet in practice, maintaining sample purity entails artfully navigating the blurred lines between "sample" and "not sample." These unpredictable and unfolding social relations between project staff and residents of sample villages challenge the notion that research projects are alienated from the everyday realities of their research subjects. Even as the data they collect are a metaphor for the project's inability to see the "real, existing forest for the [valuable] trees" (Scott 1998, 3), fieldworkers are entangled in the social realities they aim to capture.

For example, field teams sometimes attended funerals in the villages in the project's sample to pay condolences and give monetary donations. In the event of a death, data collection might be delayed for one day while field-workers attended the funeral. Andrews explained to his field team, "It is our duty to show them we are part of them." Fieldworkers were discouraged from just "sitting in the minibus" and encouraged to "get to know them [people living in research areas]." This advice was largely taken up; toward the end of a fieldwork day in August 2008, a parade of women dancing vigorously to the rhythm of drums surrounded our minibus, beckoning for us to join them. The women were celebrating *nsondo*, a girls' initiation ritual practiced in Yao areas. The field team members sitting on the bus left their newspapers, conversation, and mobile phones to join the dancing. The warp and woof of rural life intersected and redirected the temporalities and prescriptions of data collection on a daily basis, and treating the sample correctly was key to collecting good data. Seemingly insignificant and happenstance encounters in the field played a key role in lubricating data collection. Fieldworkers enjoyed meals offered to them by survey respondents, engaged in business transactions with local people (e.g., purchasing honey, fruit, or local chickens from purveyors, or buying bread and tea from the same tea stand over the course of one week), gave sick people rides to the hospital, helped women pound maize, played football with young people, and so on. Each of these small interactions functioned to elongate the relationships and build trust between a project and its sample.

Knowing the trees, in this case, is a prerequisite for seeing the forest. Even as the project itself focuses myopically on the sample as the unit of value, the production of this value is contingent on forging the right kinds of relations with those within and outside that unit. Further, actions in the present can enhance or compromise the ability of the project to collect good data over longitudinal time. In many cases, this entailed ensuring proper relations of exchange and obligation were maintained. I reproduce a scene from my field notes to show how minor but tactical investments in maintaining good social relations worked to ensure data collection went smoothly (not unlike the anthropologist's own directive to build rapport).

The MAYP Land Rover moves slowly through tall grasses, swimming in mud that lies beneath. Suddenly, we strike something hard. A man emerges from the bushes, yelling that the car has run over a clay pot filled with the day's relish (*ndiwo*). The supervisors quickly got out of the car and apologized to the man. He accepted their apology, but suggested they should compensate him for the broken pot. The supervisors consulted among themselves, and decided to give the man 600 kwacha ($4 USD at the time). The man received the money gratefully and we went on our way. Henry later explained the story to the researchers back at the office, and was given the 600 kwacha he paid the man out of his own pocket.

Here, the researcher validates the supervisors' decision to compensate the man for the pot, even though the broken pot was technically no one's fault. The scene illustrates how researchers' epistemic commitments become embodied by project staff members. The simple exchange of a small amount of money is an act with far-reaching consequences, at least in the eyes of the fieldwork teams, who suggested that paying the man for his lost property was a gesture of good faith and epitomized the project's ethical commitment to do no harm. Giving the money, they said, ensured that the man in question would not go back to his household or village with bad feelings for the project that could influence whether he, his family, or friends welcomed the project in the future or participated in the survey (it was unknown whether this particular man was in the sample). Aside from the formal introductions to district offices, traditional authorities, and others who can influence the tenor of data collection in a sample area, informal, improvised, and tactical social relations directed toward maintaining sample purity and treating the sample with respect played a central role in enabling smooth data collection in the present and the future.

Conclusion

This chapter has emphasized that good data do not lie passively in wait to be collected by fieldworkers. Instead, the shared imaginary of data compels fieldworker and respondent to meet face to face, and clean data are imagined and materialized by standards translated into the field by fieldworkers. In zooming in on some of the hundreds of research encounters that transpire every day in the field, we see that data are cooked and cleaned in multiple stages as they travel to the office or enter a database: raw data, indeed, are an imagined fiction (Gitelman 2013). Data's value is produced in the frictions that arise when the abstract epistemic investments that define clean data are translated into the particular spaces and embodied social relations of the messy field and in the messy editing practices undertaken by fieldworkers as they handle data before they reach the office. Indeed, the numbers produced are artifacts of the situated negotiations of survey research worlds more than they count or document rural realities.

The pieces of information recorded by fieldworkers like Janet, Tapika, Ishmael, Henry, Collins, and Edward, having subsequently passed through the hands of supervisors and data clerks, are now ensconced in the ordered and sterile space of the database. How do these aggregated data now traverse the boundary between producers and users? How do they reach the audiences who arbitrate their value as evidence for policy or other uses? Chapter 5 traces the next step in data's life course: its re-presentation and ordering in venues ranging from policy meetings to journal articles to conferences.

FIVE

WHEN NUMBERS TRAVEL

The Politics of Making Evidence-Based Policy

Chifundo, lead MAYP supervisor, hands me the keys to the project storage room, from which I am meant to fetch pens and clipboards for fieldworkers. As I push open the heavy wooden door, made too big for its frame by the dampness of the rainy season, I am immediately struck by the large volume of paper all around me: hundreds of completed surveys (collected last year) are stuffed into boxes piled on sagging shelves. The papers are yellowing, dusty, and covered in spider webs and the room smells musty and damp. The back room, attached to MAYP's field office, is a storehouse for raw data; each survey contains fading pencil and pen marks that have by now undergone data cleaning and been converted into codes ensconced in MAYP's growing database and enlisted into claims as evidence. Months later, I have a similar experience standing amid boxes of completed surveys in LSAM's storeroom (see figure 5.1). While boxes full of surveys are the forgotten detritus of data collection in years past, they index present and future temporalities in which the information they contain now circulates in different, cleaner form.

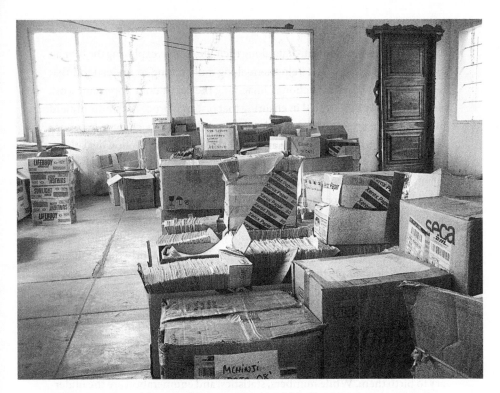

FIGURE 5.1. Boxes of completed surveys in LSAM field office storage room. Photo by Joshua Wood.

Meanwhile in the main room of the field office, data entry clerks sip sugary tea from blue plastic cups as they tap diligently at the keyboards of project-owned laptops. Next to each clerk is a marked-up survey collected the previous day by field teams: their labor is converting the pen marks—raw information provided by respondents—into neater and tidier entries typed into a growing database. A few weeks later, after all information has been entered and data collection has wound down, the makeshift field office will be locked up until the next round of data collection, and project employees will seek out the next job in their project-to-project livelihood strategy. The end of fieldwork—packing up and leaving a rural field site—is a logical bookend to the opening scene of chapter 1, which foregrounded the immense work required to set up and carry out field research under difficult and remote conditions. Yet the life course of data does not end in a dusty store room: in their repackaging as statistics and numbers, data are immortal, their future travels and uses yet unknown.

We have thus far traveled with data along their life course, exploring the human and nonhuman actors that help them along and coming to understand that even though raw data are fictional, imagining they exist does important work for demographers interested in ensuring that research proceeds smoothly and numerical data attain disciplinary quality standards. This chapter examines what happens to data after they are collected in the field. Following others, I critically examine evidence amid the rise of evidence-based rhetoric as the default language for conceptualizing the link between research and action in global health and other scientific worlds (Goldenberg 2006; Lambert 2009; Adams 2013; Biehl and Petryna 2013, 8; Fan and Uretsky 2016). In particular, I take interest in evidence-based policy, which, in the public and expert imagination, is an important site into which data are absorbed as evidence to justify claims about the distribution of resources and political energy to national (or international) problems such as the HIV epidemic. As others have shown, evidence-based global health rhetoric privileges and presumes a certain kind of evidence: good, clean numbers. This book has shown that numbers contain multitudes; in their life course, they not only represent but constitute and reflect the particular social worlds and infrastructures necessary to birth them. While numbers, statistics, and enumeration are the underlying objects and processes by which knowledge meets particular "rules of verification and falsification" in global health research worlds, it is important to understand how, why, and under which conditions specific numbers become facts and evidence (Foucault 2008, 36). Critical accounts of numbers and enumeration paradoxically often take for granted the authority, rule, and hegemony of numbers as a form of evidence, yet, as this chapter shows in detail, numbers do not stand alone but require cultural, social, and other scaffolding and negotiation to be propelled through the world (Knaapen 2013). Further, as this chapter suggests, sometimes good numbers fail to convince their audiences of their validity, and data lose out to other criteria. Evidence not only reflects the ideological or epistemological conventions of those who produce it but is verified and achieves circulation via aesthetic and performative gestures and within located social relations. Responding to Gieryn's (1999) call for detailed examinations of local and episodic constructions of science in its downstream sites of consumption after it leaves the laboratory, field, or office, this chapter probes the cultural boundaries of surveys and their product—data—in several sites where numbers are enlisted into stories and knowledge claims as evidence.

Thus far, we have observed that quantitative health data are produced by heavily negotiated social relations that, in essence, cook reality to fit templates for research. The unreliability and contingency of numbers we usually take at face value is clear. In this chapter, I move away from survey projects in the field to focus on where and how quantitative and other evidence travels beyond sites where it is collected. I then present two extended vignettes to analyze how data in their finished form (as statistical evidence) are negotiated in unfolding social relations in downstream sites, just as they have already been in the field. In the first case, I show how numbers drawn from consultants' careful literature review were altered and took different form when they made it into national AIDS policy. In the second, I show how well-collected and scientifically validated numbers about the prevalence of HIV among men who have sex with men (MSM) in Malawi failed to travel or to convince their audiences. I illustrate that the use and evaluation of data may sometimes rest less on whether it is good or bad by epistemic standards than on users of data cooking numbers toward their own ends. While this sounds insidious, it is my hope that this chapter will instead show that the numbers underlying evidence-based claims in the policy-research nexus are never stable and always subject to processes of cooking, even in finished form.

To accomplish these dual objectives, I draw on interviews and conversations with demographers, policy makers, and bureaucrats, as well as participant observation at conferences and meetings where numerical data figured heavily in discussions and debates about the AIDS epidemic in sub-Saharan Africa.[1] I also read policy, gray literature reports produced by NGOs or other organizations outside formal publication channels, and journal articles to analyze the role and performances of quantitative data within them. The analysis of evidence in this chapter is enacted against the backdrop of the rest of the book, although the evidence analyzed below is not drawn directly from the databases of the survey projects discussed in chapters 1–4. The first vignette ("The Black Box of Culture in AIDS Policy") traces the travels of data I helped collect during my time with LSAM in 2005 as a cosupervisor of the Cultural Practices Study mentioned in the introduction, showing how it was mobilized toward diverse ends in its travels between 2005 and the present. The vignette explores how and why nonexistent (ghost) numbers became a good enough evidence base to inform national AIDS policy. The second vignette ("The Case of an Unsavory Risk Group") analyzes statistical evidence—based on data collection overseen by a Malawian NGO and a major research university in the United States—of high HIV prevalence among MSM, showing how, despite its merits, it failed to inform national AIDS policy until many years later. Throughout, I foreground the continued ways in which data are cooked as they move along a life course that stretches from the office of survey design to the downstream sites where they take form as evidence. While statistics like those discussed here are often considered to be the final representative form of knowledge (clean, cooked according to scientific standards), it will become clear that in their circulation through diverse spaces, they continue to undergo transformations and critical evaluation from their audiences. How are numbers operationalized in downstream sites by their users? How is their context of production foregrounded or obscured, and to what ends, as they are enlisted into representational projects? Evidence's validity and authority—rather than being inherent to it—are performed as it travels across boundaries between actors attuned to different goals at multiple scales of policy-research bureaucracies, this chapter suggests.

The second half of the chapter analyzes the rhetoric of a policy-research gap, discussed by my informants, common to global health worlds. I argue that gaps such as this are not merely an empty space or failed communication between researchers and policy makers. Rather, this gap is best conceived as a confluence of multiple and competing interests and frictions that is full of pre- and misconceptions, which determine not only the kinds of evidence that gain authority in the policy-research nexus, but also the efficacy (or not) of translation between the two spheres (Apthorpe 1997, 55).

The sites discussed herein—conferences, presentations of findings, meetings, and policy itself—are conceptualized as stages, or places where performances of knowledge take place. Centering my analysis on the scripts, props, supporting actors, and aesthetic and generic features that propel evidence in its travels through networks and spaces that define the scientific community (including demographers and others who produce and circulate numerical data) and its overlap with policy worlds, I show that evidence making is a process that transpires within social relations, and reflects and calls into being norms and standards that arbitrate whether evidence is good or bad. In examining the stories that numbers tell in specific places, it will be clear that they project and point to pasts and futures, and index a world outside the spaces they circulate within.

What Is Evidence?

The circulation of numbers such as those produced by LSAM, MAYP, and other kinds of research projects is central to the global health apparatus; these quantitative data knit together people and institutions in diverse sites and with diverse interests. Numbers, anthropologists have shown, are the primary form of authoritative evidence for making policy decisions, funneling resources, and measuring health-related phenomena at the national, regional, and international levels. Recent initiatives to make survey and census data publicly and widely available mean they are potential forms of evidence accessible to diverse researchers, policy makers, and activists (Zuberi 2005; McCaa et al. 2006).[2] Numbers convert lives, deaths, and social phenomena into portable forms that circulate widely and can be made to tell important stories about, for example, the AIDS epidemic in Malawi. Most centrally, numbers are the evidence base for international and national policy and have gained new authority, for example, as indicators that determine which interventions should be funded or measure how well countries manage aid in a climate fixated on aid effectiveness and, increasingly, return on investment (Segone 2004; Cornish 2015; Erikson 2016). The rhetoric of policy-relevant and evidence-based policy has trickled into national-level documents, including in Malawi. The government-produced 2015 Malawi AIDS response progress report, for example, explicitly notes that the recommended strategies and interventions it proposes were "informed by research evidence" (GoM 2015, 3), and the Malawi HIV Prevention Strategy (2015–2020) terms itself "evidence-based" (NAC 2014, 11), as such policy documents have for many years now.

Media representations, policies, government statements, and public discussions rely on numbers to bolster the claims and stories they circulate. The political power of numbers lies in their ability to go unquestioned, to be taken for granted, and to shape narratives that carry with them the power to cast certain citizens as backward, to direct resources here versus there, and to insulate institutions and governments from accusations of resource mismanagement (Briggs and Mantini-Briggs 2003; Briggs and Hallin 2007; Redfield 2013, 113–114). In an era of indicators, numbers may also act to challenge the authority or status quo of governments or to reinforce northern paternalism and imperialism. They help powerful people determine which lives count or are worth saving or improving (Packard 1989; Petryna 2002; Nguyen 2010, 163; Nelson 2015). Even as national priorities and concerns around HIV in Malawi have shifted since the early days of the epidemic (see the introduction), the role of numbers in giving these stories credibility and authority has remained consistent. Projects such as LSAM have, over time, incorporated shifting and diverse concerns into their surveys, coming up with new and better ways to measure or count them along the way. Data collection happens again and again, adjusting to meet the time-sensitive needs, funding cycles, and fads of global health practitioners and institutions. The changing form of LSAM's survey questions since the late 1990s, for example, mirrors shifts in international policy and research priorities over time.[3]

Scholarship in critical global health studies has tracked the rise of evidence-based global health, showing how numbers act as a universal currency and play expedient and often unquestioned roles in how we (think we) know about health problems such as AIDS in Africa (Erikson 2012; Biehl and Petryna 2013; Adams 2016a). As Adams (2013, 57) suggests, "For evidence to say anything valid about 'how to prevent or treat a known health problem,' it must speak the language of statistics and epidemiology." To this end, in what follows, I examine some of the processes through which raw data come to speak this language (or not) and become real (or not) in the eyes of actors in the policy-research nexus in Malawi.

From its earliest etymology, "evidence" has carried connotations of transparency, obviousness, conspicuousness, and clarity: evidence seems to need nothing but itself to stand in as proof for belief or claims. Yet its etymology likewise carries meanings associated with displays or appearances from which inferences may be drawn; evidence is an indication, trace, or token (from the Oxford English Dictionary, online). The duality of meaning points to evidence as a thing to be taken at face value and a thing whose face value relies on shared interpretive frameworks. As suggested in the introduction and chapter 1, demographers form a "population-based epistemic community" that constitutes an array of actors located in policy institutions, government health and aid ministries, census and development bureaus, a range of family planning and development NGOs, and academic centers of demography and public health (Halfon 2006, 794). These actors conceive of, speak of, and theorize the world in similar ways and form a sociotechnical network that stabilizes, coordinates, and disciplines ways of talking about AIDS and other population-based issues. The surveys we have become familiar with in prior chapters—as documents and tools of scientific measurement—are not always present when such actors come together but help establish discourse and action by forging rituals of knowledge making, methods, and legitimate sources of inference (Halfon 2006, 785).

Serving as the underlying template for good data, the survey reflects and constitutes the standards by which the quality of data—and, later, evidence— will be arbitrated. For demographers leading projects like LSAM, MAYP, and GSIP, formal avenues of face-to-face communication such as policy meetings, meetings of the Population Association of America, the International Union for the Scientific Study of Population, and the Union of African Population

Scientists, journals such as *Population and Development Review, Studies in Family Planning, International Family Planning Perspectives,* and *Demography,* and documents such as demographic and health survey country reports are central sites in which the data they collect in the field aspire to become good evidence for claims made about the lives of rural Malawians (Halfon 2006, 794–795). These venues in and through which quantitative data circulate—what I term the policy-research nexus—are bounded by and reproduce population-based epistemic investments (Riles 2000, 3). Data are used to make evidence and this evidence is located, embodied, and reflective of the interests and social positions of those who enlist it into knowledge claims (Mosse 2004; Cornish 2015, 274). However, appeals to the authority of evidence, particularly quantitative evidence, obscure the subjective elements of knowledge production.

Evidence-based policy making presumes its foil. "Evidence" carries connotations of transparency, accountability, objectivity, and neutrality. Policy not based on evidence, then, is presumed to be mired in or tainted by power relations, corruption, ideology, and arbitrariness (Timmermans and Berg 2003). Further, the assumption that numbers stand alone as representative of reality overlook the complex scaffolding that propels them and enrolls supporters to the claims they bolster. In what follows, I begin in two different downstream sites in the policy-research nexus: national HIV/AIDS policy and a district-level local research dissemination meeting. In each, I present a claim about the HIV epidemic in Malawi that relies on data collected long before the claims were made. I aim not only to trace the lives of the numerical data that seem to inform such claims but also come to understand why, whether, and how claims find traction and enjoy further circulation or not.

Ghost Numbers, or When Data Lose Out: The Black Box of Culture in AIDS Policy

In 2009, Malawi's National AIDS Commission (NAC) published "National HIV Prevention Strategy: 2009–2013." The strategy notes that "harmful cultural practices" are one of the "well-documented factors that facilitate the . . . spread of HIV in Malawi" (NAC 2009, 10), and reducing risk of HIV transmission through harmful cultural practices is itemized as a strategic approach for HIV reduction (29). In the portion of the strategy that discusses the action plan for implementation, harmful cultural practices and beliefs again surface as important sites of intervention and education activities to be implemented by key organizations including NGOs and the Ministry of Health (42). This has important effects, especially considering that the action plan calls for provision of material and financial support to structures that will mobilize against harmful practices and promote positive ones (52). Indeed, the strategy describes itself as a tool for "planning, implementation, monitoring and evaluating and resource mobilization for HIV prevention interventions." It is also self-consciously "evidence-based" and "data-driven" (1).

Malawi's recent National HIV and AIDS policy, for 2011–2016, also lists "harmful cultural practices" as a major "risk factor that fuel[s] the HIV and AIDS pandemic" (NAC 2010, 8). A look at Malawi's 2015 AIDS Response Progress Report indicates that "harmful cultural practices" are a "human rights violation that promotes HIV transmission" (NAC 2015a, 26) and notes that such practices were a major theme in information, education, and communication materials distributed in the country in 2013–2014. Documents such as Malawi's Prevention Strategy, HIV and AIDS Policy, and AIDS Progress Reports play a key role in performing Malawi's priorities and commitments to both its citizens and outside states and donors, and in determining flows of money and energy during the time periods covered. Malawi, not unlike other donor-dependent countries, is notable for "the multiplication of policy documents and an absence of real (implementable and implemented) policies beyond the very short term" (Booth et al. 2006, ix). Nonetheless, in policy documents covering the past decade, "harmful cultural practices" finds a consistent place in the local Malawian expert imagination of the epidemic (Watkins and Swidler 2012, 5). Drawing on my ethnographic work in both 2005 and 2007–2008, this section takes the claim that harmful cultural practices are a major driver of the epidemic in Malawi as a starting point and aims to excavate the nature of the evidence that supports it. I focus on how information related to the claim was gathered, what was perceived as credible evidence by different actors in the policy research nexus, and how and why information was ignored, reinterpreted, and distorted, and by whom.

Preparing policy documents is a long and complicated process that requires gathering of data relevant to policy narratives and statements ahead of time. Policy analysts have shown that the ideal model of policy making—where good research evidence makes its way directly into policy—rarely materializes (Walt 1994; Crewe and Young 2002; Hutchinson 2011), and, as is examined later in this chapter, my informants perceived a policy research gap, and suggested that research findings too rarely made it into policy. Nathanson (2007) argues that the credibility and authority of knowledge and its potential transfer into policy are contingent on political regimes in place, the maneuverings and interests of knowledge brokers, and conjunctions of timing and opportunity. Scholars and local critics have documented overuse or privileged use of foreign or expatriate consultants in the policy-research nexus of the global South, which likely reinforces the gap between policy makers and researchers: the latter are presumed to possess higher-order expertise to evaluate, inform, or bolster local policy. Further, the construction of evidence discussed above as neutral, objective, desirable, and transparent maps onto racialized hierarchies informed by the postcolonial politics of collaboration in places such as Malawi, hierarchies that still structure talk and rhetoric in development, global health, and aid worlds (Crewe and Axelby 2013, 79).

There are significant material stakes in winning a consultancy and, as we saw in chapter 1, a culture of moonlighting draws local experts away from basic research and university-level teaching and toward high-paying consultancies. Consultancies are advertised in Malawi national newspapers and often recruit both Malawian and foreign consultants. In the period leading up to preparation of Malawi's 2009 National HIV Policy, the NAC hired two consultants to collaborate to review literature and collate the evidence that would inform the policy.

In June 2008, I sat around a table with five other people: Dr. Richard Castells, the American epidemiologist mentioned in the introduction and an expatriate consultant hired to evaluate HIV prevention strategies in Malawi; his Malawian coconsultant demographer Blessings Chimanda; and American graduate students in biology, demography, and sociology affiliated with LSAM. Richard was in Malawi for a short time and sought information from the other individuals present, all of whom—including the author—had spent more time on the ground in Malawi than he had. Castells's and Chimanda's findings would inform the NAC's National HIV Prevention Strategy for the coming years, which was, at the time, in preparation.

Richard kicked off the discussion with a series of queries through which he sought to ascertain the role of risky cultural practices in fueling the epidemic. While Dr. Castells would review and collate, in collaboration with Blessings, a boatload of documents, reports, and studies on HIV in Malawi before finalizing his report back to the NAC, this meeting was a chance for him to seek information in person from a group of individuals who might contest or reinforce the dominant narrative threading through such documents. His question about cultural practices was unsurprising, given researchers' and policy makers' interest in how traditional rituals, practices, and norms might exacerbate the spread of HIV at the time; included in this category were a wide range of activities under the sign "culture," ranging from traditional male circumcision rituals to widow inheritance to *fisi* to erotic dancing at ceremonies to *kulowa kufa*.[4] Further, during my time in Malawi in 2007–2008, cultural practices were often in the national newspapers' headlines, and featured prominently in discussions I had with Malawian policy makers and NGO staff, who told stories about intractable harmful cultural practices in the villages (Page 2014; Esacove 2016). Journalists captured public attention through sensationalized representations of the traditional beliefs and practices of the country's rural residents, who were consistently portrayed by radio and newspapers as wearing a "veil of ignorance" and being "killed by attitudes and . . . lack of knowledge" about AIDS, for example (Chandilanga 2008; Mpaka 2008).

As the anthropologist at the table, I was skeptical of the equation of culture and risk for reasons that will become clear as this section unfolds. I stated that I thought the focus on cultural practices was overblown and worked to draw attention away from other more pressing issues and from the failures of government-led and foreign-influenced policies, structures, and interventions by placing blame on backward culture and society's most vulnerable (Briggs and Hallin 2007). On the heels of my statements, Blessings, the Malawian coconsultant, counterargued that there is significant evidence that cultural practices were fueling Malawi's epidemic. When Castells asked him for citations they could enlist as evidence in writing the report for NAC, Chimanda stated that "a number of studies have been done" and verbally noted studies implemented in recent years by NAC, the Malawi Human Rights Commission (MHRC), and UNICEF. Positioned as he was as a local expert hired for his knowledge of matters such as these and, as a Malawian, more expert on Malawian culture than others at the table, Blessings's claim became the final word—at least that afternoon—on cultural practices: he had tentatively been extended epistemic authority by those present, winning this particular credibility contest (Gieryn 1999).

The validation of Blessings's claim as evidence—after all, it is unlikely that Castells would proceed to closely read the studies for himself given the time constraints placed on consultants—that culture should be a central site of national and international intervention worthy of funding and scrutiny relies on the few studies on the link between HIV risk and cultural practices that had been completed prior to our conversation that day. Although none had documented a link between engaging in a harmful cultural practice and contracting HIV, it was these studies that stood in as evidence to support a claim that gained momentum. The most well-known and comprehensive study of cultural practices in Malawi at the time of our meeting in 2008 was a 2006 report by the MHRC referenced by Blessings, titled "Cultural Practices and

Their Impact on the Enjoyment of Human Rights, Particularly the Rights of Women and Children in Malawi." While this 137-page report focuses on the threats that practices related to marriage, initiation, funerals, and chieftancy pose to the human rights of participants, it also presumes that such practices have a role in transmitting HIV.

In the section discussing male initiation, for example, the report suggests that the practices associated with initiation are "quite risky" in the face of the epidemic (MHRC 2006, 107); the researchers, however, did not collect HIV-test data to support this claim, making the claim about HIV transmission quite a flimsy one as judged by typical standards for evidence operative in global health worlds. The study was, as the authors suggest, based on both "quantitative and qualitative data"; the former was collected via a structured survey administered to 262 respondents in nine districts, purposively sampled to capture ethnic identity differences. The qualitative data, meanwhile, drew from a total of ninety-nine focus group discussions held across all the districts sampled. Although the survey administered contained only close-ended questions, the bulk of numbers cited in the long report capture what percentage of respondents mentioned specific cultural practices as familiar (e.g., "polygamy," 98.1 percent; *jando*, 16.5 percent, pp. 14–16).[5] The report's appendix includes the survey itself and illustrates that respondents were asked whether each of six cultural practices (in the case of practices related to rites of passage) were "found in [their] home area" (125). In this sense, the bulk of the long report relies heavily on claims made by respondents in the focus group discussions, citing throughout the perception on the part of respondents that various cultural practices pose risks for HIV, for example: "Most respondents were of the view that dances such as *mtungo* and *magolowazi* should be abolished because they promoted promiscuity and . . . the spread of STIs, including HIV/AIDS" (35).[6] Although this evidence would normally not pass muster in the eyes of demographers, epidemiologists, or policy makers under the spell of the hegemony of numbers, the MHRC report has enjoyed long citational life to this day and, as we will see, in the case of Blessings's claim above became one key part of the solid foundation for policy making in 2008–2009.

The MHRC report, and those few others that have been published in its wake, references two other studies that are often mentioned in discussions of risky culture in Malawi: a study of a single village in Lilongwe District (UNICEF 2001) and a study based on focus group discussions with village leaders in a single district (Phalombe) carried out in 1997. The latter presumed a link between cultural practices and risk of HIV transmission: the study was meant to provide a basis for advocating behavior change (Kornfield and Namate 1997, v). Again, none of the studies meant to draw a connection between cultural practices and HIV risk-tested people for HIV, nor did they ascertain the presence of other negative health conditions, such as sexually transmitted infections.

In justifying his claim about risky culture, Blessings also mentioned a study of cultural practices implemented by NAC in 2005. Though the findings of this research were never officially published, Blessings (and others in research worlds in Malawi) would have had access to it via word of mouth or knowledge of the study. Incidentally, I was involved in collecting data for this study alongside the 2005 wave of LSAM's data collection in three Malawian districts. It is worth returning briefly to my field notes and documentation of the context and processes of data collection in 2005 so that we can best understand the nature of some of the data that became evidence in our conversation three years later around the table in 2008. The Cultural Practices Study was funded by NAC and drew on the resources—particularly transportation and fieldworkers with LSAM experience—being used by LSAM during its 2005 fieldwork season in three districts. Its main objective was "to identify the extent and type of high risk cultural practices that increase transmission of STIs including HIV/AIDS" and it also sought to "explore how communities have modified risky cultural practices."[7] In its focus on "cultural guardians," the study presumed—like many projects in Malawi and elsewhere in Africa—that involving these persons in AIDS-related interventions was imperative, reflecting, I suggest, global public health's obsession with culture as simultaneously a stumbling block and possible enhancement to global designs (see also West 2016, 114–119). The data were to be collected from respondents via administration of a survey. The proposal noted that the data would act as a complement to existing sets of quantitative data drawn from sources such as Health Information Management Systems, Community Health Sciences Unit, NAC, and National Statistical Office (NSO).

The fieldwork for the project was headed by a Malawian demographer, Dr. Chirwa, but field activities were largely overseen by Malawian field supervisors and the author, who, at the time, was a graduate student in anthropology. Fieldwork for the project unfolded on a tight schedule. For example, in one site, Balaka District, two interviewers—who had previously worked with LSAM—interviewed a wide spectrum of "cultural guardians" from June 25 to July 13, 2005, and interviews were first translated from multiple languages into English (Chewa, Yao, Sena, etc.) and then transcribed by five transcribers (including the author). By July 13, fifty-five interviews had been conducted in total in Balaka, one of the three districts in which fieldwork would be undertaken.[8] These persons included chiefs, deputy chiefs, *ngaliba* (male circumcisers for initiation rituals, *jando*), *azamba* (traditional birth attendants), *chitonombe* (counselor in charge of initiation camp), *asing'anga* (traditional healers), and so on. Some individuals in each of these categories were interviewed according to a predesigned interview guide with questions that were meant to lead to an understanding of the dimensions of the cultural practice in question and to ascertain whether or not its practice posed risks for transmitting HIV. Male initiates who had recently undergone jando, for instance, were asked questions about the instruments used to cut them and whether they were sterilized after each initiate was cut, about whether any traditional medicine was used to heal their wounds, and about whether parents or others in their communities pressured them to go for initiation. In an interview with a male initiate, the interviewer (I) makes clear his interest in unearthing cultural practices as risky, foregrounding the important role that interviewer-interviewee dynamics play in the research encounter and in the way that data takes form:

I: How many initiates use one knife [to circumcise]?
R: One per person.

I: One per person and they [initiator] throws it away?
R: Yes.

I: Maybe they used one on many people?
R: No. . . .

I: But the practice of using one knife per person happens in other [places]. Maybe they use one knife on more people or after using it on one person they put the knife in hot water? . . .
R: No! I should say all [initiators] practice these methods [of using one knife per person]. . . .

I: Do you see any dangers of initiations?
R: The practice has no dangers because it is good for a person to be initiated. . . .

I: Is circumcision risky?
R: Yes! Because sometimes [initiators] make a mistake and cut the head of the penis. . . . [9]

Here, the interviewer embodies the researchers' interests in unearthing or discovering that male initiation is risky for HIV transmission, and is likely invested in presenting himself to the respondent as modern and educated. In the transformation of the boy's experience into data, the object of culture is itself produced as a visible entity that can be studied (Langwick 2011, 284). Kaufulu (2008) helpfully illustrates, in reflecting on his position as an outsider interviewing cultural guardians among the Sena of Malawi, how research instruments and perceptions of researchers by informants answering questions about cultural practices moralized in the era of AIDS often lead to scripted responses, a form of cooked data in their own right.

Although the initiate clearly states that the initiator uses one knife per boy, the interviewer probes three times: it seems that he presumed that the initiate did not initially tell the truth. Further, although the interviewer assumes that the dangers of initiation would be related to HIV, the initiate's response to his question about whether circumcision is risky circumvents HIV altogether, citing a story he heard about an initiator's knife mistakenly cutting the wrong portion of the penis. Recalling my earlier discussion of probing, we might infer that the qualitative data collected are cooked in particular ways. However, my interest here is less in exposing how contingent or coercively extracted responses become data—as we have seen already—but rather in how the findings of this study and others like it became worthy of mention by Blessings in the earlier scene and worthy of citation in future reports and even policy. Certainly, his claim that culture is a major driver of Malawi's epidemic is not assigned validity based on what he claims to take as impeccable data or on claims that he had closely read the studies he cites; rather, it is his presumed status as a local expert, in possession of uniquely Malawian knowledge, that validates his claim in a particular conversation with a foreign expert.

This scene adds new depth to the concept of local expertise in global health research worlds: as we have followed data in their life course, we have likewise witnessed how and when certain individuals are deemed expert and on what matters. For example, in chapters 2, 3, and 4, we saw that while Malawian fieldworkers are considered experts in translating the needs of the project into the field, their advice and knowledge are rarely influential on the top-down templates that govern research (e.g., their criticisms of survey questions often went unaddressed by demographers). Similarly, while Malawian researchers are valorized as local experts in the context of survey design meetings described in chapter 1, the kind of expertise they proffer rarely influences the vision, design, and organization of a survey project. In the case of Blessings, however, we observe that on the matter of culture in particular, he is assigned expertise that helps propel cultural practices into national policy and ensures his claims are taken seriously. This series of examples reiterates, then, just how slippery local knowledge or local expertise are: these formations only gain credibility, value, or influence within sets of social relations, and the particular form they take reflects power asymmetries and the shifting value and meanings that global health assigns to the local or cultural.

COOKING CULTURE IN THE POLICY-RESEARCH NEXUS

Blessings's investment in the claim that culture is risky for the spread of AIDS became much more important months later, when it surfaced again on a different stage. Months after their meeting in Balaka, Castells's and Chimanda's findings—the results of the consultancy—were presented to two audiences by two different people: (1) to an audience of Malawian policy makers and government officials by Blessings; (2) to a regional audience by a Malawian researcher not involved in the consultancy. Prior to these presentations, Richard furnished Blessings with slides and graphs assembled from their joint findings about key drivers of Malawi's epidemic—none of which had to do with harmful cultural practices, but rather with the relevance of other potential routes of HIV transmission. The slides did have numbers, based on models that characterized the different routes of transmission (e.g., sex with sex workers, serodiscordant couples), and the percentage of new HIV infections attributable to each route of transmission, termed the HIV Modes of Transmission Model (Case et al. 2012; Shubber et al. 2014).

However, Richard later learned—after leafing through the slideshow Blessings attached to an e-mail message—that in their translation from the skeleton form of a presentation into the actual PowerPoint slides used by Blessings when he presented the results to NAC, the findings had changed.[10] Blessings, he said, had filled in the blanks by featuring his own view of the primary routes of infections: specifically, Blessings identified culturally accepted intergenerational sex as a key driver of the epidemic, despite the fact that this was not a route of transmission considered in the model. When Richard shared the slides with a demographer more familiar with the Malawian context than he was, she responded, "When it comes down to mismatches between what the data say and what the conventional wisdom is (or what Blessings believes, which is probably close to the same thing), the *data lose*."[11] Yet, even as Blessings's PowerPoint presentation may have misrepresented numerical evidence amassed about the epidemic's routes of transmission, the information it contained was propelled into other spheres: it was later presented to more Malawian stakeholders by another Malawian demographer at a regional AIDS conference.

One slide in Blessings's PowerPoint presentation, titled "Risk Factors (Drivers)," lists nine drivers, ostensibly based on the statistical data presented on the prior slides and gathered through the research and literature review he and Castells collaborated on. Three drivers, however, stand out because they are not borne out by the data (numbers) presented on other slides: intergenerational sex, transactional sex, and culture. The numerical data show that none of the three was a significant driver of the epidemic. For intergenerational sex, a few slides later, when the actual numbers are presented, less than 1 percent of women aged fifteen to seventeen had nonmarital sex with a man who was ten or more years older. Similarly, only 5 percent of men fifteen to forty-nine years old reported that they bought sex in the past year. Most interesting for the purposes of this section, however, is the slide's claim that culture is a driver of the epidemic.

On another slide, titled "Initiation Rites," Blessings presents a bar graph of "male adolescents who have ever had sex by circumcision status" to support his claim that those who have been circumcised are more likely to be sexually active compared to those who have not. Though the slide fails to cite the source of the numerical data that indicate, for example, that 77 percent of males ages fifteen to nineteen who have been circumcised have had sex, while only 53 percent of those uncircumcised have, some sleuthing on my part discovers they are drawn from a 2007 article published in the *African Journal of Reproductive Health*, which draws on data collected in 2004 by the Protecting the Next Generation: Understanding HIV Risk among Youth (PNG) project conducted by the Guttmacher Institute, a reproductive health nonprofit organization, in five African countries between 2002 and 2006 (Munthali and Zulu 2007). To locate the origin of the data source cited in the 2007 article, I dug up the PNG report itself, which describes the two-pronged sources of data for the project. Quantitative data were based on the 2004 Malawi National Survey of Adolescents, a nationally representative household survey organized by Malawi's NSO (4,031 adolescents, ages twelve to nineteen), whose survey document contained a section titled "Sociocultural Practices" that asked respondents twenty-one questions about participation in initiation, circumcision status (men and women), age at circumcision, and experience with scarification (PNG 2004). Qualitative data, meanwhile, were based on eleven focus group discussions with fourteen- to nineteen-year-olds in 2003 and 102 in-depth interviews, also collected in 2003.

A slide titled "Initiation Rites" also contains a claim—sans accompanying graph this time—that "80% of the women and 60% of the men in [the] South undergo initiation ceremonies." Considering this is on the slide prior to the data taken from the PNG project and its 2004 survey, the numbers should ostensibly match those solicited by the corresponding question (no. 1001) from the same survey: "Have you ever participated in a puberty or initiation rite?" While Blessings's general claim that initiation is most common in the southern region of Malawi is correct, the precise numbers on the slide do not correspond to the data collected by question no. 1001: according to the 2004 data set, 43 percent of males and 57 percent of females in the South underwent circumcision. Whether or not the numbers on the slide are blatantly cooked—it is difficult to tell without direct citation of a source—the inclusion of this evidence on the slide is curious, considering that, as other documents have shown, many initiation ceremonies do not directly involve sexual intercourse or actual circumcision anyway (20 percent of males living across Malawi have been circumcised, while only 2 percent of women have undergone any type of circumcision (which may include actual cutting or not), even as many participate in initiation ceremonies of various kinds (Munthali and Zulu 2007).[12] A few slides later, Blessings presents a bullet list of other cultural practices including polygamy, wife inheritance, bonus wives, fisi, and kulowa kufa; again, I reiterate that in this era of evidence-based decision making and policy, at the time of his presentation, there was no quantitative data linking any of these practices directly to HIV transmission risk.

Despite the lack of any quantitative data on the correspondence of cultural practices with HIV transmission, "cultural practices" made it into the National HIV Prevention Strategy published by NAC (2009), suggesting that Blessings was not alone in disregarding evidence. To recapitulate, the strategy notes that "harmful cultural practices" are one of the "well-documented factors that facilitate the . . . spread of HIV in Malawi" (10), and reducing risk of HIV transmission through harmful cultural practices is itemized as a strategic approach for HIV reduction (29). This strategy was ostensibly at least partly informed by the research prepared by Blessings and Richard Castells as consultants to the evidence-based policy-making process. I do not suggest that Blessings's PowerPoint presentation was the sole reason "harmful cultural practices" appears in the policy. Indeed, the rhetoric of harmful cultural practices appeared across multiple discursive spaces, including media, religious, development, and donor worlds, due in part to its familiarity and because it is, as Watkins and Swidler (2012) argue, a realm of intervention that everyone can agree on. Notes on a series of consultations spearheaded by NAC in mid-2008, for example, indicate that actors ranging from community-based organizations to people living with HIV/AIDS to human rights groups yielded feedback—meant to inform the 2009 strategy—that harmful cultural practices were furthering the spread of HIV and should be modified or eradicated.[13] Nonetheless, we can safely conclude that quantitative data to substantiate the claim that they are linked to risk of contracting HIV did not exist at the time of the policy's authorship (nor do they now). Further, even as the rhetorical investment in evidence-based policy has intensified since 2009, "harmful cultural practices" continue to find space in Malawi's national policy, despite continued absence of a study or studies that have directly linked cultural practices to HIV risk.[14]

While anthropologists and critics of global health's number-centrism have clearly demonstrated the power of numbers to travel widely and be imbued with confidence and authority, the example of Blessings, Richard, and the cooked PowerPoint slides indicates that the means and criteria by which evidence is assessed might prove more central to whether or not evidence becomes real than stand-alone good numbers. In this case, evidence relies on ghost numbers that remain invisible. First, Blessings is assigned credibility as a local expert by Dr. Castells in their initial meeting. Next, in preparing the slide show to be presented to NAC that reports on their research findings, Blessings has some latitude in determining the content of the slides. Whether Blessings fudged or cooked the data in his presentation is not my interest; rather, I aim to show how a claim not founded in quantitative data makes it to its final downstream site (policy documents). A close analysis of Blessings's slides indicates that the text written on the slides does not always align with the numerical data, graphs, and evidence. Nonetheless, the cultural practices claim makes it to the next stage in the policy-research nexus, perhaps because it aligned so well with what Watkins and Swidler (2009) have termed "conventional wisdom": the commonplace and widely circulating narratives that surround "African AIDS," including that backward culture fuels the epidemic in a geographic space that continues to stand in for the untamable and the premodern (Patton 1990, 77–97; Comaroff 2007, 197; Watkins and Swidler 2012). In discussing the case of ghost numbers, I do not suggest that more quantitative data should have been collected, or even that the policies discussed here are not evidence based. Instead, I aim to show that numbers, and evidence more broadly, do not stand alone, waiting to be enfolded into policy: they are helped along a life course and altered by social relations and transactions along the way.

As others have shown, culture becomes an anxious and moralized site of contestation and claims making in times of social upheaval, political uncertainty, and epidemics, often working to scapegoat society's most vulnerable or to rhetorically protect or distinguish certain groups in society from others (Forster 1994; Briggs and Mantini-Briggs 2003; Kogacioglu 2004; Peters, Kambewa, and Walker 2010; Biruk 2014a; Page 2014). As a Malawian,

Blessings was likely afforded some measure of credibility and authority when speaking in front of an audience of fellow Malawians, all or most of whom it is likely were known to him, considering the small size and tightly knit nature of policy-research worlds in Malawi, as discussed in detail in chapter 1. As a trusted speaker and knower, Blessings's claims were bolstered, as well, by their lack of novelty: even before his presentation, it is likely that his audience expected to hear about harmful cultural practices. The phrase had, by 2008, become a buzzword (even with its own acronym, HCP), a kind of packaging or lingua franca that encased evidence and propelled it forward. The familiar form of PowerPoint slides with their graphs and numbers—the aesthetic props of dissemination in the policy-research nexus—distracted audience members from any potential disjuncture between the numbers themselves and the claims Blessings was making (the text on the slides).

As the comprehensive literature review of an unpublished report on the matter of cultural practices (primarily initiation) and HIV risk in Malawi prepared by a consultant and others for an international organization (2015) and made available to the author suggests, the evidence linking cultural practices to abuse of young people's human rights and to risks to their sexual health (such as HIV infection) is largely anecdotal, a word whose deployment immediately signals "non–evidence based." Evidence in the global health nexus is always already presumed to be quantitative. The 2015 report, however, goes against the grain and against the conventional wisdom about cultural practices by refuting the link between such practices and HIV that has been taken for granted in Malawi since the early 2000s (Page 2014). The study of 645 youths across six districts collected information on respondents' sexual and reproductive health histories, focusing on indicators such as history of STIs, contraceptive use, HIV test history, HIV status report, and so on.[15] Their findings are clear: "across all SRH [sexual and reproductive health] indicators, there were no significant differences between those who had been initiated and those who had not, suggesting that initiation ceremonies in Malawi do not have a positive or negative effect on the sexual and reproductive health of youth." It remains to be seen, in the coming years, whether the conventional wisdom of cultural practices will retain its momentum or fizzle out in the continued absence (or, perhaps, future presence) of numerical evidence, especially considering the trend whereby policy cites itself in a recursive and reproductive fashion year after year (Esacove 2016).

When Numbers Fail: The Case of an Unsavory Risk Group

In the case above, I note that a knowledge claim made it into policy in the striking absence of numbers to prove it: evidence in the form of the few studies on the link between such practices and HIV was cited and recited in a kind of evidentiary palimpsest beneath which were not good numbers but rather what we might term ghost numbers. This example helps challenge anthropologists' and others' assertions of the hegemony of numbers as the primary source of evidence in global health worlds. As they have well shown, numbers are less real, stable, and certain than they are taken to be and often fail to measure well the realities they claim to represent. Yet, as we have seen in peeling away the palimpsest underlying cultural practices rhetoric as it appears in policy, evidence is not *always* rooted in numbers, whether good, bad, or imperfect.

The case of the rhetoric of harmful cultural practices is a particularly useful lens through which to observe how social and cultural scaffolding and framing operate to define and propel evidence through spaces we might code as number-centric. The same data can wear many costumes and carry many meanings and agendas (Hodzic 2013, 100). Blessings becomes a spokesperson who is charged with not only presenting but translating evidence that stands in for and points outward to the real-world phenomena and people it seeks to represent. His slides contain miniaturized artifacts—numbers—that carry the outside inside and, in the process, make that outside make sense to a specific audience (Callon 1986). In what follows, I juxtapose this story with a quite different scenario, one where numbers—good numbers by demographic standards—are available and present, but nonetheless fail to convince their audiences and lose momentum in the world, ultimately preventing meaningful inclusion of a risk group (MSM) in national AIDS policy.

In October 2008, I attended an NAC-sponsored conference in northern Malawi, held at a posh hotel. In the years leading up to 2008, NAC had publicly stated its commitment to finding novel ways to disseminate research findings to Malawian citizens, and this conference was a pioneering effort.[16] This commitment emerged from ongoing discussions, particularly at the 2005 Research Council Meeting, that centered on how to ensure that community-based organizations (CBOs), coded as the grassroots, might best benefit from the information collected by government and outside research endeavors. As the research officer at NAC put it, NAC wished to allow people "who do not have the opportunity or means to attend the national meetings" to "hear" what was said there, behind closed doors.[17] The conference's main objective was to "discuss key findings of surveys . . . conducted in the country [Malawi]." A diverse group of individuals representing the grassroots was invited to this first meeting: chairpersons of CBOs, members of district AIDS coordinating committees, district HIV programming officers, and so on, all drawn from in and around the northern district where it was held. In order to ensure that financial barriers did not prevent these people from attending, NAC paid for participants' accommodation and transport.[18]

About forty people attended the conference, and the presenters included NAC's research officer and a collection of Malawian, American, and Canadian demographers and other AIDS researchers.[19] Amid the various Power-Point presentations that researchers shared with the audience, one, given by a researcher-activist stood out. Felix, cofounder of a human rights NGO in Malawi, presented findings from a cross-sectional study of the behaviors of MSM in Malawi. As Felix set up his presentation and projected its title on a slide, the audience chuckled. The member of an AIDS prevention CBO sitting next to me mumbled under his breath, "There are none of these MSM here [in Malawi]!" This claim—alongside similar sentiments expressed by other audience members throughout Felix's presentation—directly contradicted Felix's central claim: that "MSM are more significant in Malawi's epidemic than ever imagined."

Felix, expecting negative reactions to his presentation, came equipped with numbers as his major source of evidence. He began his presentation by locating his findings in a larger landscape of comparative quantitative data on MSM in other nearby countries. Aware that his audience might be unfamiliar with the acronym "MSM," he explicitly defined it. Next, he presented the statistical evidence to support his claims about MSM vulnerability and risk. Explaining that the data came from a larger four-country study, he led the audience through the numbers on his slides: HIV seroprevalence for MSM in Malawi was around 21 percent. Accompanying this statistic were absolute numbers and the confidence interval for the data (42/200, 95 percent confidence interval). Felix elaborated on the gravity of the situation for MSM in Malawi. They faced, for example, low access to health care (only 10 percent had disclosed to health professionals that they were MSM), and MSM's high perception of AIDS as their main health risk was cited as evidence that interventions should be targeted at this risk group. Finally, Felix's data indicated that MSM were often beaten, raped, or afraid to come out. Numbers—the primary props in Felix's presentation—were framed by a set of accompanying scripts and actors drawn from other contexts: for example, new infections in MSM comprised 10–15 percent of the global AIDS burden.

Taken together, all of these numbers aspired to status as evidence that prevalence of HIV in MSM in Malawi is higher than generalized national prevalence, which was, at the time, around 12 percent. Other statistics presented alongside prevalence data drew on findings from a structured survey with respondents and aimed to bolster his claim that social stigma against MSM makes them invisible and excludes them from prevention messages targeted at other risk groups in Malawi. Felix called for sensitization of policy makers, HIV/AIDS key players, and other stakeholders, and for research that would explore sexual behaviors, practices, and social stigma experienced by MSM in Malawi. In addition, Felix suggested Malawi was far behind its near neighbors in accepting LGBT persons and achievement of human rights.

The numerical evidence cited in Felix's presentation to this audience was drawn from a multicountry study of MSM living in Malawi, Namibia, and Botswana. Participants in all three countries were recruited by community organizations working with this population who utilized snowball sampling to, in the case of Malawi, source 202 MSM-identified males for HIV screening and administration of a structured survey instrument. Notably, although the study was approved by the IRB of Johns Hopkins University, ethical approval was sought locally from the NAC in Malawi, but no response was given after many months, a fact that the authors of published research on the study and Felix himself attributed to possible aversion to the politically unsavory material of the study in a homophobic country (Baral et al. 2009). Symbolically, this chain of events stands in to demonstrate the noncommitment at the national level to issues related to MSM as a risk group.

In front of the audience at the conference, Felix's evidence failed. While those present, for the most part, were not policy makers and had very little influence over whether or how evidence might make it into policy, they nonetheless stood in for the commodified grassroots to whom evidence in the policy-research nexus should circulate and represent. First, the degree of departure of his claim from prior, tacit knowledge held in common by those in the audience was significant. When Felix described the main avenue of transmission for MSM (anal sex), for example, audience members responded with visible shock and moral outrage, calling anal sex unnatural and expressing disgust. "That doesn't happen here!" one woman shouted from the back. While audience members persisted in establishing Malawi as a decent nation where homosexuality does not exist, Felix tried to diffuse their outbursts with his numerical evidence. Nonetheless, the numbers on the screen challenged powerfully held convictions that served as a moralized and staunch evidence base for the counterclaim that MSM do not exist within Malawi.

In mobilizing this moral evidence, audience members employed two main tactics to discredit Felix's numbers: (1) attacking the credibility or motives of the researcher; and (2) questioning the quality of the evidence itself. Felix was asked twice to disclose his sexual orientation and accused of harboring a hidden political or other mission. Attacking the evidence he presented, one man called the presentation "hearsay," asking, "How can you put this on paper? What is your *proof*?" The calling into question of this evidence drew on personal experience of the audience members, who insisted that they had never seen or heard of men having sex with men. A pastor in the audience stood up and began loudly preaching against homosexuality, calling the MSM research "unscriptural," and suggesting that it was upon seeing MSM that God burned down Sodom and Gomorrah. It was clear—in the rhetoric—that Felix's numerical proof of MSM HIV prevalence, carrying with it the assumed route of same-sex transmission, offended the moral and religious convictions of most of those present. The emotional politics of homophobia, we might suggest, make its propagators "impervious to arguments and evidence" that might unravel their affective investments in the status quo (Ioanide 2015, 6).

Although this presentation generated the most conversation in the halls of the conference venue that day, it was by far the most conclusively invalidated by the audience. Despite the quality of Felix's numbers—by the epistemic standards of demographers or epidemiologists, and reflected by their publication in peer-reviewed journals—they did not gain traction in the room but fell flat. Despite this poor reception, an NAC officer approached Felix after the presentation and suggested he apply for NAC monies to do more studies. Over lunch, however, Felix shared that he had already submitted materials to NAC for their review but had not heard back from them for many months. Historically, he elaborated, the government had been very unsupportive of efforts to educate and mobilize MSM. As mentioned earlier, the study he was presenting was possible only because he relied on the cooperation, funding, and influence of an elite foreign university. While NAC endorses evidence-based policy and typically takes numbers as the pinnacle of evidence, they stalled in disbursing support or money to Felix, capitalizing on their ability as a public trust to publicly endorse transnational causes or fads but privately exert power over where pooled donor monies would flow once they arrived in Malawi.[20]

Importantly, however, the rejection of Felix's evidence gave the same knowledge claim legitimacy on other stages where it likewise sought to enroll supporters. Though his paper met a similar reception when he presented it a few months earlier at a conference in Lilongwe, Malawi's capital, he also said the paper had "really helped [him] move around." Felix had, in 2008 when we first met, recently traveled to workshops in Mexico, Geneva, Zambia, South Africa, and so on to present his findings to audiences there. Because MSM and HIV was a hot topic for epidemiologists and global health researchers and practitioners, Felix was frequently abroad in the United States for trainings associated with the multicountry study the NGO was implementing: we met up a number of times when he was visiting major northeastern American cities in 2009 and 2010. Following the 2009 global attention to the arrest, conviction, and ultimate release of a Malawian same-sex couple, Felix and his NGO garnered increasing support from outside funders and organizations, achieving a kind of agency through local victim-hood or suffering (Hoad 1999). Soon after the event, Felix said, "After all this publicity, NAC can no longer ignore our evidence. . . . They have to pay attention!"[21]

Though "people engaged in same-sex sexual relations" were first mentioned in Malawi's National HIV/AIDS Policy (NAC 2003) in 2003—albeit only cursorily—they were not allocated funds for prevention or treatment by the NAC until 2013. When NAC delayed disbursing the NGO's first payment installment, Felix had to warn them he would go "directly to the Global Fund" if he didn't receive it soon. By 2014, a survey and HIV-test study of MSM driven by respondent-driven sampling (RDS) was under way in Malawi, headed by the NGO and funded and supported by an American research university, UNAIDS, and PEPFAR. In July 2014, the NGO was negotiating with another major American research university to set up a research partnership that would also include capacity building and educational exchanges for local staff. However, according to Felix, although NAC is very interested in the data from the RDS study—it is important for national AIDS bodies to present good evidence to donors that they are working on and with key populations—they had not provided the NGO with, for example, a car to help with the rural sampling.[22] Further, in 2014, the NGO was lobbying for inclusion of lubricants in the national list of essential drugs because they are crucial to preventing HIV/AIDS transmission among MSM.[23] When NGO staff were invited to comment on the draft of Malawi's most recent National Strategic Plan, they made comments throughout the document to draw attention to this need; an officer at the NGO had to aggressively push for the "lubrication question" to be put on NAC's agenda in July 2014. The policy document that resulted from these discussions does suggest that lubricants will be targeted at "key populations" (NAC 2014, 45).

The failure of Felix's numbers demonstrating the gravity of the HIV epidemic among Malawian MSM to convince both grassroots and national-level audiences, who dismissed them and dragged their feet in responding to their call, respectively, pokes a hole in the hegemony of statistics in convincing, swaying, or impressing audiences. Indeed, even if the numbers attained validity when measured by epistemic standards, their circulation was either blocked or slowed through spaces in the policy-research nexus in which moral commitments trumped epistemic goodness. Felix's numbers did not come to inform policy meaningfully until the political context was fertile to accept them. Since 2008, when he first presented data from the study of MSM to national audiences, his NGO has intensified their evidence-based activism, relying primarily on foreign partners to fund and support research on HIV in MSM populations that will produce data and information that can be used to lobby for more inclusive policies, more funding, and so on (Wirtz et al. 2013). This strategy has borne fruit, at least partly due to Malawi's dependency on donors and international actors who are sympathetic to the cause of gay rights in Malawi and in the wake of NAC-gate, a scandal that compelled the state organization to make explicit in proposals to the Global Fund its commitment to key populations including LGBT persons living in Malawi (Wroe 2012; Chanika, Lwanda, and Muula 2013; Biruk 2014a).[24] Thus MSM are marginalized but not marginal to the global AIDS response, largely due to the role of international actors in developing and diffusing the MSM category, which produces an array of social relations and transactions in the policy-research nexus (McKay 2016; see also van de Ruit 2012, on the category "orphan" in South Africa).

The Policy-Research Gap

Thus far, this chapter has taken interest in how, where, and why data become evidence, and, in particular, how quantitative data make their way (or do not) into policy in the era of evidence-based policy. I have shown, through the presentation of the case of Blessings's ghost numbers and Felix's failed numbers, the processes—external to the data itself—that determined whether and when data became evidence that could justify decisions whether or not to include cultural practices and MSM, respectively, in national policy as sites of intervention and attention. While it is clear that "numbers are god"—as a Malawian colleague at the Centre for Social Research told me in 2007—in global health worlds, they also require specific cultural and social scaffolding or packaging in order to perform their "god trick," that is, to appear completely and autonomously detached from their context of production or from the subjects who handle and use them (Haraway 1988, 582).

Evidence, especially in the form of statistics, is often used to rationalize action or intervention, and its construction often eliminates the background factors and processes that elevate it to be taken seriously or for granted. As Goldenberg (2006, 2623) suggests, biases that underlie the processes that characterize evidence's context of discovery are often eradicated from the "purifying process of the context of justification." A closer ethnographic look at the everyday, mundane ways in which two kinds of claims made it into national AIDS policy indicates, however, that the path between the office where numbers are made from raw data collected in the field and the downstream sites of the policy-research nexus is not straightforward. In the case of cultural practices, for example, we observe how a knowledge claim continues to find its way into national policy, despite the absence of high-quality data that we might expect would be needed to justify its inclusion. Evidence, in this case, takes the form of ghost numbers. Meanwhile, in the case of the long noninclusion of Malawian MSM in national policy, we observe how the presence of well-collected, clean numerical data failed to serve as convincing evidence in front of audiences ranging from local community-based organizations to national-level policy makers. In both cases, numbers—even as they are now outside the hands of data collectors—continue to be cooked as they move further along their life course and into policy or papers. Numbers, despite their power, are not endowed with fixed authority but are enlisted into ongoing contests of credibility between social actors and within performative contexts. Notably, credibility contests in the policy-research nexus not only arbitrate the value of numbers or other evidence by assessing their proximity or distance from shared scientific standards, but also reveal the ever-shifting interests of the actors who enlist them into claims.

In the examples presented thus far, the ideal of good research making its way into national policy often faces challenges when it enters the local networks and social relations of the policy-research nexus: there is a gap, I suggest, between research and policy, confounding the underlying assumption of evidence-based policy making, as articulated nicely by an officer at Malawi's NAC: "[Policy and research] is a constant back and forth. Back and forth."[25] Yet this officer, and many other Malawian and foreign researchers, donors, and policy makers, agreed that the policy-research gap was a major problem in need of attention. Closing the gap was very much on the minds of actors in global health worlds in 2008 and continues to be up to the present. This gap is conceived of as a space of nontranslation, a chasm of sorts, between policy makers and researchers, between those who would use and those who produce data. Closing this gap has been prioritized in international and na-

tional research and development agendas. For example, the National HIV/
AIDS Action Framework (GoM 2004, 35–36) active in 2007–2008 included
in its budget funds for research and development, and the relevant section
of the framework emphasizes dissemination of research findings that can inform programming and interventions, evaluating policy making and program
development in light of research findings, and presenting summaries of au-
thenticated HIV/AIDS research to decision makers and policy makers. This
investment, monetary and rhetorical, aims to build bridges between research
and policy via dialogue, translation, and dissemination of information.

Dialogue between policy makers and researchers is framed as a key anti-
dote to the gap. The investment in dialogue often results in forums such as
conferences, advisory boards, partnerships, or workshops where both sides
in the policy-research nexus can effectively communicate, share information,
and network, despite their differences. Members of both sides articulated the
nature of the gap between them. A clinical researcher, Dr. Hanson, for a major
tropical medicine research collaboration between a European university and
Malawi's College of Medicine, suggested, "Malawi's no different to the U.K.
in that policy makers want quick answers . . . their focus is not on scientific
rigor; their focus is on access to some information that will allow them to
make a decision quickly. . . . I think the policy makers see [researchers as] a
lot of ivory tower–type people who lack a perspective on real life, and probably academic researchers see policy makers as sort of politically driven, affected by winds of change, people who just shoot from the hip."[26]

His comments on the differences he sees between policy makers and
researchers serve two functions. First, they reinforce the gaps between policy and practice or policy and research. As he explains it, the needs, interests, and orientations of policy makers and researchers are divergent. The
former are "affected by the winds of change" and "shoot from the hip" and
the latter "lack a perspective on real life," stuck as they are in an "ivory tower."
The kinds of expertise inherent to each category of person relies on binaries
similar to those that differentiate the foreign and Malawian collaborators
with MAYP and LSAM we encountered in chapter 2: whereas policy makers
and those preoccupied with the real world might collate or refer to studies or
research in their policy making, they are not the ones who engage in the intellectual labor necessary to produce good data and may even be unable to differentiate between good and bad data. His comments suggest similar dynamics
between researchers and policy makers in the United Kingdom and Malawi,
but they also index the inequalities between Malawian researchers who feel
they are mere rubber stamps on proposals and foreign researchers who enjoy

the time and resources necessary to engage in basic academic research. Further, while research in Malawian global health worlds often carries an implicit association with foreigners, policy denotes the nationally bounded container of Malawi and refers to the technocrats who aim to govern it.

Later, Hanson reflected explicitly on what he termed the "policy-research gap": "What we don't have is a good, frequent dialogue between ourselves and policy makers. There's an initiative . . . to develop research infrastructure [and] to improve the communication back and forth between policy makers and researchers. . . . But of course it has to be two ways. We [the project] try to send representatives [to relevant conferences] whenever possible. I hope our science communication officer we just hired will open some of those channels."[27] The differential habitus of the ideal-type researcher and policy maker he mentions contributes, then, to the lack of dialogue between the two. The closed channels that impede effective back-and-forth between them are framed by Hanson—and my other informants—as a problem in need of solutions to open channels and close the gap. In the case of his project, a technical working group meant to improve communication, a research capacity-strengthening initiative, and the research partnership itself were cited as initiatives to improve communication. These efforts mirror the capacity building of projects such as LSAM and MAYP, indicating that the policy-research gap is likewise a gap between wealthy projects and researchers and Malawian collaborators, whether researchers or policy makers.

On the other side of the gap, policy makers likewise identified a communication problem. One self-identified Malawian policy maker called Mr. Manda, whose main task is compiling and synthesizing research studies to inform policy, told me, "[There is] antagonism between policy makers and researchers. Researchers [in the past] were sort of standing aloof. . . . 'We are the academicians' and what have you. [There is] very little effort to involve the policy makers, but nowadays . . . when you are setting the research agenda, the policy maker[s] are [involved]. Everybody is involved. So when a piece of work [research] is done, it's something the policy maker was already looking for. So it's easy now to get [research] into policy."[28] He provided a specific example of how research gets into policy: "This afternoon we are leaving for Mangochi [a lakeside town in Malawi]; we are going for a think tank meeting because we want to develop an HIV prevention strategy. What should the country do in terms of HIV prevention? . . . We [draw on] different studies that have been conducted, such as an intensive study that covered all areas of HIV in Malawi. We will use . . . a number of research documents pertinent to the development of a good HIV prevention strategy."[29]

Manda's characterization of the policy-research gap resonates with Dr. Hanson's: researchers "stand aloof," which creates antagonism with the more practically minded policy makers. He notes, however, that this antagonism is on the decline and suggests that policy makers are now more meaningfully involved in ensuring that research will be useful prior to its execution. Interestingly, the idiom he uses for research ("a piece of work") points to commissioned research, which implies direct communication between researcher and end user, who directs the kinds of questions and methods necessary to answer a specific question. He suggests that he and his fellows at the think tank meeting will draw on "different studies" and "research documents" in charting a way forward for Malawi's HIV/AIDS fight. It is important to note, however, the diverse kinds of research and studies carried out in Malawi and by whom.

As discussed in chapter 1, many Malawian experts, including faculty members at the universities, find work moonlighting as project consultants. Such consultancies pay handsomely and, as Dr. Mponda suggested, are easier to secure and more quickly carried out than the kinds of research conducted by LSAM or MAYP, for example. A researcher hired to evaluate whether an NGO's home-based care intervention is working or not, or to conduct a literature review of a certain topic, for example, has a short deadline by which to complete the labor and submit a tangible report. These commissioned studies are more accessible to those who will be meeting in Mangochi than the published papers of LSAM, which find homes in academic peer-reviewed journals locked behind paywalls.[30] The form of the peer-reviewed article does not necessarily compel policy implications or recommended interventions by researchers, except perhaps as an afterthought in the concluding paragraph, as is evident in two published articles that draw on data collected by LSAM and GSIP in 2004–2006 and 2007–2008, respectively (Hennink and Stephenson 2005). Angotti et al. (2009, 6) suggest that confidential, convenient (door-to-door) HIV testing should be widely implemented to increase testing acceptance, and Baird et al. (2011) gesture toward policy makers in concluding paragraphs subtitled "Concluding Discussion and Policy Implications." Both journals, *Social Science and Medicine* and the *Quarterly Journal of Economics* were only accessible to the author via password.

Many of those present at the meeting in Mangochi have likely worked as consultants to many different projects, and are more likely to draw on that knowledge and experience—or that of close friends and colleagues who have done the same with other organizations—than they are to draw on findings that have been validated by rigorous disciplinary standards governing peer-review publication but are largely inaccessible to them, as both producers and consumers of knowledge who often face "nondiscursive" impediments to having their work published by journals based in the West (Canagarajah 1996). Finally, the very form of the commissioned report makes it easily accessible to people like Manda who must quickly get a sense of the field in his role as a policy maker. When one has little time, executive summaries and short reports are much more useful than jargony and lengthy research write-ups, though there is no guarantee that even the most efficiently packaged studies will be read or will come to inform policy (Justice 1986; Hennink and Stephenson 2005; de Waal 2015).

In recent years, there has been increased interest in creating synergy between researchers and policy makers, and in training the latter to quickly assess whether evidence is good or bad (e.g., the Knowledge Transition Platform in Malawi, a partnership between a medical and research NGO and Malawi's Ministry of Health; Berman et al. 2015). Finally, this kind of research, carried out and written up rapidly, accumulates quickly and circulates more easily than the more familiar long peer review process. Reports such as those to be studied in Mangochi are known as "gray literature," documents that are not formally published, not peer reviewed, transient in nature, and difficult to locate due to lack of an archive or incentive to preserve them (Gray 2013). Nonetheless, this gray literature would be highly accessible to local policy makers, many of whom might in fact be incentivized to attend meetings and workshops funded by donors where results are distributed. Conversely, noncommissioned (academic) research such as that of LSAM and MAYP is limited in its distribution to peer-reviewed journals or academic conferences, neither of which Malawian researchers nor policy makers are likely to have access to.[31]

The lack of a central storehouse in 2008 for research findings made accessing studies a piecemeal affair, even for a consultant hired to collate and review research on Malawi conducted in a set time frame and to identify gaps in need of attention (Mwapasa 2006). It is clear that policy is informed by evidence, but that what counts as evidence in the policy-research nexus is a social artifact, reflective of the social positions, interests, and economic constraints of those who craft it in social relations. As Feierman (2011) has shown for the case of clinicians working, respectively, in African government and American university hospitals, different concepts of evidence are not a result of culture but of the material conditions under which evidence can be put into action.

Closing the Gap?

Even as my informants across the policy-research nexus acknowledged the policy-research gap, they also invested time, energy, and funds in closing the gap. The connotations of the gap, as well, are capacious and exceed its reference solely to the chasm between the researchers and policy makers I met. Indeed, the gap speaks more generally to the divide between theory and practice, basic and applied research, and wealthy and poor countries. The NAC Zonal Conference where Felix's numbers failed, for example, is a symptom of government efforts to make their results more accessible to a broader range of participants, including those most affected by the knowledge and policies usually presented behind closed doors. As we saw in chapter 3, researchers are increasingly held accountable by their research subjects, who call upon them to share the information they collect, to invest more meaningfully in communities where they work for long periods of time, and so on. Academic research projects such as LSAM have made efforts to share the data they collect more meaningfully, to build the capacity of their local collaborators, and so on. For example, LSAM researchers consistently present findings at local AIDS conferences sponsored by NAC and the National Research Council. In March 2016, LSAM—with the help of funding from the Economic and Social Research Council—held a conference at the University of Malawi's College of Medicine on how longitudinal research might inform health and family policies after the peak of the AIDS epidemic. The conference included international and Malawian researchers, and focused on presentation of evidence that was "of potential importance for policy makers to develop new policy agendas to address . . . shifting health and demographic patterns."[32]

With help from a research project he consulted with, a senior colleague at the University of Malawi was funded to spend four months as a visiting scholar at a U.K. university. Though this opportunity was meant to allow him time to work on "[his] own projects" and have at his disposal the library and other resources of a major university in the global North, he recalled how his faculty host failed to make him feel welcome. He said he was given an office, but that it was largely useless to him because he didn't receive his school identification card for weeks and couldn't access the Internet on campus. He said he spent much of the four months seeking company with fellow Malawians not affiliated with the university but living nearby.[33] Endeavors such as these, and the many others like them, indicate the continued emphasis on closing the gap, networking, increasing dialogue, and information sharing and attempts to bring LSAM's findings in front of policy makers rather than storing them behind passwords in elite demographic journals. As mentioned earlier, LSAM's data are likewise publicly accessible for use.

Formal initiatives to close the gap—increased workshops, conferences, meetings, committees, and novel forms of data sharing—might paradoxically serve to exacerbate it: While these efforts appear to convincingly fill or shrink the gap, their effects are likely largely cosmetic, because they fail to address the larger structural politics that produce global health worlds as lopsided sites of collaboration and partnership. As Riles (2000) has shown, the discursive premium placed on networking is so high that quantity is emphasized over quality of such human connections. Klenk, Hickey, and MacLellan (2010, 954) subjected a large research network to social network analysis, finding that the benefits of belonging were unevenly distributed among different collaborators. This, too, is the case in global health research worlds, where one's relative benefit from and investment in research itself reflects one's position in a larger social field. Indicators used by NAC or research projects to measure improvements in communication and dialogue between policy makers and researchers include numeric counts of fora engaging policy makers and researchers. The fundamental knowledge structures that marginalize researchers in the global South, produce policy makers as mere wonks unable to properly assess or enlist good numbers or evidence, and maintain hierarchies of knowledge and power in global health worlds are not addressed by such broad metrics focused on countable measures of success.

Creating dialogue depends firmly on both parties being on equal footing. Policy makers' and researchers' different interests and habitus reflect the terrain of the social field in which they are formed, further visibilized by the politics of knowledge production in the policy research nexus. Foreign researchers for LSAM and MAYP, for example, are first authors on publications in prestigious journals in demography or economics, continue to attract funds for innovative research proposals, and make substantial decisions regarding data collection in Malawi. Malawian researchers, meanwhile, are second or third authors at best on such academic papers, flit from project to project and consultancy to consultancy, lack skills and time to write competitive proposals of their own, and become glorified policy makers. To measure to what degree the policy-research gap is shrinking, NAC also deploys indicators to count the number of policies that are informed by evidence. Yet even as policy may enfold more evidence, the specific nature of the evidence is left unevaluated, and the persistent gaps between North and South, academic journals and gray literature, and academic and applied research are reproduced even as indicators and metrics may perform their amelioration.

As this chapter has shown, the evidence produced by research does not come to those who would use it fully formed. Instead, it is cooked through interested performances and relations. Numbers indeed have a hegemonic grip on the imagination of actors ranging from demographers to policy makers, but numbers require packaging, props, framing, and translation to travel across boundaries and communities of practice or knowledge (Peterson 2009, 42). Whether numbers or other data become evidence is not just a factor of their epistemological rigor (Behague et al. 2009). Hodzic (2013) traces the interconnected and dispersed mechanisms of policy authorship by uncoupling acts of writing and interpretation of evidence from sovereign subjects. Whether our interest is in how numbers travel (or do not) into policy, or in how numbers are assembled in the field and travel to the office, nobody is fully in control (Hodzic 2013, 104); instead diverse actors along data's life course leave their mark on data that are variously described as cooked, clean, raw, or dirty. While evidence carries connotations of transparency, neutrality, and objectivity, and presumes clean data, this chapter has shown that evidence, quantitative or not, is as cooked in its sites of consumption as it is in its sites of production.

ANTHROPOLOGY IN AND OF
(CRITICAL) GLOBAL HEALTH

This book has considered data's social lives, focusing on how quantitative data reflect and cohere the social worlds from which they emerge. In tracing data's life course—beginning with the formulation of the survey in the office through the collection of data in the field and ending in the downstream sites where data aspire to become evidence—I have centered the many actors who help data along their life course, with particular focus on the knowledge work and expertise of fieldworkers. In the process, I have attempted to problematize assumptions of researchers from the colonial period to the present that fieldworkers are merely instrumental and interchangeable, unskilled cogs in larger research infrastructures. While such representations cast fieldworkers as unreliable and prone to mistakes that threaten to mess up or dirty data, I argue it is the innovative, ad hoc, and important body of expertise they develop as they live from project to project that makes research work.

Cooking data, usually leveled as an accusation against those who occupy the lowest rungs in survey worlds, presumes its opposite: raw data. This book has suggested that data that are clean or free of any social and cultural impurities is a fiction, but one that nonetheless undergirds demographers' dreams of high-quality data. From survey design to data collection to presentations of statistics at conferences or in policy, assembling data that will eventually become evidence is a process that reflects and reproduces demographers' culture and values, and their interest in clean, high-quality data. Cooking data, however, is a figure that helps us better understand survey research worlds as a space where liberties and necessity overlap, where standards for data collection are reinvented and modified, and where data come into being and gain meaning. Taken together, the chapters of the book show that survey projects I spent time with in 2007–2008 succeeded: by their own standards, they are good projects that managed to produce data evaluated as high quality upon completion (Krause 2014). Further, these data will inevitably come to justify more research projects in the future. Global health projects march onward, largely taking as their justification that no one can be against improving human health outcomes or reducing mortality from preventable diseases. Global health is reproduced—in its own and in popular narratives—as a progressive movement rooted in good evidence and with benevolent intentions.

Like many of its contemporaries in the genre of critical global health studies, this book was conceived with the assumption that the final account would manifest the insights of an ethnographer of global health science skeptical and suspicious of the intentions and politics of global health: it would act as a critique of the kinds of global and universalizing projects that have become anthropological fodder in the wake of Ferguson's (1994) *The Anti-politics Machine*. Yet even as this book has been critical of numbers and survey projects, it does not aim to represent the world better than they do but rather to show what kinds of worlds come about through numbers, raw, cooked, or otherwise. Medical anthropologists proffered their expertise on culture and local people to colonial governments and others to expedite local populations' adoption of biomedicine; the discipline's place in contemporary global health has likewise long been to broker cultural knowledge, to translate between insiders and outsiders, or to give advice on how to make global projects work better (Baer 1990; Scheper-Hughes 1990). In the shift from colonial health to global health, the role of the anthropologist, too, has shifted: from provision of local knowledge or culture as things to be altered or replaced by biomedicine, to provision of local knowledge or culture as necessary context for global health's interventions and science. Anthropologists were called upon, for example, to share their expertise—and attain "relevance"—during the 2014 Ebola epidemic, largely to help bring knowledge of context to global health's urgent importation of templates, logics, and technologies (Beisel 2014; Henry and Shepler

2015; Benton 2017). Yet applying our expertise on culture to real-world problems sits alongside what Eve Sedgwick (2003, 141) terms a "negative" orientation to our objects of study, a critical impulse to expose, for example, global health's shortcomings, problematic logics, and hierarchies of knowledge, and to foreground its historical continuities with colonial health projects. In other words, for some anthropologists, the enduring call to provide necessary context for interventions or projects may be more worthy of critique than response; being useful sits in tension with being critical.

The rhetoric and form of anthropological theorizing today—and the payoff of ethnographic evidence itself—often presumes the anthropologist's privileged access to interpretive and critical modes of knowing better (say, about how to improve health outcomes or how to effectively measure this improvement) than the informants: The ideal-type medical anthropologist's role in global health seems to be to hold tensions contingently together, forge shaky order from them, and say something useful about them. Yet our informants today are not always or only the traditional healers, villagers, or chiefs whom global health sees as its subjects, but rather the clinicians, scientists, intermediaries (such as fieldworkers, community health volunteers, nurses), and health officials who devise and implement projects. Like neoliberalism, global health and its effects have become objects of study and frameworks for understanding our other objects of study in anthropological work (Ortner 2016, 51).

The conjugation of critical with global health necessitates shifts in the anthropologist's method, theory, and location that have important consequences for knowledge production. It is the easy juxtaposition of anthropology and demography, of anthropologists and global health scientists, and of qualitative and quantitative knowledge that makes critique the purview of the anthropologist. Following Foucault (1997b), critique is a practice invested in maintaining and performing a distance and difference from its objects. This difference is rooted in disciplinary norms for what counts as good data. The anthropologist fortunate enough to have access to grants or other funds has the privilege of slow time: he or she can spend a year or two in the field, while the projects being studied (global health) are constrained by funds that devalue long-term fieldwork, by disciplinary norms for data collection and analysis, and by the questions they are interested in answering. This is evident in the fact that my time in the field was too long to be able to spend time with only one project: in the time I was in Malawi, I was able to do fieldwork with four projects that remained in the field only as long as they needed to collect timely data (a few months each). Survey projects such as the ones in this book are governed by norms of timely data, by the need for standardized data, and by an investment in clean data. Anthropologists, on the other hand, take their time, celebrate messy or dirty data, and see questions not as conclusively answerable (especially with numerical data alone) but as provocative of new questions. The anthropologist surrenders control of the field, while the demographer seeks to control the field even from afar. Surveys collect data in standardized form; they order it as they digest it into databases. Anthropologists, meanwhile, chew on data for a long time, only ever coming to contingent order after dwelling in their raw field notes.

In general, literature authored by anthropologists of global health embodies critique in two main ways: (1) through para-ethnography or studying of global health experts, logics, and spaces of interventions such as clinics, laboratories, NGOs, humanitarian organizations, and hospitals characteristic of the projectification of the global South (Rottenburg 2009; Wendland 2010; Bornstein and Redfield 2011; Fassin 2012; Geissler 2013a; Whyte et al. 2013; Adams 2016a; McKay 2018); and (2) through fine-grained analyses of the effects or failures of state and other health projects on the ground, with particular attention to foregrounding the suffering and trauma of the world's downtrodden and precarious (Farmer 2004; Biehl 2005; Knight 2015; Wool 2015; Briggs and Mantini-Briggs 2016).

Both strands presume the anthropologist as critic, ontologically reliant on the compulsion to make visible that which dominant systems and practices of intervention, representation, power and knowledge eclipse. This project inevitably reproduces, even as it is conscious of, the temporal and spatial politics of anthropological knowing. Adams and Biehl (2016, 124) suggest that critical global health "begins from the idea that ethnographic methods can highlight the conceptual and practical conundrums arising from contested notions of evidence and efficacy. The 'global' of global health must thus be interrogated as both a political accomplishment and a means of producing other kinds of evidence." Implicit in the call for anthropologists to interrogate the global in global health is, again following Foucault (1997b, 327), a call to detach oneself from it. As anthropologists of this global health, we necessarily produce Others in our projects of critique (Fabian [1983] 2002), and often neglect to explicitly acknowledge the ways in which we, too—as critics—are produced along the way. For those of us who "study up," for example, our difference— our ability to see more or better than our subjects or our audiences—rests on the kind of slow research that gains value in juxtaposition to the fast-paced, sloppy, universalizing, and generalizing imperatives of global health's dominant, quantitative ways of knowing (Nader 1972; Adams, Burke, and Witmarsh 2014). For those of us whose political interests lie in representing in words or images the suffering of the world's most vulnerable folks, escaping the weight of our discipline's legacy of speaking for others, of complicity with power structures, and of reproducing stereotyped versions of suffering others remains a herculean task (Butt 2002; Robbins 2013; Biruk 2016; Prince 2016).

Like the PowerPoint presentations, policy jargon, databases, and articles from demography journals featured in this book, this ethnographic study finds its place in a disciplinary genre of knowledge whose boundaries are continually reproduced and patrolled by its members. Like the numbers that are the currency of demographers, ethnographic representations gain value because they fit into a particular niche and reflect the values and interests of an epistemic culture that is so intimately linked to our aspirations to be good anthropologists that we may fail to see its operations: this is the blind spot of critique. Though *Writing Culture* (Clifford and Marcus 1986) ushered in an era of anthropologists studying themselves as they study others, the moment of the anthropology of global health is a fitting one in which to consider the social lives of our own data and to ask what kinds of selves we become as we make it. What particularities and dilemmas might the rise of the global health slot in anthropology bring for ethnographic method, theory, and the ethnographer (Biruk 2014b)? What does the invitation of anthropologists to the global health table portend for how we theorize, represent, and value our selves, writing practices, methods, and analytics? How can we maintain a critical orientation to global health's projects without being merely critics—if this is our goal? (Henry and Shepler 2015, 21; Puig de la Bellacasa 2011).

In what follows, I present two vignettes drawn from my field notes, turning the lens on myself and tracing the social lives of my ethnographic data. I take up some of the long-standing concerns of anthropologists—complicity, the field, and usefulness—considering them from the perspective of a contemporary ethnographer of global health. I hope this conclusion, read alongside the rest of the book, might raise some productive questions about doing anthropology in and of global health, and about the state of critique in anthropology more broadly.

Inventing the Field: A Fieldworker among Fieldworkers

John, Victor, and I left the RAM office around midday to map Anglican churches near the border of Mulanje District, inquiring along the way with people we passed. We were attempting to set up interviews for the next day with church leaders and their congregants, and RAM was in need of more Anglican-identified persons in its sample. The directions people gave us led us to churches that were not Anglican, but we ended up finding one and meeting with the church secretary, where we booked an appointment for interviews with church elders and worshippers two days later. On the way home from the field, we stopped at a bottle store, where we enjoyed a beer and shot billiards in front of a blaring TV playing South African music videos. "Don't tell Dr. Smith," they told me conspiratorially.[1]

This excerpt from my field notes captures a bit of fieldwork that usually does not appear in demographic or ethnographic representations: RAM supervisors and I take a break from fieldwork, siphoning time from the project without the knowledge of researchers. As I pen this conclusion, I am acutely aware of my affective orientation to the field: nostalgia for time well spent with people who have remained good friends and fond recollection of the adventurous unpredictability of data collection, which never looked the same from one day to the next. In this sense, my feelings resemble those of the fieldworkers whose rhetoric and practices literally create the field from which data will be collected. In this field, I was an object of ethnographic curiosity: I was a fieldworker among fieldworkers, and my presence in the field was a result of the resources and imperatives of survey projects, as much as it was the result of anthropological grants and training.

Having a beer at the Amazon bottle store and many other actions we partook of during long fieldwork days—playing bao with villagers, drinking tea in tearooms, shopping at traveling secondhand clothing markets, listening to or dancing to music emanating from crackling minibus speakers, buying local chicken to cook for dinner, lingering over long lunches of beef and chapatti, reading newspapers—are minor deviations from the order of things and do not appear to muck up or dirty data as they travel their life course. What interests me here is not exposing the ways in which field teams make do and find ways of making fieldwork more bearable, often by siphoning time and resources from projects: indeed, this siphoning is minor and largely irrelevant to the quality of data collected, and researchers often turn a blind eye to it. However, scenes such as these raise questions about the role and relationship of the ethnographer to her subjects, who constitute the slippery entity "global health." While much of this book has focused on the experiences of middlemen or mediators in survey research worlds, we see clearly in the bottle store scene that the anthropologist, too, occupies a liminal and mediating space in such worlds.

While anthropologists have long deconstructed the politics, affects, and intimacies that influence our accounts and re-presentations, few have explicitly considered how their ethnographic encounters manufacture knowledge, produce theory, and make new subjects (White and Strohm 2014). It is unsurprising that this book has largely narrated the experiences of fieldworkers. While few have closely examined this set of actors (allowing me to carve out a space for my scholarly work), it is important, as well, to note that my sympathies largely lie with fieldworkers: these were the people I spent most days with, empathized with, learned the most about and from, and found it easiest to befriend. It is through such relations, everyday practices, and conversations that I coconstructed the field that is at the core of this book even as I, at the time, felt committed to preserving my field as different from that of demographers and fieldworkers. My field was a space of critique, while theirs, I told myself, was one of business as usual. Yet I found myself primarily among other fieldworkers, who, like me, were engaged in their own critical projects that stemmed from their precarious and ambivalent position within global health's structures. The distribution of critique—as a form of interpretive labor—among different fieldworkers (those working for projects and myself, the anthropologist), however, is uneven. As others have shown, marginalized groups are persistent critics who tirelessly theorize their position in power structures, even if their interpretive labor is less legible than anthropological critique in academic circuits of recognition (Collins [1990] 2008).

The field has long been the purview of anthropologists, a spatial anchor for their trajectory of work, the site of theorizing or generalizing outward, the place where they were insiders, and, most importantly, the place on which they were experts (Wagner 1981 Fabian [1983] 2002; Gupta and Ferguson 1997; Marcus 1998; Weston 2008). Historically, for example, anthropologists are conjoined in narrations of our discipline with their field sites or regional specialty (and job advertisements are enduring artifacts of the persistence of a geographically bounded field). I hope this book has helped to further destabilize this space as a natural or taken-for-granted anchor of knowledge production and, in the process, our modes and methods of inquiry (Faubion and Marcus 2009). My field was very clearly not my own: it was a crowded place of multiple actors and interests in which I found myself entangled for some time. While such entanglements are not new, the nature of ethnography amid and within global health perhaps makes more visible the ethnographer's reliance on and complicity with the people, resources, logics, and technologies that make up the "global" she critiques (Street 2014). During my time with MAYP, for example, I resided in a house (that also served as the field office) paid for by MAYP with a demographer who was leading data collection as my roommate. As I saw how the field became a rhetorical container of culture and difference for the demographers and fieldworkers I spent time with, I also recognized that my metamethodology—following along with projects—came to likewise produce and legitimate this unit of knowledge production. As Simpson (2016, 327) reminds us, the roots of anthropological methods lie in the ethnological grid, the kinship chart, and other categories that contained and controlled difference to make it manageable for their needs: as an anthropologist among the demographers, too, I walked the same paths and employed ways of seeing similar to those of my fellow fieldworkers, effectively bounding and making manageable the field in which my potential data resided.

Rather than collecting genealogies of rural Malawians or making lists of local plants used in traditional healers' medicaments like my disciplinary (m)ancestors, however, I made marks in red pen on hundreds of surveys, typed up transcripts from focus groups, organized log books, dislodged project SUVs from mud, printed consent forms, helped fix flat tires, helped lead training sessions, and so on. Rather than living in a tent, alone on a beach like our old friend Malinowski, I lived at run-down inns or simple houses, sometimes alone, but more often alongside or with survey projects' staff members. Rather than staying in a single village for a year or more, in the spirit of global ethnography, I followed along with peripatetic projects without losing sight of how such projects reconfigured and remade the people and places they interacted with (Erikson 2011). All of this has consequences for the relationship between the anthropologist and global health today and for what kind of expertise the anthropologist is expected to have and provide. While the aspiration of anthropology to know what is really going on, whether in the spirit of applying that knowledge, of critique or of both, would seem to rely on a different relationship to the field than that of survey teams in the thick of it, what does it mean that the labor and locations of our fieldwork often overlap, are parasitical on, or reproduce the logics and practices of those we study in new and evolving ways (Neely and Nading 2017)? While I would argue that anthropologists have almost always been parasitical on other projects, the potential disjuncture between the kinds of expertise on culture demographers, clinicians, or development workers continue to expect us to possess and the kinds of expertise we feel comfortable sharing illustrates how anthropology's enduring place in the "savage slot" (Trouillot 2003) rubs awkwardly against its occupation of something like the global health slot (Biruk 2014b). For example, while this book has shown in detail how survey projects (which resemble in some important ways hundreds of other projects operating in Africa) do not so much intervene, treat, or change the contexts they enter into as they coconstitute them, the anthropologist is still expected to provide the kinds of cultural knowledge that can enhance or fit into culturally relevant programs and plans that take context for granted and reify the tropes of local and global. Further, this niche seems to presuppose that anthropologists have privileged access to a truer representation of the local than do others, even as they—in contrast to demographers—have long willingly acknowledged that their informants lie or share information tactically, not unlike some of the survey informants we have met in this book (Metcalf 2002).

On Being Useful

> Dr. Payson has asked me to help MAYP prepare a fact sheet to distribute to villagers. She sent the draft via e-mail and asked me to have the supervisors take a look at it and provide feedback on how to make it more relevant to villagers. The fact sheet is one page and contains basic statistical information about those surveyed by MAYP as part of their 2007 baseline survey in Salima. It includes, for example, facts such as "5 percent of young women and men live in households with a flush toilet," "43 percent of young women and men are currently in school," and "99 percent of the sample speak Chichewa." The sheet also contains three graphs. The first is a bar graph showing highest schooling level completed by gender and the other two are pie graphs indicating living arrangements and religious affiliations, respectively. When I showed it to MAYP supervisors, they suggested that the bar graph would not be understood by villagers and that the facts listed could contain more context and interpretation.[2]

In addition to recording field notes for my own use down the line, I often provided project researchers with feedback I thought might be useful to them. For example, I informed LSAM and MAYP researchers that people in the field (including not only villagers in the sample but also district officials) often suggested they wished to hear back from projects about what they found after analyzing all the surveys. When I accompanied the LSAM field supervisors and American data collection supervisor to the district offices in Mchinji to meet with the district commissioner and introduce the project, for example, he inquired whether LSAM would be sharing the results so "district staff [could] find out what [they found]."[3] That same day, when we visited the police station to inform them of our presence, the officers likewise inquired whether LSAM would tell them what they found. The district commissioner complained that they never heard anything about the results of all this research, even as the projects came back to the same villages year after year. In response to similar critiques, MAYP decided to design a simple fact sheet to be distributed to the district offices and shared with traditional authorities or respondents in future waves of survey research. Via e-mail correspondence with the MAYP principal investigators in the United States, I was asked to provide feedback on this draft fact sheet, in collaboration with fieldwork supervisors. In addition to the supervisors' feedback documented above, I also suggested that the researchers aim to break down the statistics further to the level of neighborhood, since people in the district espoused strong neighborhood identities.

As an anthropologist among the demographers, I felt acutely the need to be useful. I took on a role as a project fieldworker and engaged in the daily labor practices associated with this role to carry my weight and not to be a burden. (I also had to negotiate between being the eyes and ears of demographers and my loyalties to fieldworkers.) In this sense, I helped produce high-quality data—the very numbers anthropologists are rightfully suspicious of. In the field notes excerpt above, we see another way in which I was invited to make myself useful to projects. I helped brainstorm ways that they might more effectively build trust with respondents over time. Yet, having read chapter 3, the reader can infer that what rural Malawians really want from projects is not a mere fact sheet, even if they do say they want to know what the research finds. These calls for results, for hearing back about the data they provide, act as an idiom in which participants express their deeper frustrations with lopsided interactions between wealthy researchers and poor villagers, and with the lack of change they see in their communities. Like the critique of the gift of soap, the call for more information is a symptom of how global health research inevitably reproduces the asymmetries it seeks to redress.

All this said, then, it is unclear whether I can claim making fact sheets as an example of something useful I did in the field. Despite the long duration of my fieldwork and hundreds of pages of field notes collected in 2007–2008, nor can I adequately or quickly answer the simple question demographers often ask when they hear me present my work: "So, what can we do better?" This question reflects the long history of anthropologists' collaboration with medicine and public health, particularly in African contexts, and aims to embrace the nuanced, contextual, and cultural information that is the purview of the anthropologist as a way to improve numbers, fine-tune data collection, figure out why people are not taking medicines, and collect input from target populations (McKay 2018). Yet thirty years after Justice (1986) provided anthropologists concrete suggestions for presenting their findings more effectively to planners, we continue to fail by others' and our own standards: our work has not really revolutionized medicine, global health, or development. In fact, by these metrics, the critical development studies and medical anthropology literature—much of which has, since the 1990s, documented how grand projects fail—is also an archive of anthropologists' own continued failure to be useful in the strong sense we may aspire to.

Perhaps amid all this hand-wringing about failure and not being useful, the moment of critical global health studies might prompt us to ask not how we might succeed but rather what kinds of rewards the failure to be useful can offer to us as a discipline (and to global health more broadly) (Halberstam 2011). What can we learn from our own supposed failure to be useful amid what Kingori and Sariola (2015) term the "museum of failed [HIV] research," for example? Global health, demography, and other projects rooted in quantitative data, timeliness, and standardization presume success to be measurable. Anthropology—and in particular its critical relationship to global health—can help us retheorize failure and its relationship to knowledge production. The enduring potential of an ethnographic mode of critique, I suggest, lies in the figure of the fieldworker, betwixt and between, fetishizing neither the convincing logics and success stories of global health, nor overstating the (possibility of) resistance or counteractions of those in its belly. The fieldworker—whether the anthropologist or Malawian data collector at the center of this book—is well aware of the ambiguities and blind spots on which dichotomies like success/failure, global/local, quantitative/qualitative, and outside/inside are built, and negotiates them carefully without resolving or settling them as he or she lives from project to project.

As long as they have been expected to improve or fix misconceived health projects, anthropologists have struggled to escape their disciplinary habitus and writing practices. Margaret Read, for example, was the official anthropologist on the Nyasaland Survey in the late 1930s. Carried out in the very same geographic territory as some of the surveys discussed in this book, the survey was the result of new colonial enthusiasm around systematic, survey-based research into nutrition and its implications for colonial development. The surviving papers suggest its grand ambitions: "The results of the Survey will be of value to everyone interested not merely in the nutrition but in the general welfare of backwards peoples not only in Africa but in all parts of the world" (Berry and Petty 1992, 17). Dr. B. S. Platt, trained in chemistry and medicine, was chosen to lead the survey in Nyasaland, one of Britain's poorest dependencies. Read, at the time she was invited to join the survey, was in Nyasaland—in the field—finishing independent field research among the Ngoni as part of her course of study in anthropology at the London School of Economics. Read and Platt's relationship was full of tension and disagreement that centered on the former's investment in ethnographic data, as it sat uneasily with the latter's interest in careful quantitative measurement of land held, crops planted, labor expended, and food eaten. The quantitative investments and methods underlying Platt's survey took easy precedence over Read's slower-form anthropological study, which ended up being a wholly unintegrated appendage to Platt's main report (not very useful, we might say). Read's study, like qualitative data today, was framed, in the words of a Malawian sociologist and colleague of mine reflecting on anthropology, as a mere "side dish" to survey or quantitative data, echoing Justice's (1986, 148) informants in Nepali health bureaucracies who saw sociocultural information as soft data. The well-documented tensions between Platt and Read are perhaps a factor less of clashing personalities than of their habitus as a demographer and an anthropologist and their celebratory and suspicious relationship to quantitative data, respectively (cf. Brantley 2003).

The Colonial Office's interest in knowing about rural African nutrition stemmed from a desire for data that described local conditions before initiating development efforts, a precursor to today's evidence-based policy. In fact, Platt's goal as the head of the survey was to utilize the data collected in the service of future development projects. He was enthusiastic about this agenda, proposing a development project in the form of the Nutrition Development Unit even before the problematic data—dirtied by difficulties in measuring crop yields, labor, and nutritional value of foods—were analyzed (Deane 1953; Brantley 2002, 68); Berry, the appointed head of the unit, was never furnished with a copy of Platt's report and lacked access to any of the voluminous data collected, despite his repeated pleas in letters to Platt in the early 1940s (Berry and Petty 1972, 286–289). Considering the ambitions of Platt's proposed development agenda—which included agricultural education, nutritional education, maternity care and dispensaries, fisheries improvement, and provision of demonstrations outside Kota Kota District, among other things—the project was widely considered a failure and left behind few trained personnel and no infrastructure (Brantley 2002, 140–141, 152).

With hindsight, we see that the survey's ambitions to use or apply evidence to stage better interventions were not fulfilled. It left little material mark on the landscape, but, as Brantley (2002, xiii) found when she revisited survey villages in the early 1990s, villagers recalled a female researcher they nicknamed "Mwadyachiyani?" (What have you eaten?, in Chichewa) coming to fill in boxes and write down things they said. Research, then, even if it fails—in the eyes of anthropologists critical of its logics and forms, fieldworkers critical of its exploitative labor practices, or villagers critical of its failed promises— leaves an indelible, if less visible, mark on the landscapes it traverses. Research participants, fieldworkers, and the anthropologist are made and remade as they interact with data in their various forms. Data come to reflect the people and places they emerge from, and also redirect their imaginations and cultivate expectations. Rather than exposing the failures and shortcomings of global health's grand ambitions, or revealing the flaws in the evidence its practitioners spend much time and energy collecting, a less negative mode of critique might entail telling some of global health's other stories, those not only eclipsed by but constituted by the fetishization of numbers that produces more and more projects. Numbers—and the standards by which they are evaluated—not only misrepresent real worlds but make new ones. In this book, I have tried to keep data themselves at the center of the story, without losing sight of the people, places, and things that cohere around them. In this sense, I hope I have succeeded in telling another kind of story through and about medical anthropology in Africa today (Mkhwanazi 2016).

Having spent much time around anthropologists of global health (an anthropologist among the anthropologists), I am struck by our shared culture of critique and the techniques of the self it manifests. We unearth, uncover, unpack, deconstruct, expose, and bring into relief: nuancing has long been the favored activity of the anthropologist, and it is worth thinking with Healy (2017, 121) how nuance itself might be a manifestation of disciplinary virtue and distinction that risks becoming a species of "self-congratulatory symbolic violence," an aesthetic gesture or in-group performance. Yet amid all of this, we compel ourselves to be useful, presuming too much nuancing to be the opposite of utility. Pfeiffer and Nichter (2008, 412–413), for example, call upon us to be better at reaching our audiences: "In the anthropologists' traditional roles as culture brokers, we are often better positioned . . . to document and contextualize the effectiveness of health services as they impact people's lives." Hemmings (2005, 97) likewise suggests that anthropologists "need to produce evidence that their ideas can improve outcomes" and that "anthropology is failing medicine." While applied anthropology arguably occupies a marginalized position in the academic hierarchy, where theory is the goal, we nonetheless continue to witness the call for anthropologists to put their theories to good use—to intervene—especially during times of crisis and emergency such as epidemics, war, or mass displacement (Calhoun 2010).

"Documenting and contextualizing" (Pfeiffer and Nichter 2008, 413) are the stuff of ethnographic method, and the major medium in which anthropology has found a role as a complement to science and established its niche as unflagging critic amid the global health boom, as a review of the growing literature suggests (Packard 2016). As teachers, too, anthropologists speak to increased student interest in the topic and the rise of voluntourism, and find collaborators in the rising number of global health centers on university campuses (Crane 2010b; Wendland 2012; Locke 2015; Sullivan 2016). A brief look at job ads for the past few years indicates high demand for those who can comment on, engage with, or analyze global health, and public health has risen as a core area of a new global health diplomacy (Kickbusch, Silberschmidt, and Buss 2007; Adams, Novotny, and Leslie 2008; Erikson 2008). Medical anthropologists reside in a global health slot from which they circulate critiques and commentary, one that, not unlike Trouillot's (2003) savage slot, relies on and reproduces the West and the rest, or the global North and the global South, with consequences for which places and people are included in global health's embrace (Brada 2011; Meyers and Hunt 2014). Africa, as Anna West (2016) suggests, *is* global health. Yet, not unlike Margaret Read's anthropological study back in the late 1930s, our knowledge often falls on deaf ears: it is clunky, complex, and doesn't fit neatly into the number-dominated spaces of global health. From the perspective of many of those who work in global health, ethnographic data are "at best anecdotal, at worst insignificant" (Ecks 2008, S77). But how might we provoke ourselves to imagine ways of being anthropological that are not governed quite so much by either the compulsion to critique and/or to be useful in particular ways (Foucault 1997c)?

Echoing Sedgwick's (2003) observations that the dominant mode of scholarly critique is rooted in a "negative" relation to our objects of study—disavowal, distance, skepticism—Fassin (2012) considers the difficulties of maintaining critical distance for the anthropologist of, in his case, humanitarian governance. Reflecting on his dual complicity with and critique of humanitarian organizations, he calls for a mode of critique that "includes us—individually and collectively—and not one that leaves the social scientist outside [Plato's allegorical] cave" (246). Similarly, Puig de la Bellacasa (2011, 92) urges us to think of and represent sociotechnical assemblages—such as the survey project—as "matters of care" to counter corrosive critique in the study of science and technology and to engage more intentionally with their becoming(s). She suggests that we not lose sight of how a "critical cut into a thing, a detachment of a part of the assemblage, involves a re-attachment"; in other words, critical cuts should not merely expose things, but foster caring and reparative relations (97). Caring about the things we critique entails resisting knee jerk disidentifications from them in order to tend to the daily practices through which they come into being. I have aimed to briefly account for a few of the ways in which I—an outsider to survey worlds—entered into, altered, and came to care about certain things and people I encountered in demographic research worlds. The experience was humbling, and close attention to the specific dimensions of doing ethnography of global health can, I think, call into being new forms of critique that are neither wholly inside nor outside, useful nor useless, negative nor positive. Colvin (2015, 102) invites anthropologists to find ways of doing anthropology that are not limited to becoming either a "culture expert" or an unflagging critic of neoliberal science. In a controversial essay, Nyamnjoh (2015) calls for a more thoroughly evidence-based anthropology, writing against what he sees as the discipline's increasingly salvationist impulses in Africa. As an anthropologist among the demographers, I came to understand my role as a caring critic whose aim is to show how all data, including our own, depend on the underlying framework against which they are evaluated as evidence and made meaningful (Lambert 2009). This mode of critique does not aim to look beyond numbers or to dismiss them (it is doubtful that demography or global health will ever be "without numbers"; Scheper-Hughes 1997), but to take seriously the ways in which they not only measure and claim to represent but also coconstruct the worlds and relations they emerge from. This moment in which anthropologists consensually malign the rising hegemony of numbers in global health and other neoliberal audit cultures seems a particularly apt one in which to take them ever more seriously, and to seek out ways of knowing and caring about numbers, and ourselves relative to them, more deeply.

Raw and Cooked: Coda

Underlying the trajectory of this book has been my interest in opening taken-for-granted descriptors of data such as raw and cooked that circulate in demographic cultures to empirical study. We have seen that raw data are a fiction that nonetheless determine the forms, relations, and practices of survey research worlds. I have playfully written against normative definitions of cooked data as bad or flawed by arguing that it is the innovative and flexible behaviors and practices that take root in research cultures that ensure the production of good numbers. Like the numbers we take for granted produced by projects such as LSAM and MAYP, this book converts raw data (e.g., field notes) into a polished, clean form that obscures the shifting positionalities adopted by the ethnographer that are influential on all stages of knowledge production (Dilger, Huschke, and Mattes 2015). Looking across all scales of research worlds, and especially at overlooked actors such as fieldworkers, helps us to see and understand better how and why numbers gain value and authority.

The potential of ethnographies of global health lies in their ability to challenge some of the dichotomies that underlie its formation and narration: global/local, science/culture, raw/cooked, office/field, and so on. Instead, then, of viewing global health and its local sites or researchers and research subjects (or even anthropologists and demographers) as distinct or autonomous formations that come into conflict or clash, it is useful to conceive of research worlds as contact zones, or social spaces where subjects usually distant from one another are copresent and intersect for some period of time (Pratt 1992, 6–8). Survey research worlds, for example, are places produced by and reflective of actors' investments in clean data. Research subjects, researchers, fieldworkers, policy makers, and the anthropologist are constituted in and through their relations to one another and to data themselves. While this book has been critical of numbers, it does not aim to represent the world better than they do, but rather to show what kinds of worlds come about through numbers, raw, cooked, and otherwise. Demographers and anthropologists might have more in common in the age of global health than we think. Both, to start, are "dependent on [their] [O]thers to know [themselves]," whether those "Others" are target populations partitioned into samples or the demographers and fieldworkers who do that partitioning (Pratt 1992, 4). Anthropological knowledge, too, is implicated in and harnessed to the socioeconomic and political processes we so easily associate with global health (Tilley 2007, 12). The mode of critique employed in critical global health studies must leave space, as well, for explicit discussion of how anthropologists come to know and see themselves as they navigate the same global health worlds as their subjects; we should not lose sight of the dimensions of our own ever-evolving critical subjectivity.

Andrews, a longtime fieldwork supervisor, once told me, "I don't think there are any [places in Malawi] that have not yet been researched. [Researchers] are everywhere here. Even me, I've been all over Malawi doing all manners of things, all different districts, everywhere." His words validate the sense one gets from reading the growing literature in critical global health studies: that projects are everywhere, parachuting in and setting up shop. Andrews also drives home an important insight of this book: research does not merely document or shape, but rather produces and coheres new worlds, subjectivities, expertise, and expectations. Tracking these processes should be as much the concern of the anthropologist as showing how global health and its evidence fails. Research makes data, but it makes people too. From the perspective of the field, one thing seems certain: Akafukufuku abweranso! The researchers (including anthropologists) continue to come, again and again.

SAMPLE HOUSEHOLD
ROSTER QUESTIONS

No.	Question Description

FULL NAME

Q1 Family and Household members
See instructions for listing of names above

RELATIONSHIP TO RESP

Q2 What is (name)'s relationship to you?

Q3 SEX

Is (name) male or female?
[M = 1 F = 2]

ALIVE?

Q4 Is (name) alive?
If (name) is dead, when did he/she die?
If (name) is dead, strike out Q5–Q16;
do not ask Q5–Q16 for persons who have died

AGE

Q5   How old is (name)?

OR, in what year was (name)

Born

Circle age or birth year

DK = 9999

If under 1 year, then age = 0.

REG MEM OF HOUSEHOLD

Q6   Where does (name) usually live?

Q7   Did (name) sleep here last night?

NO = 0

YES = 1

MOBILITY

Q8   When did (name) move to this place?

Ask <u>only</u> if Q6=1 or Q6=2

HEALTH

Q9   Has (name) been ill in the past 12 months?

IF YES: For how long?

Q10   How would you rate (name)'s health in general?

Q11   How would you compare (name)'s

health to other people in your village who are the same age and sex?

MARITAL STATUS

<u>IF AGE ≥ 10</u>

Q12   What is (name)'s current marital status?

<u>Probe current marital status if not currently married.</u>

<u>*IF MARRIED: To another household or family member?*</u>

<u>*WRITE LINE ID OF SPOUSE*</u>

EDUCATION

<u>IF AGE ≥ 5</u>

Q13 What is the highest level of schooling (name) attended?

Q14 How many grades (in years) did
(name) complete at that level?
[enter number of years]
DK/CR = 99

WORK

<u>IF AGE ≥ 15</u>

Q15 What is (name)'s main way of earning money?

SAMPLE HOUSEHOLD ROSTER

	Full Name	Relationship to Resp	Sex	Alive?	Age	
ID	Q1	Q2	Q3	Q4	Q5	
LINE ID	NAME	CODE	CODE	CODE	AGE OR YEAR OF BIRTH	
01	(=Resp.)	1		1	age	b-year
02					age	b-year
03					age	b-year
04					age	b-year
05					age	b-year
06					age	b-year
07					age	b-year
08					age	b-year
09					age	b-year

Reg mem of household		Mobility	Health			Marital Status		Education		Work
Q6	Q7	Q8	Q9	Q10	Q11	Q12		Q13 & 14		Q15
CODE	CODE	CODE	CODE	CODE	CODE	CODE	LINE ID	CODE	YRS	CODE

INTRODUCTION: *An Anthropologist among the Demographers*

1. All project and personal names in this book are anonymized. Because Malawi is a small country, the reader may be able to ascertain which projects are discussed here. Researchers were, for the most part, amenable to being mentioned by name and having their projects mentioned by name, but I maintain anonymity as much as possible in line with my IRB protocol. Data from my field notes or events that may put any of my informants at risk in any way are not included in the book.

2. In other contexts, fabricating data has also been called curbstoning, referring to sitting on a curb and completing a survey rather than visiting respondents (Koczela et al. 2015, 414).

3. In his analysis of the term "data," Daniel Rosenberg (2013, 18, 33) suggests that by the end of the eighteenth century, data lost its meaning as the basis of argument or scriptural facts that could not be contested and gained connotations as the result rather than the premise of investigation; data today are the product of experiment, experience, or collection and carry no assumptions about veracity in their rhetorical form.

4. In other words, I seek to excavate the ways in which knowledge statements are made legible in a discursive community disciplined by its loose unification beneath the term "demography" (Foucault 1972). In shifting focus from individual sovereign knowers and thinking the subject as a function of discourse, we gain insight into the disciplining of knowers, whether demographers or anthropologists, by the weight of their learned notions of good and bad ways of knowing, writing, and thinking (Foucault [1969] 1998). Among demographers, not only was my training as an anthropologist more acutely felt, but so too did I recognize firsthand the diversity of knowers identified under the generalizing term "demographer." Some demographers view themselves as outliers in their field (just as some anthropologists do); in a presentation at the 2013 meeting of the Population Association of America, for example, demographer Susan Watkins suggested to the audience that she occupied a position betwixt and between the "tribes" of demography and anthropology. She

recounted a conversation with another demographer in which she defended the narrative data collected by twenty Malawian research assistants she employed to collect on-the-ground perspectives to complement survey data. He suggested one could not generalize from a sample size of twenty, and she retorted, "You have a sample size of four thousand, but they *lie*" (Susan Watkins, personal communication, 2013).

5. Malawi's NAC was embroiled in a scandal referred to locally as NAC-gate, which threw into question their role as the major grants subcontractor in Malawi. In late 2014, NAC was accused of funneling pooled monies from the Global Fund meant for HIV/AIDS initiatives to political intimates, not disbursing funds to NGOs shortlisted to receive them, using funds to buy unapproved vehicles, and directing funds to "ghost NGOs." In mid-2015, the Global Fund redirected $574 million in HIV/AIDS funding away from NAC and through the Ministry of Health, World Vision, and ActionAid instead. The series of events was widely reported in Malawi's national newspapers.

6. Author's field notes, July 14, 2008.

7. Field notes, July 30, 2008.

8. Here I wish to acknowledge LSAM's novel and ambitious effort to employ survey interviewers as journalists or hearsay ethnographers who record overheard conversations and observations on local AIDS discourse in notebooks analyzed by LSAM researchers. The journals project emerged out of demographers' own concerns about the quality of survey data collected by LSAM, and their analysis of the journals is generally cognizant of the limitations of the data and acknowledges the possibility that journalists might fabricate data. The author, as a graduate student, worked closely with the journals project as a thematic coder and deems the journals an interesting and valuable source of situated knowledge that provides a long-view perspective on shifts in discourse, priorities, and anxieties around HIV in rural Malawi (Watkins, Swidler, and Biruk 2011; Kaler, Watkins, and Angotti 2015). Esacove (2016), in her book-length treatment of U.S. HIV policy in Malawi, has drawn heavily on the journals as a source of information about bottom-up AIDS discourse.

9. John Caldwell (1996, 328), a leading demographer of Africa and, notably, considered an internal critic of his disciplinary fellows, suggests that methods employed by demographers "make it possible to rearrange raw data so that truths become visible," for example.

10. The DHS program collects and disseminates nationally representative data on health and population in developing nations. The DHS household surveys take interest in, for example, reproductive health, HIV/AIDS, malaria, and fertility. Malawi's 2015–2016 DHS survey, implemented by its National Statistical Office, sampled over 26,000 Malawians.

11. The African Census Analysis Project (ACAP), a collaboration between the University of Pennsylvania's Population Studies Center and African research and governmental institutions, has created a data bank that preserves previously decaying data from census rounds on the continent and has implemented capacity-building activities centered on training African researchers in data analysis techniques. In line with the interest of this book in the materiality of data, it is interesting to note

the challenges ACAP faced in recovering data from the 1977 Malawi census, held on fourteen 9-track magnetic tapes. After many rounds of failed data recovery, ACAP managed to convert the contents of the tapes into clean, usable data twenty-seven years after its collection (Zuberi and Bangha 2006).

CHAPTER ONE: *The Office in the Field*

1. Dr. Jones, interview with author, September 20, 2007, Lilongwe, Malawi.
2. Dr. Payson, interview with author, August 23, 2007, Philadelphia.
3. Dr. Payson, interview with author, January 19, 2008, Zomba, Malawi.
4. Dr. Canton, interview with author, December 14, 2007, Arusha, Tanzania.
5. Dr. Matenje, interview with author, December 14, 2007, Arusha, Tanzania.
6. Dr. Johnson, an economist based at a research university in the U.S. Midwest, however, highlighted unexpected benefits that sometimes flow from South to North. He criticized his colleagues at a major midwestern (U.S.) university working on a project with South African collaborators for "panhandling" at the South African university for sabbatical years in a desirable city (interview with author, December 15, 2007, Arusha, Tanzania).
7. Acting head of National Research Council, interview with author, November 17, 2007, Zomba, Malawi; Dr. Jones, interview, September 20, 2007, Lilongwe, Malawi. In 2006, the NHSRC began viewing the memorandum of understanding as a central text in ensuring meaningful collaboration, and looked for it when reviewing proposals. Members of the council noted that despite foreign research projects existing in Malawi since the 1970s and the increasing volume of research, Malawi has seen little material or other benefit from all of this research ("Minutes," November 18, 2005).
8. Dr. Kamwendo, interview with author, December 14, 2007, Arusha, Tanzania.
9. This list is compiled from across approved proposals shared with me by case study projects and other survey projects working in Malawi.
10. In 2006, 106 faculty on staff at all six of the constitutive colleges of the University of Malawi held a PhD degree. For 2001, the most recent date that such statistics are available prior to 2006, the number was higher, at 155 (EMIS 2006). Malawian historian P. T. Zeleza's (2002) self-description as an "academic nomad in distant lands" captures a trend by which Malawian academics either seek greener pastures than the cash-strapped and underresourced University of Malawi or spend much of their time traveling for consultancies or conferences.
11. Field notes, November 29, 2007, dinner at Ku Chawe Inn, Zomba, Malawi.
12. Dr. Chirwa, interview with author, June 17, 2008, Balaka, Malawi.
13. Field notes, Dr. Mponda, interview with author, December 1, 2008, Hotel Masongola, Zomba, Malawi.
14. Field notes, Dr. Mponda, interview with author, December 1, 2008.
15. A 1986 report on the status of research infrastructure and objectives in Malawi suggested that "given the stage of Malawi's development, the emphasis should be on technical and applied subjects—hence, the liberal arts are not a significant component of education in Malawi" (Mkandawire 1986, 26).

16. This metaphor finds geographic analogue in island-based biological or epidemio-logical studies across the globe. Researchers use islands to study mechanisms through which infection diffuses through a closed or bounded population. In 1935, colonial researchers conducted a medical survey in an "isolated community" on Chilwa Island in Zomba District, Malawi, with such a rationale (M2/14/1 1935). Since 2005, the Likoma Network Study has collected data pertaining to sexual networks and HIV transmission on Likoma Island, an eighteen-square-kilometer island in Malawi with limited transport to the mainland and a population of seven thousand. The study views Likoma as an "epidemiological laboratory" (Helleringer et al. 2009, 432). Ann Kelly (2015, 305) likewise suggests that the small size of the Gambia gave it experi-mental appeal as a contained site for research during the colonial era.

17. After finishing his doctoral degree, the first joined the UN International Labour Organization, while the second joined the Development Research Group at the World Bank.

18. The survey instrument is a compilation of questions submitted by researchers af-filiated with a project. For example, six months prior to LSAM's sixth round of data collection in 2010, the lead demographer invited members of the research group to submit questions on "a topic [they] wish[ed] to analyze." However, he noted that "competition for space on the questionnaires will be fierce" and that those interested in submitting new questions should be aware that the 2010 surveys would contain most of the same questions from the 2008 instruments to facilitate longitu-dinal analysis (e-mail correspondence, December 10, 2009).

19. It is now conventional to refer to these teams as HIV Testing and Counseling, but I retain the acronym used in 2007–2008 in this book.

20. Field notes, May 22, 2008.

21. For examples of vignettes used to measure constructs ranging from women's travel autonomy to work limitations to HIV risk, see the Anchoring Vignettes Website compiled by political scientist Gary King (http://gking.harvard.edu/vign).

22. Andrews, interview with author, training sessions, July 28, 2008, Balaka, Malawi.

23. By now, male circumcision in Malawi is widely known by the medicalized acronym VMMC (voluntary male medical circumcision). In 2007, the WHO and UNAIDS recommended making VMMC part of the HIV prevention package in countries with a generalized epidemic, and scale-up of VMMC occupies a central position in Ma-lawi's most recent National HIV and AIDS Strategy (NAC 2014; Sgaier et al. 2014). Radio and other campaigns have made the acronym familiar to most Malawians, though in 2008, the acronym would have been largely unknown in rural areas.

CHAPTER TWO: *Living Project to Project*

1. Field notes, RAM training session, July 9, 2008, Blantyre, Malawi.

2. Nonetheless, the tour guide role is likewise assigned to fieldworkers by foreign researchers. Lead RAM supervisor John complained to fellow supervisor Victor that he felt like the American researchers treated him like a "chauffeur." They asked him to drive them to the grocery store or to check e-mails at Internet cafes, for example.

Victor agreed and joked that John should be paid as a driver in addition to a supervisor (field notes, July 7, 2008).

3. The director of one such firm explained that his small office was drowning in CVs dropped off by college graduates looking for project-to-project work amid high levels of unemployment even for the most educated Malawians (field notes, February 28, 2008).

4. Unless otherwise noted, direct quotations and observations in this chapter come from fieldwork trainings, meetings and other forums in which I interacted with fieldworkers and researchers.

5. "Doing business" implied also its foil: farming. As historian John McCracken illustrates, upon settling in what is now Malawi in the late eighteenth century, Yao men focused their energies on trade, leaving farming largely to women. Masculinity was often associated with leaving or "going outside" for trading purposes. This speaks to the early connections of Yao with the Swahili coast and trading networks (McCracken 2012, 27–29).

6. Dionne (2014) performs a quantitative analysis of LSAM job applications in 2010 and notes that contrary to fieldworkers' perspectives, research assistants' regional background was not a significant predictor of employment.

7. Only 2.2 percent of fifteen- to twenty-four-year-old Malawians successfully passed their Malawi Schools Certificate of Education (MSCE) exams at the end of secondary school (IFPRI 2002, 56).

8. Unpublished training manual authored by fieldworkers and distributed to the HIV VCT team for LSAM, May 2008.

9. Field notes, training session, May 21, 2008.

10. Though this is generally accurate, it depended on the specific project's hiring practices. While MAYP, RAM, and GSIP projects hired interviewers who were urban, more cosmopolitan, and college educated, LSAM—as mentioned above—made a point of hiring fieldworkers from local sample areas to bring some financial benefit to the surrounding communities. There was much discussion as to whether this model was better or worse than one that brings in strangers to conduct intimate interviews (see chapter 4 for further discussion on interviewer effects in survey projects). Nonetheless, the fieldworkers hired locally tended to be very similar to the people they were interviewing; in some cases, their relatives (or even, in one case, the actual individual) were in the research sample. Across the projects, however, the production of difference during the training sessions was consistent.

11. The appearance and dress of data collectors and enumerators was at the center of one critic's lambasting of the "worthless data" collected by enumerators hired from the U.S. Works Progress Administration relief rolls to administer a consumer purchasing survey in 1935: "Many housewives refused to talk to the enumerators; for, as one woman stated, the man who was called to obtain the data was 'unshaven and so dirty and ragged' that she would not allow him to enter the house—certainly she would not allow him to take an inventory of the refrigerator" (Hartkemeier 1944, 164). In her words, we might infer the disdain held for the largely poor and unskilled listed on the relief rolls by both the persons they were meant to interview and critics of the quality of the data themselves.

12. Though LSAM fieldworkers were working in contexts familiar to them, they provided similar responses to the survey questions (and in discussions) about fieldwork.

13. The fieldworkers' implicit association of Chewa with "real Malawi" is unsurprising, in light of postindependence president Hastings Kamuzu Banda's advancement of the Chichewa language and promotion of Chewa culture as the cornerstone of nationhood during his thirty years of rule (Kaspin 1995; Vail and White 1989).

14. In 1952, Goldthorpe (1952, 163–165) assigned his undergraduate students at Makerere University in Uganda an essay assignment in which they reflected on the "difficulties of doing a census among [their] people." The language used foregrounded the "wildness" and "primitiveness" of the spaces where a census would be administered.

15. Incidentally, this local knowledge is generally inaccurate, according to the statistics collected by LSAM; the data indicate that there is a single man in the project sample in these districts with seven wives (e-mail correspondence with LSAM principal investigator, March 19, 2011).

16. Training manual distributed to the HIV VCT team for LSAM; May 2008.

17. Although Malawian small-scale farmers tend to produce enough maize to feed their household for the year, the need for cash to buy items such as soap, sugar, relish, salt, or washing powder often motivates villagers to sell their maize to government or private middleman buyers in the boma, or local town center. In most cases, this means that the same household will have to buy back maize later in the season when it runs out, and at a higher price than they sold for.

18. "Silly villager stories" are commonplace, as well, at conferences and workshops. At a 2005 research dissemination meeting, for example, a presenter whose paper discussed women's understanding of menopause suggested some women were afraid that if they got pregnant they would give birth to a lizard, generating laughter among the audience members, and acting to draw a line in the sand between the scientific, rational elites present at the meeting and the villagers in the field (LSAM demographer's field notes, November 12, 2005).

19. Whereas we might assume that sensitive questions (such as "How many sexual partners did you have this year?") administered in face-to-face settings might lead respondents to underreport the number of partners, fieldworkers often assumed the opposite, particularly about male respondents. They would return to the fieldwork van after an interview and joke about how a respondent claimed to sleep with what was deemed by field teams to be a "ridiculous number."

20. Andrews, interview with author, July 30, 2008. It should be noted, however, that even as supervisors complained about the azungu checkers, they also felt overburdened by the imperative to submit checked surveys at the end of each workday. Many had to check over dinner or before bed; their fatigue likely compromised their ability to check accurately and comprehensively. In discussions with the supervisors about azungu checkers, their perceptions of my own competence as a checker were higher; they explained that because I spent every day with the teams and checked hundreds of surveys, I had picked up some basic facts from them.

21. Interview with Dr. Smith, June 1, 2008, Blantyre, Malawi.

22. In media and policy circles in mid-2000s Malawi, "traditional cultural practices" (including, e.g., male initiation rituals, norms around sexual debut at an early age, etc.) were discursively linked to HIV risk (Esacove 2016). The Malawi Human Rights Commission (MHRC, 2006) produced a report on this link. For a critical analysis of this discourse, see Peters, Kambewa, and Walker (2010) and chapter 5 of this book.

23. While some foreign researchers relied heavily and uncritically on fieldworkers' local knowledge, others did not. One researcher's impression of local knowledge could differ drastically from another's. I noted that researchers who were more skeptical supervised their field staff more intensively and had longer experience working in Malawi.

24. The 2008 Malawi Population and Housing Census was conducted June 8–28, 2008. It employed 13,000 enumerators and 3,400 supervisors (National Statistical Office, 2008).

25. Fluency in English was a bottom-line requirement for employment by research projects (as mentioned in interviews by researchers for biomedical and social scientific projects in Malawi).

26. Field notes, August 12, 2008.

27. Interview with author, December 2, 2008.

28. Interview with author, May 7, 2008.

29. Field notes, July 28, 2008, and August 2008.

30. Field notes, June 5, 2008.

31. Field notes, LSAM staff meeting, July 23, 2008.

32. Field notes, July 30, 2008.

CHAPTER THREE: *Clean Data, Messy Gifts*

1. Anthropologists and others critique informed consent as ethical benchmark, suggesting that a consenter's low education or poor financial position can enfold coercion into consent (Kelly 2003; Moniruzzaman 2012). Mfutso-Bengo and Masiye (2011) trouble the antirelational autonomy that grounds consent.

2. Discussion with parents of respondent in MAYP sample, field notes, February 26, 2008.

3. Not all projects gave soap, and some gave no gifts at all. Interviews with researchers leading projects outside this study's purview but in Malawi suggested they used chitenje, Coca-Cola, and other tokens as gifts. Emphasis on gifts being small was consistent. Standards for gift giving have shifted since 2008: some projects give mobile phone airtime, others small amounts of money, and so on. Notably, while gifts have been used in the survey projects discussed here, the Demographic and Health Surveys, World Bank Living Standards Measurement Study, census, and other enumerative efforts do not give gifts.

4. There are hierarchies of desirability around soap, with some being considered luxury soap and others poor or cheap soap; LSAM and MAYP disbursed the latter.

5. Dr. Payson, MAYP principal investigator, interview with author, July 9, 2008.
6. Former Malawian ethics board member, interview with author, November 20, 2009, New Orleans, LA.
7. In his influential essay *The Gift*, Mauss ([1922] 1967) draws on examples of gift-giving behavior from across societies to describe three obligations inherent to exchanges: to give, receive, and return gifts. This triple obligation reflects shared moral codes between transactors such that a primary function of the gift is to solidify social bonds and maintain social ties. Gifts also carry the power to undermine or cut social bonds, as when persons involved in their transaction fail to adhere to tacit rules around gifting. Mauss argues that although gifts appear to be given freely, they are actually given in an interested way, primarily to open a relationship between two people or groups who become mutually indebted to one another through ongoing transactions. The soap gift is peculiar, since there is no pretense of its being freely given (its transaction is governed or compelled by research ethics), and since the intention of its givers is to foreclose future obligation between themselves and its recipients.
8. Commentary on sugar, money, soap, and gifting in general in this section of the chapter is drawn from field notes where I recorded conversations with foreign and Malawian researchers and Malawian fieldworkers during fieldwork with MAYP (January–March 2008) and LSAM (June–September 2008). Quotations from research participants are drawn from a set of semistructured interviews I conducted during the same period with informants in LSAM and MAYP's samples.
9. Field notes, June 28, 2008.
10. Interview with author, Matukuta village, August 24, 2008, Balaka District.
11. Field notes, August 5, 2008.
12. Grace, interview with author, July 26, 2008, Chipapa, Balaka District.
13. Andrews, interview with author, September 22, 2008, Zomba, Malawi.
14. This logic of compensation also manifests in elite worlds, where individuals refuse to attend workshops or conferences that do not offer per diems. On "perdiemitis," see Ridde (2010), Conteh and Kingori (2010), and Soreide, Tostensen, and Skage (2012).
15. LSAM supervisor, interview with author, July 5, 2008.
16. Research participant, interview with author, July 26, 2008.
17. Traditional authority, interview with author, December 4, 2007, Zomba District.
18. Dr. Pierson Ntata, interview with author, February 8, 2008; Chinsinga (2011).
19. Tiwonge, interview with author, August 25, 2008, Nkumba, Balaka District.
20. Field notes, February 19, 2008, Salima District.
21. Interview with author, August 18, 2008, Chopi village, Balaka District.
22. E-mail correspondence with MAYP principal investigators, February 14–15, 2008.

CHAPTER FOUR: *Materializing Clean Data in the Field*

1. Enumeration areas are units of geographic space canvassed by national census enumerators. They can contain part of a village, a whole village, or several villages, estates, trading centers, or part of an urban area. Enumeration areas are efficient and useful units of data collection for survey projects, because data collected can

be compared with data collected by government surveys and other projects that likewise use these units. At the time of my fieldwork, there were 12,631 demarcated EAs in Malawi.

2. Data entry clerks for LSAM were often rewarded with incentives after a month of entering data eight hours per day if they entered data accurately and with few input errors. These incentives complemented their standard salary of 1,500 kwacha (about $11 USD at the time) per day.

3. Respondents' critiques of the project's beans exercise as childish or a form of child's play should be situated in a longer history whereby colonial ethnopsychiatrists analogized the adult African mind with the European child's (McCulloch 1995, 83; Keller 2007, 27; Anderson, Jenson, and Keller 2011). Imperial presumptions that Africans were simpleminded and possessed a "primitive mentality" laid the groundwork for the claim that they had little regard for the future (and by exten-sion, perhaps, probabilistic forecasting): they "experience mostly the present, like children" (Fassin 2011, 229, quoting Antoine Porot, leader of the Algiers School of Psychiatry, 1952). Colonial psychiatry assumed that the "African mind" displayed inept logic and lacked the capacity for abstract thought (Vaughan 1991, 35). In this sense, we note the way in which traces of the "African mind" surface in the design and administration of a survey exercise meant to translate probability from an abstract concept to a simple one via a childish tactile activity or game.

4. The beans were also a source of practical frustration on a daily basis. Interviewers sometimes forgot their bean dish and often lost some of their ten beans while out in the field.

5. One respondent refused to complete Section 15 of the survey because he thought it was a competition. He recalled that the last time someone came asking about expectations and numbers, some people won and others lost. He was referring to the lottery cash transfers project described in chapter 3.

6. Supervisors relished the opportunity to share stories of research teams being tricked by respondents. Stories were drawn from past experience in the field and were often told and retold; in this way, they acted as refresher lessons that reminded fieldworkers to be ever vigilant for lying or cunning respondents.

7. In a classic early volume on population in Africa, *The Demography of Tropical Africa*, van de Walle (1968, 13) generalizes about the problem of age recall: "All African demographic surveys share the problem of trying to record the ages of people who do not know their exact ages and are not fundamentally interested in knowing them."

8. The fieldworkers' bottom-up observations about the codes they were provided to represent marital status on the household roster resonate with demographers' own anxieties about how best to capture and define marriage trends across cultural and geographic contexts where terms and definitions are nonuniform or are interpreted differently (van de Walle 1993, 120–125).

9. Supervisors were asked to track and periodically evaluate the performance of their interviewers in the field. The more callbacks an interviewer accumulated, the more likely he or she was to be ranked poorly (and, possibly, to lose his or her job).

10. Madiega et al. (2013, 25), in a study of fieldworkers associated with an HIV trial in western Kenya, document how fieldworkers lie about their identities, as well— posing as missionaries or visiting relatives, for example—to protect their informants from being outed as HIV-positive through association with an HIV-related project.

11. For example, though received wisdom would indicate that data are better when interviewer and interviewee are the same sex, studies have shown ambiguous evidence for this claim in the Nigerian, Ghanaian, and South Asian contexts (Choldin, Kahn, and Ara 1967; Blanc and Croft 1992; Becker, Feyistan, and Makinwa-Adebusoye 1995). In an analysis of coethnic interviewer effects on response patterns across Afrobarometer surveys administered in fourteen African countries, Adida et al. (2014) found modest but systematic effects: for example, respondents interviewed by coethnics gave different and less socially desirable answers to explicitly ethnic questions. In narrowing their analysis to South Africa, they found that racial interviewer effects swamped ethnic interviewer effects. Dionne (2014), in an analysis of LSAM data from 2010, found that interviewer coethnicity affected the ways in which respondents answered questions related to sexual behavior in Malawi.

12. In the Nyasaland Survey in the late 1930s, native recorders were asked to be similarly vigilant so as to uncover potential lies: "[He, the recorder] should make, week by week, a list of the various foodstuffs which are in season or obtainable and are likely to be used as snacks. He should also *keep his eyes open* as to what extras are being eaten, so as to be able to *check up the information being given to him*" (Berry and Petty 1992, 27–28, emphasis added).

13. Though these instructions seem nitpicky, concerns over inconsistent writing practices have long preoccupied demographers and survey administrators. El-Badry (1961), for example, shows how enumerators' failure to record a "o"—instead leaving the space blank or using a dash—for childless women in population censuses affects quality and accuracy of data.

14. Importantly, Namoyo's incredulity at being asked whether she had, for example, solar panels or a metal roof is stricken from the pages of the survey, which record only her "no" responses. In this sense, her deprivation and poverty do not come to figure as data, and take form as nonknowledge that becomes a kind of public secret among research teams, who often felt sympathetic toward their respondents, even as the ethics and temporalities of field research did not allow them to intervene or explicitly address the suffering they encountered (as we saw in chapter 3) (Geissler 2013b).

15. What a project sees is highly dependent on whom it includes in its sample. From the mid-1980s, for example, monitoring the HIV epidemic relied on sentinel-surveillance data, often collected from pregnant women at antenatal clinics. These data have been noted to contain several biases: the exclusion of men from the sample, the inclusion of only pregnant women who are also sexually active in the sample, and the selective location of clinics in the sample (Brookmeyer 2010). The large-scale survey projects discussed in this chapter provide an alternative vision that is not restricted to a selected subpopulation.

16. Field notes, February 2008.

17. Like many of the instructions and forms implemented from above, this tool became the subject of jokes among field teams. One day the driver of a field vehicle was driving poorly, and an interviewer joked that he should drive more safely, or "someone will have to do a verbal autopsy on *us!*"

18. Ganyu is a form of casual or piecework labor usually exchanged somewhat reciprocally between peasant households. Rural Malawians engage in ganyu to cushion themselves, often (but not exclusively) during the hunger months or lean months (*njala*) when the majority of rural households run out of food before the next harvest begins. Scholars have variously interpreted rates of ganyu in a given year as a measure of vulnerability or a form of social capital (Kerr 2005; Dimowa, Michaelowa, and Weber 2010). In the wake of the 2001–2003 famine, for example, ganyu became a key source of income, especially for rural women and youth (Bryceson 2006, 2012).

19. Field notes, February 28, 2008.

20. This practice meant scouts were sometimes not qualified for the job; supervisors frequently complained that their scout knew nothing about the local area or was lazy (one was often found sleeping under trees). However, well aware of the need to keep chiefs happy for the sake of smooth data collection, teams would not fire scouts hand-picked by a chief, but would instead hire an assistant scout to work with the primary scout.

CHAPTER FIVE: *When Numbers Travel*

1. Insights in this chapter are drawn primarily from field notes, interviews, and conversations I participated in at the following conferences: the Union of African Population Scientists conference in Arusha, Tanzania (December 10–14, 2007), the Review of the National HIV and AIDS response in Lilongwe, Malawi (October 1–3, 2007), the first annual NAC Zonal Quarterly Review and Dissemination Workshops in Mzuzu, Malawi (November 24, 2008), the 2008 Malawi National Research Council meeting in Lilongwe, Malawi (March 11–14, 2008), and the National Symposium on HIV/AIDS in Lilongwe, Malawi (June 30–July 1, 2014).

2. Prime examples of this effort to increase use and dissemination of data are the African Census Analysis Project and the Integrated Public Use Microdata Series, based at the University of Pennsylvania's and the University of Minnesota's population studies centers, respectively. DevInfo, a database endorsed by the United Nations Development Group, is a storehouse of socioeconomic data from all over the world.

3. The initial survey, administered by LSAM in 1998, contained fewer sections and much less detail than the 2008 version. The 1998 survey's questions were heavily weighted toward family planning topics, reflecting a new emphasis at the time—in the wake of the 1994 International Conference on Population and Development—in national policies on reproductive health and family planning (Oucho, Akwara, and Ayiemba 1995; Kekovole and Odimegwu 2014).

4. Widow inheritance, often crudely glossed as "sexual cleansing," entails the widow of a recently deceased man being "inherited" (including sexual relations), usually

by a relative. An MHRC (2006) study found that the practice was described by respondents to the survey mostly as a thing of the past. *Afisi*, the Chewa word for hyena, refers to a figure, male or female, who is glossed as a cleanser and associated with both procreation and initiation. In the former case, when a man and woman are unable to conceive a child, a man's colleague or relative may have sexual relations with her, with any resulting child being considered her husband's. In the second case, young girls are said to be encouraged to engage in sexual relations with a man following exit from initiation camps. This practice is known as *kuchotsa fumbi* or cleaning the dust. Kulowa kufa (welcoming/entering death, or death has entered) entails an afisi sleeping with a woman whose husband has died, or vice versa. While dominant interpretations of kulowa kufa claim its function is putting to rest the spirit of the deceased, Kaufulu (2008), in an unpublished undergraduate dissertation, suggests—drawing on interviews in Nsanje District—that the practice functions to reestablish lost balance, via dispelling a kind of "heaviness" that resides in objects and individuals in the immediate vicinity of a death. Further, he helpfully demonstrates how this and other cultural practices are often lumped together in the era of AIDS, although there are important differences and meanings between them and their various component parts. Analyzing linguistic meanings behind Chewa terms for the practices described in this note, he shows how "cleanser" is often a crude and inaccurate translation for the person termed afisi.

5. Jando is a Yao male initiation ceremony involving circumcision.

6. Mtungo and magolowazi are wedding dances at which people invited by both bride and groom drink beer and dance together. Magolowazi also refers to dancing, but carries connotations of young people sneaking off into the bushes to have sexual intercourse in secret.

7. Text drawn from the research proposal for "Mapping Cultural Practices Related to Sexual and Reproductive Health Outcomes and HIV Transmission," 2005, made available to the author.

8. Memo, "Field Report," internal correspondence between field teams and principal investigator, Dr. Chirwa, dated September 30, 2005.

9. Interviewer and male initiate, interview transcript excerpt, Cultural Practices Study, NAC, June 30, 2005, Balaka District.

10. The draft of the prevention strategy that Castells sent to Blessings, for example, actually stated—in a section on modes of transmission and epidemiological evidence—that "the proportion of HIV transmission attributed to [cultural] practices is relatively small."

11. Author's research notes and e-mail correspondence, October 2008 and January 2009.

12. Since 2007, I have attended many policy meetings, human rights conferences, and HIV meetings where the topic of female circumcision has come up, often resulting in debate among those present as to whether it happens in Malawi, which seems to be a kind of open question answered primarily by speculation.

13. Notes on Regional Workshop on HIV Prevention Strategy (central, south, north Malawi), consultations with children living with HIV, and consultations with

human rights and gender group in mid- to late August 2008, made available to the author.

14. They also receive continued attention elsewhere. Page (2014, 180–181) notes that foreign-funded life skills curriculum materials in Malawian secondary schools from 2004 to 2008 featured activities that constructed cultural practices as risky. In 2010, Malawi passed legislation that would make subjecting a child to a social or customary practice harmful to the health or general development of the child a crime punishable by ten years' imprisonment (GoM 2010). The draft HIV bill, currently under review, likewise criminalizes a list of 18 "harmful [cultural] practices." Harmful cultural practices continue to receive ample media coverage: a recent article representative of others that appear in national newspapers and authored by a Malawian journalist was headlined "Harmful Cultural Practices Resurface and Threaten Malawi's HIV Response" (Ganthu 2016).

15. The American demographer who collaborated on the study of cultural practices and youth sexual reproductive health initially proposed (in response to the international organization's call for proposals) the collection of biomarkers as well, but this portion of the research program was deemed unnecessary or irrelevant by the proposal review committee and, so, dropped from the plan. The published findings thus use self-reported HIV status and the other indicators as proxy or indirect measures of sexual and reproductive health (author's e-mail correspondence with demographer-consultant, January 21, 2016).

16. Research officer, NAC, interview with author, April 28, 2008, Malawi.

17. Research officer, interview, April 28, 2008.

18. Invitations were sent by NAC to district assemblies and CBOs they funded in the region, asking them to send a representative to the Zonal Conference. Attendees were also provided with a 2,500 kwacha ($18) per diem, for a total of 7,500 kwacha ($54) over the three days.

19. Detail, quotations, and descriptions in this section are drawn from my field notes, October 22, 2008.

20. Malawi's NAC was embroiled in a scandal referred to locally as "NAC-gate," which threw into question their role as the major grants subcontractor in Malawi. In late 2014, NAC was accused of funneling pooled monies from the Global Fund meant for HIV/AIDS initiatives to political intimates, not disbursing funds to NGOs short-listed to receive them, using funds to buy unapproved vehicles, and directing funds to ghost NGOs. In mid-2015, the Global Fund redirected $574 million in HIV/AIDS funding away from NAC and through the Ministry of Health, World Vision, and ActionAid, instead. The series of events was widely reported in Malawi's national newspapers.

21. Felix, field notes, December 2010, Baltimore, MD.

22. Conversation with researchers, field notes, June 30, 2014.

23. Lubricant was in great demand among MSM in Malawi and very difficult to source. One day a large truck rumbled into the driveway of the NGO offices in Lilongwe and off-loaded 124,000 units of lube "from the American people" funded by USAID. Staff were excited, but lamented that the costs of transporting it to the many places it was needed should also be offset by funding (field notes, June 18, 2014).

24. According to the most recent HIV/AIDS Strategic Plan, "key population" refers to populations where the most HIV-positive individuals can be identified and linked to treatment. The strategy mentions MSM alongside female sex workers, prisoners, adolescents and youth, estate workers, and mobile groups such as truckers and fish buyers/sellers (NAC 2014, 5). The 2014 strategy is, notably, also the first to explicitly mention "transgendered persons," which emerged from debates about which groups should be considered key populations in Malawi during a small workshop attended by members of civil society organizations, foreign researchers, members of government ministries, and the author (field notes, July 2, 2014, Lilongwe).

25. Officer, NAC, interview with author, April 28, 2008, Lilongwe.

26. Dr. Hanson, senior clinical researcher, interview with author, April 1, 2008, Blantyre, Malawi.

27. Hanson, interview, April 1, 2008.

28. Mr. Manda, interview with author, April 28, 2008, Lilongwe.

29. Manda, interview, April 28, 2008.

30. At the time of my research, Internet access in Malawi, even in institutions such as the University of Malawi, was very limited, unreliable, and spotty. Smartphones, which have since proliferated as the major portal of mass Internet access in Malawi, were then unavailable. When I was working as an instructor at Chancellor College September–December 2008, it was close to impossible to access the Internet. Power outages were frequent, and the copy machines were often broken or lacked paper.

31. It should be noted that all projects discussed in this book have made attempts to distribute their findings to policy makers and local researchers. For example, LSAM put together packets that aimed to present the collated findings of studies emanating from their data sets in a quick and easy format: the first page was a two-line summary of each study, and the next pages were abstracts. Also, LSAM furnished local actors with USB keys with the full papers on them.

32. Call for papers, "Frontiers of Longitudinal Research in Malawi," January 28, 2016.

33. Faculty member at the University of Malawi, interview with author, January 12, 2013.

CONCLUSION: *Anthropology in and of (Critical) Global Health*

1. Field notes, July 7, 2008.

2. Taken from fact sheet draft, MAYP, May 22, 2008; field notes and e-mail correspondence, February 27–28, 2008.

3. Field notes, May 15, 2008.

PUBLISHED SOURCES

AAPOR. 2003. "Interviewer Falsification in Survey Research: Current Best Methods for Prevention, Detection, and Repair of Its Effect." Oakbrook Terrace, IL: American Association for Public Opinion Research. https://www.aapor.org/AAPOR_Main /media/MainSiteFiles/falsification.pdf.

adams, jimi, Philip Anglewicz, Stephane Helleringer, Christopher Manyamba, James Mwera, Georges Reniers, and Susan Watkins. n.d. "Identifying Elusive and Eager Respondents in Longitudinal Data Collection." Unpublished manuscript.

Adams, J. W., and A. B. Kasanoff. 2004. "Spillovers, Subdivisions, and Flows: Questioning the Usefulness of 'Bounded Container' as the Dominant Spatial Metaphor in Demography." In *Categories and Contexts: Anthropological and Historical Studies in Critical Demography*, edited by S. Szreter, H. Sholkamy, and A. Dharmalingam. Oxford: Oxford University Press.

Adams, Vincanne. 2013. "Evidence-Based Global Public Health: Subjects, Profits, Erasures." In *When People Come First*, edited by João Biehl and Adriana Petryna. Durham, NC: Duke University Press.

Adams, Vincanne, ed. 2016a. *Metrics: What Counts in Global Health*. Durham, NC: Duke University Press.

Adams, Vincanne. 2016b. "Metrics of the Global Sovereign." In *Metrics: What Counts in Global Health*, edited by Vincanne Adams. Durham, NC: Duke University Press.

Adams, Vincanne, and João Biehl. 2016. "The Work of Evidence in Critical Global Health." *Medicine Anthropology Theory* 3 (2): 123–126.

Adams, Vincanne, N. J. Burke, and I. Witmarsh. 2014. "Slow Research: Thoughts for a Movement in Global Health." *Medical Anthropology* 33 (3): 179–197.

Adams, V., T. E. Novotny, and H. Leslie. 2008. "Global Health Diplomacy." *Medical Anthropology* 27 (4): 315–323.

Adida, Claire L., Karen E. Ferree, Daniel N. Posner, and Amanda L. Robinson. 2015. "Who's Asking? Interviewer Coethnicity Effects in African Survey Data." Working Paper

No. 158. *Afrobarometer*. http://afrobarometer.org/sites/default/files/publications /Working%20papers/afropaperno158.pdf.

Aiga, Hirotsugu. 2007. "Bombarding People with Questions: A Reconsideration of Survey Ethics." *Bulletin of the World Health Organization* 85 (11): 823–824.

Alderman, Harold, Jere Behrman, Hans-Peter Kohler, John A. Maluccio, and Susan Watkins. 2001. "Attrition in Longitudinal Household Survey Data." *Demographic Research* 5 (4): 79–124.

Andaya, Elise. 2009. "The Gift of Health: Socialist Medical Practice and Shifting Material and Moral Economies in Post-Soviet Cuba." *Medical Anthropology Quarterly* 23 (4): 357–374.

Anderson, Benedict. 1991. "Census, Map, Museum." In *Imagined Communities: Reflections on the Origin and Spread of Nationalism.* New York: Verso.

Anderson, Ronald, Judith Kasper, Martin R. Frankel, et al., eds. 1979. *Total Survey Error: Applications to Improve Health Surveys.* San Francisco: Jossey Bass.

Anderson, Warwick. 2008. *The Collectors of Lost Souls: Turning Kuru Scientists into Whitemen.* Baltimore, MD: Johns Hopkins University Press.

Anderson, Warwick, Deborah Jeson, and Richard C. Keller. 2011. *Unconscious Dominions: Psychoanalysis, Colonial Trauma, and Global Sovereignties.* Durham, NC: Duke University Press.

Andreas, Peter, and Kelly M. Greenhill, eds. 2010. *Sex, Drugs and Body Counts: The Politics of Numbers in Global Crime and Conflict.* Ithaca, NY: Cornell University Press.

Anglewicz, Philip, jimi adams, Francis Obare, Hans-Peter Kohler, and Susan Watkins. 2009. "The Malawi Diffusion and Ideational Change Project 2004–06: Data Collection, Data Quality, and Analysis of Attrition." *Demographic Research* 20 (21): 503–540.

Anglewicz, Philip, and Jesman Chintsanya. 2011. "Disclosure of HIV Status between Spouses in Rural Malawi." *AIDS Care* 23 (8): 998–1005.

Angotti, Nicole, A. Bula, L. Gaydosh, E. Kimchi, R. Thronton, and S. Yeatman. 2009. "Increasing the Acceptability of HIV Counseling and Testing with Three C's: Convenience, Confidentiality and Credibility." *Social Science and Medicine* 68 (12): 2263–2270.

Appadurai, Arjun. 1996. "Number in the Colonial Imagination." In *Modernity at Large: Cultural Dimensions of Globalization.* Minneapolis: University of Minnesota Press.

Apthorpe, Raymond. 1997. "Writing Development Policy and Policy Analysis Plain or Clear: On Genre and Power." In *Anthropology of Policy: Critical Perspectives on Governance and Power,* edited by C. Shore and S. Wright. New York: Routledge.

Arendt, Hannah. 1958. *The Human Condition.* Chicago: University of Chicago Press.

Asdal, Kristin. 2008. "Enacting Things through Numbers: Taking Nature into Account/ing." *Geoforum* 39: 123–132.

Ashforth, Adam. 2014. "When the Vampires Come for You: A True Story of Ordinary Horror." *Social Research* 81 (4): 851–882.

Attanasio, Orazio P. 2009. "Expectations and Perceptions in Developing Countries: Their Measurement and Their Use." *American Economic Review* 99 (2): 87–92.

Baer, Hans. 1990. "The Possibilities and Dilemmas of Building Bridges between Critical Medical Anthropology and Clinical Anthropology: A Discussion." *Social Science and Medicine* 30 (9): 1011–1013.

Baird, S., E. Chirwa, C. McIntosh, and B. Ozler. 2011. "Cash or Condition? Evidence from a Cash Transfer Experiment." *Quarterly Journal of Economics* 126 (4): 1709–1753.

Ballestero, Andrea. 2012. "Transparency Short-Circuited: Laughter and Numbers in Costa Rican Water Politics." *PoLAR* 35 (2): 223–241.

Bank, Andrew, and Leslie J. Bank, eds. 2013. *Inside African Anthropology: Monica Wilson and Her Interpreters.* Cambridge: Cambridge University Press.

Baral, Stefan, Gift Trapence, Felistus Motimedi, Eric Umar, Scholastika Iipinge, Friedel Dausab, and Chris Beyrer. 2009. "HIV Prevalence, Risks for HIV Infection, and Human Rights among MSM in Malawi, Namibia, and Botswana." *PloS ONE* 4 (3): e4997.

Barnes, Sandra. 1986. *Patrons and Power: Creating a Political Community in Metropolitan Lagos.* Bloomington: Indiana University Press.

Bayart, Jean-François. 1993. *The State in Africa: The Politics of the Belly.* London: Longman.

Becker, S., K. Feyistan, and P. Makinwa-Adebusoye. 1995. "The Effect of Sex of Interviewers on the Quality of Data in a Nigerian Family Planning Questionnaire." *Studies in Family Planning* 26 (4): 233–240.

Beguy, Donatien. 2016. "Poor Data Affects Africa's Ability to Make the Right Policy Decisions." African Population and Health Research Center, August 22. http://aphrc.org/post/7313.

Behague, D., C. Tawiah, M. Rosato, T. Some, and J. Morrison. 2009. "Evidence-Based Policy-Making: The Implications of Globally-Applicable Research for Context-Specific Problem-Solving in Developing Countries." *Social Science and Medicine* 69 (10): 1539–1546.

Beisel, U. 2014. "On Gloves, Rubber and the Spatio-temporal Logics of Global Health." *Somatosphere*, October 6. http://somatosphere.net/2014/10/rubber-gloves-global-health.html.

Bell, Kirsten. 2014. "Resisting Commensurability: Against Informed Consent as Anthropological Virtue." *American Anthropologist* 116 (3): 511–522.

Benatar, Solomon R. 1998. "Global Disparities in Health and Human Rights: A Critical Commentary." *American Journal of Public Health* 88 (2): 295–300.

Benson, Todd. 2002. *Malawi: An Atlas of Social Statistics.* Zomba, Malawi: Government Statistical Office, Government of Malawi, and Washington, DC: International Food Policy Research Institute (IFPRI).

Benton, Adia. 2015. *HIV Exceptionalism: Development through Disease in Sierra Leone.* Minneapolis: University of Minnesota Press.

Benton, Adia. 2017. "Ebola at a Distance: A Pathographic Account of Anthropology's Relevance." *Anthropological Quarterly* 90 (2): 495–524.

Berman, Joshua, Collins Mitambo, Beatrice Matanje-Mwagomba, Shiraz Khan, Chiyembekezo Kachimanga, Emily Wroe, Lonia Mwape, Joep J. van Oosterhout, Getrude Chindebvu, Vanessa van Schoor, Lisa M. Puchalski Ritchie, Ulysses Panisset, and

Damson Kathyola. 2015. "Building a Knowledge Translation Platform in Malawi to Support Evidence-Informed Health Policy." *Health Research Policy and Systems* 13: 73.

Berry, Veronica, and Celia Petty, eds. 1992. *The Nyasaland Survey Papers, 1938–1943.* London: Academy.

Biehl, João. 2005. *Vita: Life in a Zone of Social Abandonment.* Berkeley: University of California Press.

Biehl, João, and Adrian Petryna. 2013. *When People Come First: Critical Studies in Global Health.* Princeton, NJ: Princeton University Press.

Biemer, Paul P., and Lars E. Lyberg. 2003. "Errors Due to Interviewers and Interviewing." In *Introduction to Survey Quality.* Hoboken, NJ: Wiley.

Bignami-Van Assche, Simona. 2003. "Are We Measuring What We Want to Measure? Individual Consistency in Survey Response in Rural Malawi." *Demographic Research* 1 (3): 77–108.

Bignami-Van Assche, Simona, Georges Reniers, and Alexander A. Weinreb. 2003. "An Assessment of the KDICP and MDICP Data Quality: Interviewer Effects, Question Reliability and Sample Attrition." *Demographic Research* 1 (2): 31–76.

Biruk, Crystal. 2012. "Seeing Like a Research Project: Producing 'High Quality Data' in AIDS Research in Malawi." *Medical Anthropology* 31 (4): 347–366.

Biruk, Crystal. 2014a. "Aid for Gays: The Moral and the Material in 'African Homophobia' in Post-2009 Malawi." *Journal of Modern African Studies* 52 (3): 447–473.

Biruk, Crystal. 2014b. "Ebola and Emergency Anthropology: The View from the Global Health Slot." *Somatosphere*, October 3. http://somatosphere.net/2014/10/ebola-and-emergency-anthropology-the-view-from-the-global-health-slot.html.

Biruk, Crystal. 2016. "Studying Up in Critical NGO Studies Today: Reflections on Critique and the Distribution of Interpretive Labor." *Critical African Studies* 8 (3): 291–305.

Biruk, Crystal. 2017. "Ethical Gifts? An Analysis of Soap-for-Data Transactions in Malawian Survey Research Worlds." *Medical Anthropology Quarterly*, April 7. doi:10.1111/maq.12374.

Bishop, Cortlandt F. 1893. *History of Elections in the American Colonies.* New York: Columbia College.

Bisika, T. J., and P. Kakhongwe. 1995. "Research on HIV/AIDS, STDs, and Skin Disease in Malawi: A Review." Zomba, Malawi: Centre for Social Research.

Blanc, A. K., and T. N. Croft. 1992. "The Effect of the Sex of Interviewer on Responses in Fertility Surveys: The Case of Ghana." Paper presented at the annual meeting of the Population Association of America, Denver, Colorado, April 30–May 1, 1992.

Bledsoe, Caroline. 2002. *Contingent Lives: Fertility, Time and Aging in West Africa.* Chicago: University of Chicago Press.

Bledsoe, Caroline H. 2010. "Sociocultural Anthropology's Encounters with Large Public Data Sets: The Case of the Spanish Municipal Register." *Anthropological Theory* 10 (1–2): 103–111.

Bledsoe, Caroline H., René Houle, and Papa Sow. 2007. "High Fertility Gambians in Low Fertility Spain." *Demographic Research* 16 (12): 375–412.

Bleek, W. 1987. "Lying Informants: A Fieldwork Experience from Ghana." *Population and Development Review* 13 (2): 314–322.

Bolton, P., and A. M. Tang. 2002. "An Alternative Approach to Cross-Cultural Function Assessment." *Social Psychiatry and Psychiatric Epidemiology* 37 (11): 537–543.

Booth, David, Diana Cammack, Jane Harrigan, Edge Kanyongolo, Mike Mataure, and Naomi Ngwira. 2006. "Drivers of Change and Development in Malawi." Working Paper 261, Overseas Development Institute.

Bornstein, Erica. 2012. *Disquieting Gifts: Humanitarianism in New Delhi.* Palo Alto, CA: Stanford University Press.

Bornstein, Erica, and Peter Redfield, eds. 2011. *Forces of Compassion: Humanitarianism between Ethics and Politics.* Santa Fe, NM: SAR Press.

Bourdieu, Pierre. 1986. "The Forms of Capital." In *Handbook of Theory and Research for the Sociology of Education,* edited by J. G. Richardson. New York: Greenwood.

Bowden, A., and J. A. Fox-Rushby. 2003. "A Systematic and Critical Review of the Process of Translation and Adaptation of Generic Health-Related Quality of Life Measures in Africa, Asia, Eastern Europe, the Middle East, South America." *Social Science and Medicine* 57 (7): 1289–1306.

Bowker, Geoffrey. 2005. *Memory Practices in the Sciences.* Cambridge, MA: MIT Press.

Bowker, Geoffrey C., and Susan Leigh Star. 1999. *Sorting Things Out: Classification and Its Consequences.* Cambridge, MA: MIT Press.

Boyer, Dominic. 2005. "The Corporeality of Expertise." *Ethnos* 70 (2): 243–266.

Boyer, Dominic. 2008. "Thinking through the Anthropology of Experts." *Anthropology in Action* 15 (2): 38–46.

Brada, B. 2011. "Not Here: Making the Spaces and Subjects of 'Global Health' in Botswana." *Culture Medicine Psychiatry* 35 (2): 285–312.

Brantley, Cynthia. 2002. *Feeding Families: African Realities and British Ideas of Nutrition and Development in Early Colonial Africa.* Portsmouth, NH: Heinemann.

Brantley, Cynthia. 2003. "Ben and Maggie: Consuming Data: Reassessing Scientific and Anthropological Evidence: Historical Perspective on Nutrition Studies." In *Sources and Methods in African History: Spoken, Written, Unearthed,* edited by Toyin Falola and Christian Jennings. Rochester, NY: University of Rochester Press.

Briggs, Charles L., and Daniel C. Hallin. 2007. "Biocommunicability: The Neoliberal Subject and Its Contradictions in News Coverage of Health Issues." *Social Text* 25: 43–66.

Briggs, Charles L., and Clara Mantini-Briggs. 2003. *Stories in the Time of Cholera: Racial Profiling during a Medical Nightmare.* Berkeley: University of California Press.

Briggs, Charles, and Clara Mantini-Briggs. 2016. *Tell Me Why My Children Died: Rabies, Indigenous Knowledge, and Communication.* Durham, NC: Duke University Press.

Brives, Charlotte. 2013. "Identifying Ontologies in a Clinical Trial." *Social Studies of Science* 43 (3): 397–416.

Brookmeyer, R. 2010. "Measuring the HIV/AIDS Epidemic: Approaches and Challenges." *Epidemiological Review* 32: 26–37.

Brown, Hannah. 2015. "Global Health Partnerships, Governance, and Sovereign Responsibility in Western Kenya." *American Ethnologist* 42 (2): 340–355.

Bryceson, Deborah Fahy. 2006. "Ganyu Casual Labour, Famine, and HIV/AIDS in Rural Malawi: Causality and Casualty." *Journal of Modern African Studies* 44 (2): 173–202.

Bryceson, Deborah Fahy. 2012. "Ganyu in Rural Malawi: Transformation of Local Labour Relations under Famine and HIV/AIDS Duress." In *Fractures and Reconnections: Civic Action and the Redefinition of African Political and Economic Space*, edited by J. Abbink. Berlin: LIT Verlag.

Bulmer, Martin, and Donald P. Warwick. 1983. "Data Collection." In *Social Research in Developing Countries*, edited by M. Bulmer and D. P. Warwick. New York: Wiley.

Burke, Timothy. 1996. *Lifebuoy Men, Lux Women: Commodification, Consumption, and Cleanliness in Modern Zimbabwe*. Durham, NC: Duke University Press.

Butt, Leslie. 2002. "The Suffering Stranger: Medical Anthropology and International Morality." *Medical Anthropology* 21 (1): 1–24.

Caldwell, John. 1996. "Demography and Social Science." *Population Studies* 50 (3): 305–333.

Caldwell, John, and Pat Caldwell. 1987. "The Cultural Context of High Fertility in Sub-Saharan Africa." *Population Development Review* 13 (3): 409–437.

Calhoun, Craig. 2010. "The Idea of Emergency: Humanitarian Action and Global (Dis)-order." In *Contemporary States of Emergency: The Politics of Military and Humanitarian Interventions*, edited by Didier Fassin and Mariella Pandolfi. New York: Zone.

Callon, Michel. 1986. "Some Elements of a Sociology of Translation: Domestication of the Scallops and the Fishermen of St Brieuc Bay." In *Power, Action, and Belief: A New Sociology of Knowledge?*, edited by J. Law. New York: Routledge.

Canagarajah, A. Suresh. 1996. "Nondiscursive Requirements in Academic Publishing, Material Resources of Periphery Scholars, and the Politics of Knowledge Production." *Written Communication* 13 (4): 435–472.

Carael, Michel, and Judith R. Glynn, eds. 2008. *HIV, Resurgent Infections and Population Change in Africa*. New York: Springer.

Carothers, J. C. 1953. *The African Mind in Health and Disease: A Study in Ethnopsychiatry*. Geneva: WHO.

Carrier, James G. 2003. "Maussian Occidentalism: Gift and Commodity Systems." In *Occidentalism: Images of the West*, edited by James G. Carrier. New York: Oxford University Press.

Cartwright, Nancy, and Jeremy Hardie. 2012. *Evidence Based Policy: A Practical Guide to Doing It Better*. New York: Oxford University Press.

Case, Kelsey K., Peter D. Ghys, Eleanor Gouws, Jeffrey W. Eaton, Annick Borquez, John Stover, Paloma Cuchi, Laith J. Abu-Raddad, Geoffrey P. Garnett, and Timothy B. Hallett. 2012. "Understanding the Modes of Transmission Model of New HIV Infection and Its Use in Prevention Planning." *Bulletin of the World Health Organization* 90 (11): 831–838.

Casley, Dennis J., and Krishna Kumar. 1988. *The Collection, Analysis, and Use of Monitoring and Evaluation Data*. A joint publication of the World Bank, IFD, and FAO. Baltimore, MD: Johns Hopkins University Press.

Chandilanga, Herbert. 2008. "Tearing a Veil of Ignorance." *The Nation*, March 5.

Chanika, Emmie, John Lwanda, and Adamson S. Muula. 2013. "Gender, Gays and Gain: The Sexualized Politics of Donor Aid in Malawi." *Africa Spectrum* 48 (1): 89–105.

Chinsinga, Blessings. 2011. "Exploring the Politics of Land Reforms in Malawi: A Case Study of the Community Based Rural Land Development Programme (CBRLDP)." *Journal of International Development* 23 (3): 380–393.

Chirwa, Wiseman Chijere. 1997. "Migrant Labour, Sexual Networking and Multi-partnered Sex in Malawi." *Health Transition Review* 7 (3): 5–15.

Choldin, Harvey M., A. Majeed Kahn, and B. Hosne Ara. 1967. "Cultural Complications in Fertility Interviewing." *Demography* 4 (1): 244–252.

CIOMS. 2002. *International Ethical Guidelines for Biomedical Research Involving Human Subjects.* Geneva: Council for International Organizations of Medical Sciences.

Cleland, John, and Susan C. Watkins. 2006. "The Key Lesson of Family Planning Pro-grammes for HIV/AIDS Control." *AIDS* 20 (1): 1–3.

Clifford, James, and George Marcus, eds. 1986. *Writing Culture: The Poetics and Politics of Ethnography.* Berkeley: University of California Press.

Coast, Ernestina. 2003. "An Evaluation of Demographers' Use of Ethnographies." *Population Studies* 57 (33): 337–347.

Cohn, Bernard S. 1987. "An Anthropologist among the Historians: A Field Study." In *An Anthropologist among the Historians and Other Essays.* New York: Oxford University Press.

Collins, Patricia Hill. (1990) 2008. *Black Feminist Thought: Knowledge, Consciousness, and the Politics of Empowerment.* London: Routledge.

Colvin, Christopher J. 2015. "Anthropologies in and of Evidence-Making in Global Health Research and Policy." *Medical Anthropology* 34 (2): 99–105.

Comaroff, Jean. 2007. "Beyond Bare Life: AIDS, (Bio)politics, and the Neoliberal Order. *Public Culture* 19 (1): 197–219.

Conteh, L., and P. Kingori. 2010. "Per Diems in Africa: A Counterargument." *Tropical Medicine and International Health* 15 (12): 1553–1555.

Cooper, Melinda, and Catherine Waldby. 2014. *Clinical Labor: Tissue Donors and Research Subjects in the Global Bioeconomy.* Durham, NC: Duke University Press.

Coopmans, Catelijne, and Graham Button. 2014. "Eyeballing Expertise." *Social Studies of Science* 44 (5): 758–785.

Cordell, Dennis D. 2010. "African Historical Demography in the Postmodern and Postcolonial Eras." In *Demographics of Empire: The Colonial Order and the Creation of Knowledge,* edited by Karl Ittman, Dennis D. Cordell, and Gregory H. Maddox. Columbus: Ohio State University Press.

Cornish, Flora. 2015. "Evidence Synthesis in International Development: A Critique of Systematic Reviews and a Pragmatist Alternative." *Anthropology and Medicine* 22 (3): 363–377.

Crane, Johanna. 2010a. "Adverse Events and Placebo Effects: African Scientists, HIV, and Ethics in the 'Global Health Sciences.'" *Social Studies of Science* 40 (6): 843–870.

Crane, Johanna. 2010b. "Unequal 'Partners': AIDS, Academia and the Rise of Global Health." *Behemoth* 3: 78–97.

Crane, Johanna. 2013. *Scrambling for Africa: AIDS, Expertise and the Rise of American Global Health Science*. Ithaca, NY: Cornell University Press.

Crespi, Leo P. 1946. "The Cheater Problem in Polling." *Public Opinion Quarterly* 9 (4): 431–445.

Crewe, Emma, and Richard Axelby. 2013. *Anthropology and Development: Culture, Morality and Politics in a Globalized World*. New York: Cambridge University Press.

Crewe, Emma, and John Young. 2002. "Bridging Research and Policy: Context, Evidence and Links." Working Paper 173. London: Overseas Development Institute.

Dahl, Bianca. 2014. "Too Fat to Be an Orphan": The Moral Semiotics of Food Aid in Botswana." *Cultural Anthropology* 29 (4): 626–647.

Daston, Lorraine, and Peter Galison. 2010. *Objectivity*. New York: Zone.

Davis, Kevin E., Benedict Kingsbury, and Sally Engle Merry. 2012. "Global Governance by Indicators." In *Governance by Indicators: Global Power through Quantification and Rankings*, edited by Kevin E. Davis, Angelina Fisher, Benedict Kingsbury, and Sally Engle Merry. New York: Oxford University Press.

Day, Sophie, Celia Lury, and Nina Wakeford. 2014. "Number Ecologies: Numbers and Numbering Practices." *Distinktion: Scandanavian Journal of Social Theory* 15 (2): 123–154.

Deane, Phyllis. 1953. *Colonial Social Accounting*. National Institute of Economic and Social Research. New York: Cambridge University Press.

Deaton, A. S. 1997. *The Analysis of Household Surveys: A Microeconometric Approach to Development Policy*. Baltimore, MD: Johns Hopkins University Press.

deLaet, Marianne, and Annemarie Mol. 2000. "The Zimbabwe Bush Pump: Mechanics of a Fluid Technology." *Social Studies of Science* 30 (2): 225–263.

Delavande, Adeline, Xavier Giné, and David McKenzie. 2011. "Eliciting Probabilistic Expectations with Visual Aids in Developing Countries: How Sensitive Are Answers to Variations in Elicitation Design?" *Journal of Applied Econometrics* 26 (3): 479–497.

Delavande, Adeline, and Hans-Peter Kohler. 2007. "Subjective Expectations in the Context of HIV/AIDS in Malawi." WPS 07-06. Philadelphia: University of Pennsylvania, Population Aging Research Center.

de Leeuw, Edith D., Joop T. Hox, and Don A. Dillman, eds. 2008. "The Cornerstones of Survey Research." In *International Handbook of Survey Methodology*, edited by Edith D. de Leeuw, Joop T. Hox, and Don A. Dillman. Philadelphia: Taylor and Francis.

Demeny, Paul. 1988. "Social Science and Population Policy." *Population and Development Review* 14 (3): 451–479.

Desrosiéres, Alain. 1998. *The Politics of Large Numbers: A History of Statistical Reasoning*. Cambridge, MA: Harvard University Press.

de Waal, Alex. 2015. "Policy to Research to Policy in Difficult Places." *Humanity*, December 7. http://humanityjournal.org/blog/policy-to-research-to-policy-in-difficult-places/.

Dickert, N., and C. Grady. 1999. "What's the Price of a Research Subject? Approaches to Payment for Research Participation." *NEJM* 341 (3): 198–203.

Dilger, Hansjorg, Susann Huschke, and Dominik Mattes. 2015. "Ethics, Epistemology and Engagement: Encountering Values in Medical Anthropology." *Medical Anthropology* 34 (1): 1–10.

Dillman, Don A. 2008. "The Logic and Psychology of Constructing Questionnaires." In *International Handbook of Survey Methodology*, edited by Edith D. de Leeuw, Joop T. Hox, and Don A. Dillman. Philadelphia: Taylor and Francis.

Dimowa, Ralitza, Katharina Michaelowa, and Anke Weber. 2010. "Ganyu Labour in Malawi: Understanding Rural Households' Labour Supply Strategies." Working Paper 52. Zurich: Center for Comparative and International Studies.

Dionne, Kim Yi. 2012. "Local Demand for a Global Intervention: Policy Preferences in the Time of AIDS." *World Development* 40 (12): 2468–2477.

Dionne, Kim Yi. 2014. "The Politics of Local Research Production: Surveying in a Context of Ethnic Competition." *Politics, Groups, and Identities* 2 (3): 459–480.

Dionne, Kim Yi, Patrick Gerland, and Susan Watkins. 2013. "AIDS Exceptionalism: Another Constituency Heard From." *AIDS and Behavior* 17 (3): 825–831.

du Plessis, Elsabé, and Robert Lorway. 2016. "What Really Works? Understanding the Role of 'Local Knowledges' in the Monitoring and Evaluation of a Maternal, Newborn and Child Health Project in Kenya." In *Monitoring and Evaluation in Health and Social Development: Interpretive and Ethnographic Perspectives*, edited by Stephen Bell and Peter Aggleton. New York: Routledge.

Durham, Deborah. 2005. "Did You Bathe This Morning? Baths and Morality in Botswana." In *Dirt, Undress, and Difference: Critical Perspectives on the Body's Surface*, edited by Adeline Masquelier. Bloomington: Indiana University Press.

Ecks, Stefan. 2008. "Three Propositions for an Evidence-Based Medical Anthropology." *JRAI* 14 (s1): S77–S92.

El-Badry, M. A. 1961. "Failure of Enumerators to Make Entries of Zero: Errors in Recording Childless Cases in Population Censuses." *Journal of the American Statistical Association* 56 (296): 909–924.

Emanuel, Ezekiel J. 2004. "Ending Concerns about Undue Inducement." *Journal of Law, Medicine, and Ethics* 32: 100–105.

EMIS. 2006. "Education Statistics." EMIS Section of the Department of Education Planning, Ministry of Education and Vocational Planning. Government of Malawi.

Engel, N., I. V. Hoyweghen, A. Krumeich, and I. Hoyweghen, eds. 2014. *Making Global Health Care Innovation Work: Standardization and Localization*. London: Palgrave Macmillan.

Englund, Harri. 2002. "The Village in the City, the City in the Village: Migrants in Lilongwe." *Journal of Southern African Studies* 28 (1): 137–154.

Englund, Harri. 2006. *Prisoners of Freedom: Human Rights and the African Poor*. Berkeley: University of California Press.

Epstein, Steven. 1996. *Impure Science: AIDS, Activism, and the Politics of Knowledge*. Berkeley: University of California Press.

Erikson, Susan L. 2008. "Getting Political: Fighting for Global Health." *Lancet* 371 (9620): 1229–1230.

Erikson, Susan L. 2011. "Global Ethnography: Problems of Theory and Method." In *Reproduction, Globalization and the State: New Theoretical and Ethnographic Perspectives*, edited by Carole H. Browner and Carolyn F. Sargent. Durham, NC: Duke University Press.

Erikson, Susan L. 2012. "Global Health Business: The Production and Performativity of Statistics in Sierra Leone and Germany." *Medical Anthropology* 31: 367–384.

Erikson, Susan L. 2016. "Metrics and Market Logics of Global Health." In *Metrics: What Counts in Global Health*, edited by Vincanne Adams. Durham, NC: Duke University Press.

Esacove, Anne. 2016. *Modernizing Sexuality: US HIV Prevention Policy in Sub-Saharan Africa*. New York: Oxford University Press.

Espeland, Wendy Nelson, and Mitchell L. Stevens. 2008. "A Sociology of Quantification." *European Journal of Sociology* 49: 401–436.

Everson, Stephen, ed. 1996. *Aristotle: The Politics and the Constitution*. New York: Cambridge University Press.

Fabian, Johannes. (1983) 2002. *Time and the Other: How Anthropology Makes Its Object*. New York: Columbia University Press.

Fairhead, J., M. Leach, and M. Small. 2006. "Where Technoscience Meets Poverty." *Social Science and Medicine* 63: 1109–1120.

Fan, Elsa L., and Elanah Uretsky. 2016. "In Search of Results: Anthropological Interrogations of Evidence-Based Global Health." *Critical Public Health* 27 (2): 157–162.

Farmer, Paul. 2004. *Pathologies of Power: Health, Human Rights, and the New War on the Poor*. Berkeley: University of California Press.

Fassin, Didier. 2011. "Ethnopsychiatry and the Postcolonial Encounter: A French Psychopolitics of Otherness." In *Unconscious Dominions: Psychoanalysis, Colonial Trauma, and Global Sovereignties*, edited by Warwick Anderson, Deborah Jenson, and Richard C. Keller. Durham, NC: Duke University Press.

Fassin, Didier. 2012. *Humanitarian Reason: A Moral History of the Present*. Berkeley: University of California Press.

Faubion, James, and George E. Marcus, eds. 2009. *Fieldwork Is Not What It Used to Be: Learning Anthropology's Method in a Time of Transition*. Ithaca, NY: Cornell University Press.

Feierman, Steven. 2011. "When Physicians Meet: Local Medical Knowledge and Global Public Goods." In *Evidence, Ethos and Experiment: The Anthropology and History of Medical Research in Africa*, edited by Wenzel P. Geissler and Catherine Molyneux. New York: Berghahn.

Ferguson, James. 1994. *The Anti-politics Machine: Development, Depoliticization, and Bureaucratic Power in Lesotho*. Minneapolis: University of Minnesota Press.

Ferguson, James. 1999. *Expectations of Modernity: Myths and Meanings of Urban Life on the Zambian Copperbelt*. Berkeley: University of California Press.

Ferguson, James. 2015. *Give a Man a Fish: Reflections on the New Politics of Distribution*. Durham, NC: Duke University Press.

Finn, Arden, and Vimal Ranchhod. 2013. "Genuine Fakes: The Prevalence and Implications of Fieldworker Fraud in a Large South African Survey." Southern Africa Labour and Development Research Unit Working Paper, 115. Cape Town, South Africa: SALDRU.

Flaherty, Annette, and Walter Kipp. 2004. "Where a Bar of Soap Can Make a Difference: Family Planning Volunteers in Uganda Express Their Needs." *International Journal of Volunteer Administration* 22 (1): 27–33.

Folayan, Morenike Oluwatoyin, and Dan Allman. 2011. "Clinical Trials as an Industry and an Employer of Labour." *Journal of Cultural Economy* 4 (1): 97–104.

Forster, P. G. 1994. "Culture, Nationalism, and the Invention of Tradition." *Journal of Modern African Studies* 32 (3): 477–497.

Foucault, Michel. (1969) 1998. "What Is an Author?" in *Aesthetics, Method and Epistemology*, edited by James D. Faubion. Translated by Josuè V. Harari. New York: New Press.

Foucault, Michel. 1972. *The Archaeology of Knowledge*. Translated by A. M. Sheridan Smith. New York: Pantheon.

Foucault, Michel. (1978) 2007. *Security, Territory, Population: Lectures at the Collège de France, 1977–1978*. Edited by Michel Senellart. Translated by Graham Burchell. London: Picador.

Foucault, Michel. 1991. "Governmentality." In *The Foucault Effect: Studies in Governmentality*, edited by Graham Burchell, Colin Gordon, and Peter Miller. Chicago: University of Chicago Press.

Foucault, Michel. 1997a. "The Birth of Biopolitics." In *Ethics: Subjectivity and Truth*, edited by Paul Rabinow. New York: New Press.

Foucault, Michel. 1997b. "The Masked Philosopher." In *Ethics: Subjectivity and Truth*, edited by Paul Rabinow. New York: New Press.

Foucault, Michel. 1997c. "What Is Critique?" In *The Politics of Truth*, edited by Sylvére Lotringer. Los Angeles: Semiotext(e).

Foucault, Michel. 2003. *"Society Must Be Defended": Lectures at the Collège de France, 1975–1976*. Translated by David Macey. New York: Picador.

Foucault, Michel. 2008. *The Birth of Biopolitics: Lectures at the Collège de France, 1978–1979*. Edited by Michell Senellart. Translated by Graham Burchell. London: Picador.

Ganthu, Joseph. 2016. "Harmful Cultural Practices Resurface and Threaten Malawi's HIV Response." Key Correspondents, *AllAfrica*, January 14. http://allafrica.com/stories/201601141275.html.

Garenne, Michel. 2011. "Fifty Years of Research in African Demography: Progresses and Challenges." *African Population Studies* 25 (2): 151–167.

Geertz, Clifford. 1977. *The Interpretation of Cultures*. New York: Basic Books.

Geertz, Clifford. 1988. *Works and Lives: The Anthropologist as Author*. Palo Alto, CA: Stanford University Press.

Geissler, P. Wenzel. 2005. "Kachinja Are Coming! Encounters around Medical Research Work in a Kenyan Village." *Africa* 75: 175–202.

Geissler, P. W. 2013a. "The Archipelago of Public Health: Comments on the Landscape of Medical Research in 21st Century Africa." In *Making and Unmaking Public Health in Africa: Ethnographic and Historical Perspectives*, edited by Ruth J. Prince and Rebecca Marsland. Columbus: Ohio University Press.

Geissler, P. W. 2013b. "Public Secrets in Public Health: Knowing Not to Know While Making Scientific Knowledge." *American Ethnologist* 40 (1): 13–34.

Geissler, P. Wenzel. 2015a. "A Life Science in Its African Para-state." In *Para-states and Medical Science: Making African Global Health*, edited by P. Wenzel Geissler. Durham, NC: Duke University Press.

Geissler, P. Wenzel. 2015b. "What Future Remains? Remembering an African Place of Science." In *Para-states and Medical Science: Making African Global Health*, edited by P. Wenzel Geissler. Durham, NC: Duke University Press.

Gerrets, R. 2015a. "Charting the Road to Eradication: Health Facility Data and Malaria Indicator Generation in Rural Tanzania." In *The World of Indicators: The Making of Governmental Knowledge through Quantification*, edited by R. Rottenburg, Sally Engle Merry, and J. Muegler. New York: Cambridge University Press.

Gerrets, Rene. 2015b. "International Health and the Proliferation of 'Partnerships': (Un)-Intended Boost for State Institutions in Tanzania?" In *Para-states and Medical Science: Making African Global Health*, edited by P. Wenzel Geissler. Durham, NC: Duke University Press.

Gervais, Raymond R., and Issiaka Mandé. 2010. "How to Count the Subjects of Empire? Steps toward an Imperial Demography in French West Africa before 1946." In *Demographics of Empire: The Colonial Order and the Creation of Knowledge*, edited by Karl Ittman, Dennis D. Cordell, and Gregory H. Maddox. Columbus: Ohio State University Press.

Geschiere, Peter. 1997. *The Modernity of Witchcraft: Politics and the Occult in Postcolonial Africa*. Charlottesville: University of Virginia Press.

Gieryn, Thomas. 1999. *Cultural Boundaries of Science*. Chicago: University of Chicago Press.

Gitelman, Lisa, ed. 2013. *"Raw Data" Is an Oxymoron*. Cambridge, MA: MIT Press.

Gitelman, Lisa, and Virginia Jackson. 2013. "Introduction." In *"Raw Data" Is an Oxymoron*. Cambridge, MA: MIT Press.

Glewwe, Paul. 2005a. "An Overview of Questionnaire Design for Household Surveys in Developing Countries." In *Household Sample Surveys in Developing and Transition Countries*. New York: United Nations Statistics Division.

Glewwe, Paul. 2005b. "Overview of the Implementation of Household Surveys in Developing Countries." In *Household Sample Surveys in Developing and Transition Countries*. New York: United Nations Statistics Division.

Goldenberg, Maya J. 2006. "On Evidence and Evidence-Based Medicine: Lessons from the Philosophy of Science." *Social Science and Medicine* 62: 2621–2632.

Goldthorpe, J. E. 1952. "Attitudes to the Census and Vital Registration in East Africa." *Population Studies* 6 (2): 163–171.

Government of Malawi (GoM). 2003. *National HIV/AIDS Policy: A Call to Renewed Action*. Lilongwe, Malawi: Government of Malawi.

Government of Malawi (GofM). 2004. *National HIV/AIDS Action Framework (NAF), 2005–2009*. Lilongwe, Malawi: Government of Malawi.

Government of Malawi (GofM). 2010. Child Care, Protection and Justice Act, Action no. 22 of 2010. Lilongwe, Malawi: Government of Malawi.

Government of Malawi (GoM). 2015. *Malawi AIDS Response Progress Report*. Lilongwe, Malawi: Government of Malawi.

Graboyes, Melissa. 2015. *The Experiment Must Continue: Medical Research and Ethics in East Africa, 1940–2014*. Columbus: Ohio University Press.

Grassly, Nicholas C., James J. C. Lewise, Mary Mahy, Neff Walker, and Ian M. Timaeus. 2004. "Comparison of Household-Survey Estimates with Projections of Mortality and Orphan Numbers in Sub-Saharan Africa in the Era of HIV/AIDS." *Population Studies* 58 (2): 207–217.

Gray, Eve. 2013. "Research for Development and the Role of 'Grey Literature' in Southern African Research Production." *Ecancermedicalscience* 7 (22).

Greenhalgh, Susan. 1990. "Toward a Political Economy of Fertility: Anthropological Contributions." *Population and Development Review* 16 (1): 85–106.

Greenhalgh, Susan, ed. 1995. *Situating Fertility: Anthropology and Demographic Inquiry*. New York: Cambridge University Press.

Greenhalgh, Susan. 2004. "Making Up China's Black Population." In *Categories and Contexts: Anthropological and Historical Studies in Critical Demography*, edited by Simon Szreter, Hania Sholkamy, and A. Dharmalingam. New York: Oxford University Press.

Gross, C. 1898. "Early History of the Ballot in England." *American Historical Review* 3 (3): 456–463.

Groves, R. M. 1989. *Survey Errors and Survey Costs*. Hoboken, NJ: Wiley.

Gupta, Akhil, and James Ferguson. 1997. "Discipline and Practice: 'The Field' as Site, Method, and Location in Anthropology." In *Anthropological Locations: Boundaries and Grounds of a Field Science*. Berkeley: University of California Press.

Guyer, Jane, Naveeda Khan, Juan Obarrio, et al. 2010. "Introduction: Number as Inventive Frontier." *Anthropological Theory* 10 (1–2): 36–61.

Guyer, Jane I., and Pauline E. Peters. 1987. "Introduction." *Development and Change* 18 (2): 197–214.

Hacking, Ian. 1986. "Making Up People." In *Reconstructing Individualism*, edited by T. Heller, M. Sosna, and D. Wellbery. Palo Alto, CA: Stanford University Press.

Hailey, Malcolm. 1957. *An African Survey Revised*. London: Oxford University Press.

Halberstam, Judith [Jack]. 2011. *The Queer Art of Failure*. Durham, NC: Duke University Press.

Halfon, Saul. 2006. "The Disunity of Consensus: International Population Policy Coordination as Socio-technical Practice." *Social Studies of Science* 36 (5): 783–807.

Hammel, E. A. 1990. "A Theory of Culture for Demographers." *Population and Development Review* 16 (3): 455–485.

Hansen, Sue Ellen, Grant Benson, Ashley Bowers, Beth-Ellen Pennell, Yuchieh Lin, and Benjamin Duffey. 2010. "Survey Quality." In *Survey Research Center Guidelines for Best Practice in Cross-Cultural Surveys*. Ann Arbor: Survey Research Center, Institute for Social Research, University of Michigan. http://www.ccsg.isr.umich.edu/.

Haraway, Donna. 1988. "Situated Knowledges: The Science Question in Feminism and the Privilege of Partial Perspective." *Feminist Studies* 14 (3): 575–599.

Haraway, Donna. 1989. "Apes in Eden, Apes in Space: Mothering as a Scientist for *National Geographic*." In *Primate Visions: Gender, Race, and Nature in the World of Modern Science*. New York: Routledge.

Harkness, Janet A., Ipek Bilgen, AnaLucía Córdova Cazar, Kristen Cibelli, Lei Huang, Debbie Miller, Matthew Stange, and Ana Villar. 2010. "Questionnaire Design." In *Survey Research Center Guidelines for Best Practice in Cross-Cultural Surveys*. Ann Arbor, MI: Survey Research Center, Institute for Social Research, University of Michigan. http://www.ccsg.isr.umich.edu/.

Harpham, Trudy, Emma Grant, and Elizabeth Thomas. 2002. "Measuring Social Capital within Health Surveys: Key Issues." *Health Policy and Planning* 17 (1): 106–111.

Hartkemeier, Harry Palle. 1944. "The Use of Data Collected by Poorly Trained Enumerators." *Journal of Political Economy* 52 (2): 164–166.

Hasty, Jennifer. 2005. "The Pleasures of Corruption: Desire and Discipline in Ghanaian Political Culture." *Cultural Anthropology* 20 (2): 271–301.

Havinden, M. A., and D. Meredith. 1993. *Colonialism and Development: Britain and Its Tropical Colonies, 1850–1960*. London: Routledge.

Healy, Kieran. 2017. "Fuck Nuance." *Sociological Theory* 35 (2): 118–127.

Heimer, Carol. 2007. "Old Inequalities, New Disease: HIV/AIDS in Sub-Saharan Africa." *Annual Review of Sociology* 33: 551–577.

Helleringer, Stéphane, Hans-Peter Kohler, Agnes Chimbiri, Praise Chatonda, and James Mkandawire. 2009. "The Likoma Network Study: Context, Data Collection, and Initial Results." *Demographic Research* 21 (15): 427–468.

Hemmings, Colin P. 2005. "Rethinking Medical Anthropology: How Anthropology Is Failing Medicine." *Anthropology and Medicine* 12 (2): 91–103.

Hennink, M., and R. Stephenson. 2005. "Using Research to Inform Health Policy: Barriers and Strategies in Developing Countries." *Journal of Health Communication* 10: 163–180.

Henry, Doug, and Susan Shepler. 2015. "AAA 2014: Ebola in Focus." *Anthropology Today* 31 (1): 20–21.

Herdman, Michael, J. Fox-Rushby, and X. Badia. 1997. "Equivalence and the Translation and Adaptation of Health-Related Quality of Life Questionnaires." *Quality of Life Research* 6 (3): 237–247.

Higgs, Edward. 2004. "The Linguistic Construction of Social and Medical Categories in the Work of the English General Register Office, 1837–1950." In *Categories and Contexts: Anthropological and Historical Studies in Critical Demography*, edited by Simon Szreter, Hania Sholkamy, and A. Dharmalingam. New York: Oxford University Press.

Hill, K. 1990. "Demographic Estimation from Deficient or Defective Data." In *Demography from Scanty Evidence: Central Africa in the Colonial Era*, edited by B. Fetter. Boulder, CO: Lynne Rienner.

Hirschman, Charles. 1987. "The Meaning and Measurement of Ethnicity in Malaysia: An Analysis of Census Classifications." *Journal of Asian Studies* 46 (3): 555–582.

Hoad, Neville. 1999. "Between the White Man's Burden and the White Man's Disease: Tracking Lesbian and Gay Human Rights in Southern Africa." *GLQ* 5 (4): 559–584.

Hodzic, Saida. 2013. "Ascertaining Deadly Harms: Aesthetics and Politics of Global Evidence." *Cultural Anthropology* 28 (1): 86–109.

Hoeyer, Klaus, and Linda F. Hogle. 2014. "Informed Consent: The Politics of Intent and Practice in Medical Research Ethics." ARA 43: 347–362.

Holland, Dana. 2006. "Socializing Knowledge: The Production and Circulation of Social Science in Malawi, 1964–2004." PhD diss., University of Pennsylvania.

Holland, Dana. 2009. "Between the Practical and the Academic: The Relation of Mode 1 and Mode 2 Knowledge Production in a Developing Country." *Science Technology and Human Values* 34 (5): 551–572.

Hunnings, Gordon. 1981. *The Realization of a Dream: The University of Malawi: 1964–1974.* Limbe, Malawi: Montfort Press.

Hunter, Mark. 2010. *Love in the Time of AIDS: Inequality, Gender, and Rights in South Africa.* Bloomington: Indiana University Press.

Hutchinson, Eleanor. 2011. "The Development of Health Policy in Malawi: The Influence of Context, Evidence, and Links in the Creation of a National Policy for Cotrimoxazole Prophylaxis." *Malawi Medical Journal* 23 (4): 109–114.

Hutchinson, Sharon. 1992. "The Cattle of Money and the Cattle of Girls among the Nuer, 1930–83." *American Ethnologist* 19 (2): 294–316.

Illife, John. 2006. *The African AIDS Epidemic: A History.* Columbus: Ohio University Press.

Ioanide, Paula. 2015. *The Emotional Politics of Racism: How Feelings Trump Facts in an Era of Colorblindness.* Stanford, CA: Stanford University Press.

Jackson, John. 2012. "Ethnography Is, Ethnography Ain't." *Cultural Anthropology* 27 (3): 480–497.

Jacob, Marie-Andrée, and Annelise Riles. 2007. "The New Bureaucracies of Virtue." *PoLAR* 30 (2): 181–191.

Jacobs, Nancy. 2016. *Birders of Africa: History of a Network.* New Haven, CT: Yale University Press.

Jain, S. Lochlann. 2013. *Malignant: How Cancer Becomes Us.* Berkeley: University of California Press.

James, Wendy. 1973. "The Anthropologist as Reluctant Imperialist." In *Anthropology and the Colonial Encounter,* edited by Talal Asad. New York: Humanities Press.

Jerven, Morten. 2013. *Poor Numbers: How We Are Misled by African Development Statistics and What to Do about It.* Ithaca, NY: Cornell University Press.

Joffe, S. H. 1973. "Political Culture and Communication in Malawi: The Hortatory Regime of Kamuzu Banda." PhD diss., Boston University.

Johnson-Hanks, Jennifer. 2007. "Natural Intentions: Fertility Decline in the African Demographic and Health Surveys." *American Journal of Sociology* 112 (4): 1008–1043.

Justice, Judith. 1986. *Policies, Plans and People: Culture and Health Development in Nepal.* Berkeley: University of California Press.

Kaler, Amy. 2009. "Health Interventions and the Persistence of Rumour: The Circulation of Sterility Stories in African Public Health Campaigns." *Social Science and Medicine* 68 (9): 1711–1719.

Kaler, Amy, Susan Cotts Watkins, and Nicole Angotti. 2015. "Making Meaning in the Time of AIDS: Longitudinal Narratives from the Malawi Journals Project." *African Journal of AIDS Research* 14 (4): 303–314.

Kamuya, Dorcas M., Sally J. Theobald, Patrick K. Munywoki, Dorothy Koech, Wenzel P. Geissler, and Sassy C. Molyneux. 2013. "Evolving Friendships and Shifting Ethical Dilemmas: Fieldworkers' Experiences in a Short Term Community Based Study in Kenya." *Developing World Bioethics* 13 (1): 1–9.

Kaspin, Deborah. 1995. "The Politics of Ethnicity in Malawi's Democratic Transition." *Journal of Modern African Studies* 33: 595–620.

Kasprzyk, Daniel. 2005. "Measurement Error in Household Surveys: Sources and Measurement." In *Household Sample Surveys in Developing and Transition Countries*. New York: United Nations Statistics Division.

Kaufulu, Moses Mphatso. 2008. "*Kulowa Kufa* Cultural Practise: Its Nature, Practice and Function in an Era of HIV/AIDS." Undergraduate thesis. Sociology Department, University of Malawi-Chancellor College, Zomba, Malawi.

Kekovole, John, and Clifford O. Odimegwu. 2014. "Population Policies in Sub-Saharan Africa: Evolution, Achievements, and Challenges." In *Continuity and Change in Sub-Saharan African Demography*, edited by Clifford O. Odimegwu and John Kekovole. New York: Routledge.

Keller, Richard. 2007. "Taking Science to the Colonies: Psychiatric Innovation in France and North Africa." In *Psychiatry and Empire*, edited by Sloane Mahone and Megan Vaughan. New York: Cambridge University Press.

Kelly, Ann. 2003. "Research and the Subject: The Practice of Informed Consent." *PoLAR* 26 (2): 182–195.

Kelly, Ann. 2015. "The Territory of Medical Research: Experimentation in Africa's Smallest State." In *Para-states and Medical Science: Making African Global Health*, edited by P. Wenzel Geissler. Durham, NC: Duke University Press.

Kelly, Ann, David Ameh, Silas Majambere, Steve Lindsay, and Margaret Pinder. 2010. " 'Like Sugar and Honey': The Embedded Ethics of a Larval Control Project in the Gambia." *Social Science and Medicine* 70 (12): 1912–1919.

Kennickell, Arthur. 2015. "Curbstoning and Culture." *Statistical Journal of the IAOS* 31: 237–240.

Kenworthy, Nora. 2014. "Participation, Decentralization and Déjà Vu: Remaking Democracy in Response to AIDS?" *Global Public Health* 9 (1–2): 25–42.

Kerr, David, and Jack Mapanje. 2002. "Academic Freedom at the University of Malawi." *African Studies Review* 45 (2): 73–91.

Kerr, Rachel Bezner. 2005. "Informal Labor and Social Relations in Northern Malawi: The Theoretical Challenges and Implications of Ganyu Labor for Food Security." *Rural Sociology* 70 (2): 167–187.

Kertzer, David I. 1995. "Political, Economic and Cultural Explanations of Demographic Behavior." In *Situating Fertility: Anthropology and Demographic Inquiry*, edited by Susan Greenhalgh. New York: Cambridge University Press.

Kertzer, David I., and Dominique Arel. 2002. *Census and Identity: The Politics of Race, Ethnicity, and Language in National Censuses*. New York: Cambridge University Press.

Kertzer, David, and Tom Fricke, eds. 1997. *Anthropological Demography: Toward a New Synthesis*. Chicago: University of Chicago Press.

Kickbusch, Ilona, Gaudenz Silberschmidt, and Paulo Buss. 2007. "Global Health Diplomacy: The Need for New Perspectives, Strategic Approaches, and Skills in Global Health." *Bulletin of the World Health Organization* 85 (3): 230–232.

King, G., and J. Wand. 2007. "Comparing Incomparable Survey Responses: Evaluating and Selecting Anchoring Vignettes." *Political Analysis* 15: 46–66.

King, Nicholas B. 2002. "Security, Disease, Commerce: Ideologies of Postcolonial Global Health." *Social Studies of Science* 32 (5–6): 763–789.

Kingori, Patricia. 2013. "Experiencing Everyday Ethics in Context: Frontline Data Collectors' Perspectives and Practices of Bioethics." *Social Science and Medicine* 98: 361–370.

Kingori, Patricia, and René Gerrets. 2016. "Morals, Morale and Motivations in Data Fabrication: Medical Research Fieldworkers Views and Practices in Two Sub-Saharan African Contexts." *Social Science and Medicine* 166: 150–159.

Kingori, Patricia, and Salla Sariola. 2015. "Museum of Failed HIV Research." *Anthropology and Medicine* 22 (3): 213–216.

Klenk, Nicole L., Gordon M. Hickey, and James Ian MacLellan. 2010. "Evaluating the Social Capital Accrued in Large Research Networks: The Case of the Sustainable Forest Management Network (1995–2009)." *Social Studies of Science* 40 (6): 931–960.

Knaapen, Loes. 2013. "Being 'Evidence-Based' in the Absence of Evidence: The Management of Non-evidence in Guideline Development." *Social Studies of Science* 43 (5): 681–706.

Knight, Kelly Ray. 2015. *Addicted. Pregnant. Poor.* Durham, NC: Duke University Press.

Knoll, Megan, Lianne Soller, Moshe Ben-Shosan, Daniel Harrington, Joey Fragapane, Lawrence Joseph, Sebastien La Vieille, Yvan St-Pierre, Kathi Wilson, Susan Elliott, and Ann Clark. 2012. "The Use of Incentives in Vulnerable Populations for a Telephone Survey: A RCT." *BMC Research Notes* 5: 572.

Knorr-Cetina, Karin. 1999. *Epistemic Cultures: How the Sciences Make Knowledge.* Cambridge, MA: Harvard University Press.

Koczela, Steve, Cathy Furlong, Jaki McCarthy, and Ali Mushtaq. 2015. "Curbstoning and Beyond: Confronting Data Fabrication in Survey Research." *Statistical Journal of the IAOS* 31: 413–422.

Kogacioglu, D. 2004. "The Tradition Effect: Framing Honor Crimes in Turkey." *Differences* 15 (2): 119–151.

Kornfield, Ruth, and Dorothy Namate. 1997. "Cultural Practices Related to HIV/AIDS Risk Behaviour: Community Survey in Phalombe, Malawi." Washington, DC: USAID.

Kranzer, K., N. McGrath, J. Saul, A. C. Crampin, A. Jahn, S. Malema, D. Mulawa, P. E. M. Fine, B. Zaba, and J. R. Glynn. 2008. "Individual Household and Community Factors Associated with HIV Test Refusal in Rural Malawi." *Tropical Medicine and International Health* 13 (11): 1341–1350.

Krause, Monica. 2014. *The Good Project: Humanitarian Relief and the Fragmentation of Reason.* Chicago: University of Chicago Press.

Kriel, Antoinette, Sara Randall, Ernestina Coast, and Bernadene de Clercq. 2014. "From Design to Practice: How Can Large-Scale Household Surveys Better Represent the Complexities of the Social Units under Investigation?" *African Population Studies* 28 (3): 1309–1323.

Kuczynski, R. R. 1949. *Demographic Survey of the British Colonial Empire.* Oxford: Oxford University Press.

Kuklick, Henrika, and Robert E. Kohler, eds. 1996. *Science in the Field.* Chicago: University of Chicago Press.

Lairumbi, Geoffrey M., Michael Parker, Raymond Fitzpatrick, and Michael C. English. 2012. "Forms of Benefit Sharing in Global Health Research Undertaken in Resource Poor Settings: A Qualitative Study of Stakeholders' Views in Kenya." *Philosophy, Ethics, and Humanities in Medicine* 7 (7).

Lambek, Michael. 1993. *Knowledge and Practice in Mayotte: Local Discourses of Islam, Sorcery, and Spirit Possession.* Toronto: University of Toronto Press.

Lambert, Helen. 2009. "Evidentiary Truths? The Evidence of Anthropology through the Anthropology of Medical Evidence." *Anthropology Today* 25 (1): 16–20.

Lampland, Martha. 2009. "Reckoning with Standards." In *Standards and Their Stories: How Quantifying, Classifying, and Formalizing Practices Shape Everyday Life*, edited by Martha Lampland and Susan Leigh Star. Ithaca, NY: Cornell University Press.

Lampland, Martha. 2010. "False Numbers as Formalizing Practices." *Social Studies of Science* 40 (3): 377–404.

Langwick, Stacey A. 2011. "Healers and Scientists: The Epistemological Politics of Research about Medicinal Plants in Tanzania or 'Moving Away from Traditional Medicine.'" In *Evidence, Ethos and Experiment: The Anthropology and History of Medical Research in Africa*, edited by Wenzel P. Geissler and Catherine Molyneux. New York: Berghahn.

Latour, Bruno. 1983. "Give Me a Laboratory and I Will Raise the World." In *Science Observed*, edited by K. D. Knorr-Cetina and M. J. Mulkay. Thousand Oaks, CA: Sage.

Latour, Bruno. 1987. *Science in Action: How to Follow Scientists and Engineers through Society.* Cambridge, MA: Harvard University Press.

Latour, Bruno, and Steven Woolgar. 1979. *Laboratory Life.* Thousand Oaks, CA: Sage.

Law, John, and Marianne Elizabeth Lien. 2012. "Slippery: Field Notes in Empirical Ontology." *Social Studies of Science* 43 (3): 363–378.

Lekgoathi, Sekibakiba. 2009. "Colonial Experts, Local Interlocutors, Informants and the Making of the 'Transvaal Ndebele,' 1930–1989." *Journal of African History* 50: 61–80.

Leonard, Joan deLourdes. 1954. "Elections in Colonial Pennsylvania." *William and Mary Quarterly* 11 (3): 385–401.

Lévi-Strauss, Claude. 1969. *The Raw and the Cooked.* Chicago: University of Chicago Press.

Livingston, Julie. 2012. *Improvising Medicine: An African Oncology Ward in an Emerging Cancer Epidemic.* Durham, NC: Duke University Press.

Locke, Peter. 2015. "Anthropology and Medical Humanitarianism in the Age of Global Health Education." In *Medical Humanitarianism: Ethnographies of Practice*, edited by Sharon Abramowitz and Catherine Painter-Brick. Philadelphia: University of Pennsylvania Press.

Lorimer, Frank. 1968. "Introduction." In *The Demography of Tropical Africa*, edited by William Brass, Ansley J. Cole, Paul Demeny, Don F. Heisel, Frank Lorimer, Anatole Romaniuk, and Etienne van de Walle. Princeton, NJ: Princeton University Press.

Lorimer, Jamie. 2008. "Counting Corncrakes: The Affective Science of the UK Corncrake Census." *Social Studies of Science* 38 (3): 377–405.

Lorway, R., and S. Khan. 2014. "Reassembling Epidemiology: Mapping, Monitoring and Making-Up People in the Context of HIV Prevention in India." *Social Science and Medicine* 112: 51–62.

Loveman, Mara. 2007. "The US Census and the Contested Rules of Racial Classification in Early Twentieth-Century Puerto Rico." *Caribbean Studies* 35 (2): 78–113.

Luke, Nancy. 2006. "Local Meanings and Census Categories: Widow Inheritance and the Position of Luo Widows in Kenya." In *African Households: Censuses and Surveys*, edited by Etienne van de Walle. New York: Routledge.

Lwanda, John. 2005. *Politics, Culture, and Medicine in Malawi: Historical Continuities and Ruptures with Special Reference to HIV/AIDS*. Zomba, Malawi: Kachere.

Lyberg, Lars E., and Paul P. Biemer. 2008. "Quality Assurance and Quality Control in Surveys." In *International Handbook of Survey Methodology*, edited by Edith D. de Leeuw, Joop T. Hox, and Don A. Dillman. Philadelphia: Taylor and Francis.

Lynn, P. 2008. "The Problem of Nonresponse." In *International Handbook of Survey Methodology*, edited by Edith D. de Leeuw, Joop T. Hox, and Don A. Dillman. Philadelphia: Taylor and Francis.

Madhavan, Sangeetha, Mark Collinson, Nicholas W. Townsend, Kathleen Kahn, and Stephen M. Tollman. 2007. "The Implications of Long Term Community Involvement for the Production and Circulation of Population Knowledge." *Demographic Research* 17 (13): 369–388.

Madiega, Philister Adhiambo, Gemma Jones, Ruth Jane Prince, and Paul Wenzel Geissler. 2013. " 'She's My Sister-in-Law, My Visitor, My Friend'—Challenges of Staff Identity in Home Follow-Up in an HIV Trial in Western Kenya." *Developing World Bioethics* 13 (1): 21–29.

Maes, Kenneth. 2015. "Community Health Workers and Social Change." *Annals of Anthropological Practice* 39 (1): 1–15.

Maes, Kenneth. 2017. *The Lives of Community Health Workers: Local Labor and Global Health in Urban Ethiopia*. New York: Routledge.

Malikwa, Y. 2007. "Chiradzulu: A District of Mystery." *Pride Magazine* (Zomba, Malawi).

Malinowski, Bronislaw. (1922) 1984. *Argonauts of the Western Pacific*. New York: Routledge.

Mamdani, Mahmood. 2012. *Define and Rule: Native as Political Identity*. Cambridge, MA: Harvard University Press.

Mandala, Elias. 2005. *The End of Chidyerano: A History of Food and Everyday Life in Malawi*. Portsmouth, NH: Heinemann.

March, James G., and Herbert A. Simon. 1958. *Organizations*. New York: Wiley.

Marcus, George. 1998. *Ethnography through Thick and Thin*. Princeton, NJ: Princeton University Press.

Martin, C. J. 1949. "The East African Population Census, 1948. Planning and Enumeration." *Population Studies* 3 (3): 303–320.

Masquelier, Adeline. 2012. "Public Health or Public Threat? Polio Eradication Campaigns, Islamic Revival, and the Materialization of State Power in Niger." In *Mobility and Power in Global Health: Transnational Health and Healing*, edited by Hansjorg Dilger, Abdoulaye Kane, and Stacey A. Langwick. Bloomington: Indiana University Press.

Mauss, Marcel. (1922) 1967. *The Gift: Forms and Functions of Exchange in Archaic Societies*. New York: Norton.

Mauss, Marcel. 1973. "Techniques of the Body." *Economy and Society* 2 (1): 70–88.

May, Marian. 2008. " 'I Didn't Write the Questions!' Negotiating Telephone-Survey Questions on Birth Timing." *Demographic Research* 18 (18): 499–530.

Mba, Chuks J. 2014. "Examining the Accuracy of Age-Sex Data: An Evaluation of Recent Sub-Saharan African Population Censuses." In *Continuity and Change in Sub-Saharan African Demography*, edited by Clifford O. Odimegwu and John Kekovole. New York: Routledge.

McAuliffe, E. 1994. "AIDS: The Barriers to Behavior Change." Zomba, Malawi: UNICEF and CSR.

McCaa, Robert, Albert Esteve, Steven Ruggles, and Matt Sobek. 2006. "Using Integrated Census Microdata for Evidence-Based Policy Making: The IPUMS-International Global Initiative." *African Statistical Journal* 2: 83–100.

McClintock, Anne. 1995. *Imperial Leather: Race, Gender, and Sexuality in the Colonial Contest*. New York: Routledge.

McCook, Stuart. 1996. " 'It May Be Truth, but It Is Not Evidence': Paul du Chaillu and the Legitimation of Evidence in the Field Sciences." *Osiris* 11: 177–197.

McCracken, John. 2012. *A History of Malawi, 1859–1966*. Woodbridge, U.K.: Boydell and Brewer.

McCulloch, Jock. 1995. *Colonial Psychiatry and the African Mind*. New York: Cambridge University Press.

McFerran, A. 2003. "Vampire Hysteria Haunts Hungry Villagers of Malawi." *London Times*.

McGranahan, Carole. 2016. "Theorizing Refusal: An Introduction." *Cultural Anthropology* 31 (3): 319–325.

McKay, Ramah. 2012. "Humanitarian Histories and Critical Subjects in Mozambique." *Cultural Anthropology* 27 (2): 286–309.

McKay, Ramah. 2018. *Medicine in the Meantime: The Work of Care in Mozambique*. Durham, NC: Duke University Press.

McKay, Tara. 2016. "From Marginal to Marginalised: The Inclusion of Men Who Have Sex with Men in Global and National AIDS Programmes and Policy." *Global Public Health* 11 (7–8): 902–922.

McNicoll, Geoffrey. 1990. "The Agenda of Population Studies: A Commentary and Complaint." *Population Development Review* 18 (3): 399–420.

Meinert, Lotte. 2015. "The Work of the Virus: Cutting and Creating Relations in an ART Project." In *Para-states and Medical Science: Making African Global Health*, edited by Wenzel P. Geissler. Durham, NC: Duke University Press.

Meinert, Lotte, and Susan Reynolds Whyte. 2014. "Epidemic Projectification: AIDS Responses in Uganda as Event and Process." *Cambridge Journal of Anthropology* 32 (1): 77–94.

Mercer, Claire. 2003. "Performing Partnership: Civil Society and the Illusions of Good Governance in Tanzania." *Political Geography* 22: 741–763.

Merry, Sally Engle. 2011. "Measuring the World: Indicators, Human Rights, and Global Governance." *Current Anthropology* 52 (s3): s83–s95.

Metcalf, Peter. 2002. *They Lie, We Lie: Getting On with Anthropology*. London: Routledge.

Meyers, Todd, and Nancy Rose Hunt. 2014. "The Other Global South." *Lancet* 384 (9958): 1921–1922.

Mfutso-Bengo, Joseph, and Francis Masiye. 2011. "Toward an African Ubuntuology/ uMunthuology: Bioethics in Malawi." In *Bioethics around the Globe*, edited by Catherine Myser. Oxford: Oxford University Press.

MHRC. 2006. "Cultural Practices and Their Impact on the Enjoyment of Human Rights, Particularly the Rights of Women and Children in Malawi." Lilongwe, Malawi: Malawi Human Rights Commission.

Miller, Kate, Eliya Msiyaphazi Zulu, and Susan Cotts Watkins. 2001. "Husband-Wife Survey Responses in Malawi." *Studies in Family Planning* 32 (2): 161–174.

Mitchell, Timothy. 1991. *Colonising Egypt*. Berkeley: University of California Press.

Mkandawire, N. A. 1986. *Study on Small Countries Research: Report on Malawi*. Ottawa: International Development Research Centre.

Mkhwanazi, Nolwazi. 2016. "Medical Anthropology in Africa: The Trouble with a Single Story." *Medical Anthropology* 35 (2): 193–202.

Mmana, D. 2007. "Bloodsuckers Terrorize Chiradzulu!" *Malawi News*, September 29– October 5.

Mohler, P. P. 2006. "Sampling from a Universe of Items and the De-Machiavellization of Questionnaire Design." In *Beyond the Horizon of Measurement: Festschrift in Honor of Ingwer Bborg*, edited by M. Braun and P. P. Mohler. Mannheim: ZUMA.

Mojola, Sanyu. 2014. *Love, Money and HIV: Becoming a Modern African Woman in the Age of AIDS*. Berkeley: University of California Press.

Mol, Annemarie. 2002. *The Body Multiple: Ontology in Medical Practice*. Durham, NC: Duke University Press.

Molyneux, Sassy, and P. Wenzel Geissler. 2008. "Ethics and the Ethnography of Medical Research in Africa." *Social Science and Medicine* 67 (5): 685–695.

Molyneux, S., D. Kamuya, P. A. Madiega, T. Chantler, V. Angwenyi, and P. W. Geissler. 2013. "Fieldworkers at the Interface." *Developing World Bioethics* 13 (1): ii–iv.

Moniruzzaman, Monir. 2012. " 'Living Cadavers' in Bangladesh: Bioviolence in the Human Organ Bazaar." *MAQ* 26 (1): 69–91.

Morphy, Frances. 2007. "Uncontained Subjects: 'Population' and 'Household' in Remote Aboriginal Australia." *Journal of Population Research* 24 (2): 163–184.

Mosse, D. 2004. "Is Good Policy Unimplementable? Reflections on the Ethnography of Aid Policy and Practice." *Development and Change* 35 (4): 639–671.

Moyer, Eileen. 2015. "The Anthropology of Life after AIDS: Epistemological Continuities in the Age of Antiretroviral Treatment." *Annual Review of Anthropology* 44: 259–275.

Mpaka, Vincent. 2008. "AIDS as Suffered in Phalombe." *Daily Times*, June 19.

Mulwafu, Wapulumuka Oliver. 2011. *Conservation Song: A History of Peasant-State Relations and the Environment in Malawi, 1860–2000*. Winwick, U.K.: White Horse Press.

Munthali, A. C., and E. M. Zulu. 2007. "The Timing and Role of Initiation Rites in Preparing Young People for Adolescence and Responsible Sexual and Reproductive Behavior in Malawi." *African Journal of Reproductive Health* 11 (3): 150–167.

Munthali, G. 2002. "No Bloodhunters Around—Muluzi." *The Nation*, December 23.

Musambachime, Mwelwa C. 1988. "The Impact of Rumor: The Case of the Banyama (Vampire Men) Scare in Northern Rhodesia, 1930–1964." *International Journal of African Historical Studies* 21 (2): 201–215.

Muula, A. S., and J. M. Mfutso-Bengo. 2007. "Responsibilities and Obligations of Using Human Research Specimens Transported across National Boundaries." *Journal of Medical Ethics* 33 (1): 35–38.

Muwamba, E. 2007. "Villagers Beat up DPP Official." *The Nation*, December 19.

Mwapasa, Victor. 2006. "Planning Research Studies on the Impact of the National HIV/AIDS Response in Malawi." Malawi: National AIDS Commission.

NAC. 2003. "National HIV and AIDS Policy, 2003." Malawi: National AIDS Commission.

NAC. 2009. "National HIV Prevention Strategy: 2009–2013." Malawi: National AIDS Commission.

NAC. 2010. "National HIV and AIDS Policy, July 2011–June 2016." Malawi: National AIDS Commission.

NAC. 2014. "National HIV Prevention Strategy, 2015–2020." Malawi: National AIDS Commission.

NAC. 2015a. "Malawi AIDS Response Progress Report, 2015." Malawi: National AIDS Commission.

NAC. 2015b. "National Strategic Plan for HIV and AIDS, 2015–2020." Malawi: National AIDS Commission.

Nader, Laura. 1972. "Up the Anthropologist—Perspectives Gained from Studying Up." In *Reinventing Anthropology*, edited by Dell Hymes. New York: Vintage.

Nading, Alex M. 2013. " 'Love Isn't There in Your Stomach': A Moral Economy of Medical Citizenship among Nicaraguan Community Health Workers." *Medical Anthropology Quarterly* 27 (1): 84–102.

Nathanson, Constance A. 2007. "The Contingent Power of Experts: Public Health Policy in the United States, Britain and France." *Journal of Policy History* 19 (1): 71–94.

National Statistical Office (NSO). 2008. "2008 Population and Housing Census Preliminary Report." Zomba, Malawi: NSO.

Nations, Marilyn K., and L. A. Rebhun. 1988. "Mystification of a Simple Solution: Oral Rehydration Therapy in Northeast Brazil." *Social Science and Medicine* 27 (1): 25–38.

NCPHSBBR. 1979. "The Belmont Report: Ethical Principles and Guidelines for the Protection of Human Subjects." Washington, DC: National Commission for the Protection of Human Subjects of Biomedical and Behavioral Research.

Ndebele, P., J. Mfutso-Bengo, and T. Mduluza. 2008. "Compensating Clinical Trial Participants from Limited Resource Settings in Internationally Sponsored Trials." *Malawi Medical Journal* 20 (2): 42–45.

Neely, Abigail H., and Alex M. Nading. 2017. "Global Health from the Outside: The Promise of Place-Based Research." *Health & Place* 45: 55–63.

Nelson, Diane. 2015. *Who Counts? The Mathematics of Life and Death after Genocide.* Durham, NC: Duke University Press.

Netz, R. 2002. "Counter Culture: Towards a History of Greek Numeracy." *History of Science* 40: 321–352.

Nguyen, Vinh-Kim. 2010. *The Republic of Therapy: Triage and Sovereignty in West Africa's Time of AIDS.* Durham, NC: Duke University Press.

Nyambedha, Erick Otieno. 2008. "Ethical Dilemmas of Social Science Research on AIDS and Orphanhood in Western Kenya." *SSM* 67: 771–779.

Nyamnjoh, Francis. 2015. "Beyond an Evangelizing Public Anthropology: Science, Theory, and Commitment." *JCAS* 33 (1): 48–63.

Obare, Francis. 2010. "Nonresponse in Repeat Population-Based Voluntary Counseling and Testing for HIV in Rural Malawi." *Demography* 47 (3): 651–665.

Obare, F., P. Fleming, P. Anglewicz, R. Thornton, F. Martinson, A. Kapatuka, M. Poulin, S. Watkins, and H.-P. Kohler. 2009. "Acceptance of Repeat Population-Based Voluntary Counseling and Testing for HIV in Rural Malawi." *Sexually Transmitted Infections* 85 (2): 139–144.

Ortner, Sherry. 2016. "Dark Anthropology and Its Others: Theory since the Eighties." *HAU* 6 (1): 47–73.

Oucho, J. P. Akwara, and Elias H. O. Ayiemba. 1995. "African Population and Development Agenda from Bucharest to Cairo and Beyond." Paper No. 5. Nairobi: African Population and Environment Institute.

Owusu, D. J. 1968. "Taking a Population Census in Tropical Africa." In *The Population of Tropical Africa*, edited by John C. Caldwell and Chukuka Okonjo. New York: Columbia University Press.

Packard, Randall. 1989. *White Plague, Black Labor: Tuberculosis and the Political Economy of Health and Disease in South Africa.* Berkeley: University of California Press.

Packard, Randall. 2016. *A History of Global Health: Interventions into the Lives of Other Peoples.* Baltimore, MD: Johns Hopkins University Press.

Page, Samantha. 2014. "Narratives of Blame: HIV/AIDS and Harmful Cultural Practices in Malawi, Implications for Policies and Programmes." PhD diss., University of Portsmouth.

Patton, Cindy. 1990. *Inventing AIDS.* New York: Routledge.

Pennell, Beth-Ellen, Rachel Levenstein, and Hyun Jung Lee. 2010. "Data Collection." In *Survey Research Center Guidelines for Best Practice in Cross-Cultural Surveys.* Ann Arbor, MI: Survey Research Center, Institute for Social Research, University of Michigan. http://www.ccsg.isr.umich.edu/.

Peters, Pauline E., Daimon Kambewa, and Peter A. Walker. 2010. "Contestations over 'Tradition' and 'Culture' in a Time of AIDS." *Medical Anthropology* 29 (3): 278–302.

Peters, Rebecca Warne. 2016. "Local in Practice: Professional Distinctions in Angolan Development Work." *American Anthropologist* 118 (3): 495–507.

Peterson, Brian. 2002. "Quantifying Conversion: A Note on the Colonial Census and Religious Change in Postwar French Mali." *History in Africa* 29: 381–392.

Peterson, Kristin. 2009. "Phantom Epistemologies." In *Fieldwork Is Not What It Used to Be: Learning Anthropology's Method in a Time of Transition*, edited by James D. Faubion and George E. Marcus. Ithaca, NY: Cornell University Press.

Peterson, Kristin, Morenike Oluwatoyin Folayan, Edward Chigwedere, and Evaristo Nthete. 2015. "Saying 'No' to PrEP Research in Malawi: What Constitutes 'Failure' in Offshored HIV Prevention Research." *Anthropology and Medicine* 22 (3): 278–294.

Petryna, Adriana. 2002. *Life Exposed: Biological Citizens after Chernobyl*. Princeton, NJ: Princeton University Press.

Petryna, Adriana. 2005. "Ethical Variability: Drug Development and Globalizing Clinical Trials." *American Ethnologist* 32 (2): 183–197.

Pfeiffer, James, and Mark Nichter. 2008. "What Can Critical Medical Anthropology Contribute to Global Health?" *Medical Anthropology Quarterly* 22 (4): 410–415.

Phiri, Vincent. 2008. "Bad Weather Affects Census." *The Nation*, June 13.

Pierre, Jemima. 2013. *The Predicament of Blackness: Postcolonial Ghana and the Politics of Race*. Chicago: University of Chicago Press.

Pigg, Stacey Leigh. 1996. "The Credible and the Credulous: The Question of 'Villagers' Beliefs' in Nepal." *Cultural Anthropology* 11 (2): 160–201.

PNG. 2004. "National Survey of Adolescents, Adolescent Questionnaire." New York, Guttmacher Institute, Protecting the Next Generation Project.

Poovey, Mary. 1998. *A History of the Modern Fact*. Chicago: University of Chicago Press.

Povinelli, Elizabeth. 2011. *Economies of Abandonment: Social Belonging and Endurance in Late Liberalism*. Durham, NC: Duke University Press.

Pratt, Mary Louise. 1991. "Arts of the Contact Zone." *Profession* 91: 33–40.

Pratt, Mary Louise. 1992. *Imperial Eyes: Travel Writing and Transculturation*. New York: Routledge.

Prince, Ruth J. 2012. "HIV and the Moral Economy of Survival in an East African City." *MAQ* 26 (4): 534–556.

Prince, Ruth J. 2014. "Precarious Projects: Conversions of Biomedical Knowledge in an East African City." *Medical Anthropology* 33 (1): 68–83.

Prince, Ruth J. 2016. "The Diseased Body and the Global Subject: The Circulation and Consumption of an Iconic AIDS Photograph in East Africa." *Visual Anthropology* 29 (2): 159–186.

Prince, Ruth J., and P. Otieno. 2014. "In the Shadowlands of Global Health: Observations from Health Workers in Kenya." *Global Public Health* 9 (8): 927–945.

Prohmmo, Aree, and John Bryant. 2004. "Measuring the Population of a Northeast Thai Village." In *Categories and Contexts: Anthropological and Historical Studies in Critical Demography*, edited by Simon Szreter, Hania Sholkamy, and A. Dharmalingam. New York: Oxford University Press.

Puig de la Bellacasa, M. 2011. "Matters of Care in Technoscience: Assembling Neglected Things." *Social Studies of Science* 41 (1): 85–106.

Putzel, James. 2004. "The Global Fight against AIDS: How Adequate Are the National Commissions?" *Journal of International Development* 16: 1129–1140.

Raj, Kapil. 2007. *Relocating Modern Science: Circulation and the Construction of Knowledge in South Asia and Europe, 1650–1900.* London: Palgrave Macmillan.

Randall, Sara, and Ernestina Coast. 2015. "Poverty in African Households: The Limits of Survey and Census Representations." *Journal of Development Studies* 51 (2): 162–177.

Randall, Sara, Ernestina Coast, Natacha Compaore, and Philippe Antoine. 2013. "The Power of the Interviewer." *Demographic Research* 28 (27): 763–792.

Randall, Sara, Ernestina Coast, and Tiziana Leone. 2011. "Cultural Constructions of the Concept of Household in Sample Surveys." *Population Studies* 65 (2): 217–229.

Reddy, Deepa S. 2007. "Good Gifts for the Common Good: Blood and Bioethics in the Market of Genetic Research." *Cultural Anthropology* 22 (3): 429–472.

Redfield, Peter. 2008. "Vital Mobility and the Humanitarian Kit." In *Biosecurity Interventions*, edited by Andrew Lakoff and Stephen Collier. New York: Columbia University Press.

Redfield, Peter. 2012. "The Unbearable Lightness of Ex-pats: Double Binds of Humanitarian Mobility." *Cultural Anthropology* 27 (2): 358–382.

Redfield, Peter. 2013. *Life in Crisis: The Ethical Journey of Doctors without Borders.* Berkeley: University of California Press.

Redfield, Peter. 2016. "Fluid Technologies: The Bush Pump, the LifeStraw and Microworlds of Humanitarian Design." *Social Studies of Science* 46 (2): 159–183.

Reniers, Georges, and Jeffrey Eaton. 2009. "Refusal Bias in HIV Prevalence Estimates from Nationally Representative Seroprevalence Surveys." *AIDS* 23 (5): 621–629.

Reynolds, Lindsey, Thomas Cousins, Marie-Louise Newell, and John Imrie. 2013. "The Social Dynamics of Consent and Refusal in HIV Surveillance in Rural South Africa." *Social Science and Medicine* 77: 118–125.

Ribes, David, and Steven J. Jackson. 2013. "Data Bite Man: The Work of Sustaining a Long-Term Study." In *"Raw Data" Is an Oxymoron*, edited by Lisa Gitelman. Cambridge, MA: MIT Press.

Ridde, Valéry. 2010. "Per Diems Undermine Health Interventions, Systems and Research in Africa: Burying Our Heads in the Sand." *Tropical Medicine and International Health*, July 28. doi:10.1111/j.1365-3156.2010.02607.x.

Riedmann, Agnes. 1993. *Science That Colonizes: A Critique of Fertility Studies in Africa.* Philadelphia: Temple University Press.

Riles, Annelise. 2000. *The Network Inside Out.* Ann Arbor: University of Michigan Press.

Riley, Nancy E., and James McCarthy. 2003. *Demography in the Age of the Postmodern.* New York: Cambridge University Press.

Robbins, Joel. 2013. "Beyond the Suffering Subject: Toward an Anthropology of the Good." *JRAI* 19 (3): 447–462.

Rosenberg, Daniel. 2013. "Data before the Fact." In *"Raw Data" Is an Oxymoron*, edited by Lisa Gitelman. Cambridge, MA: MIT Press.

Rottenburg, R. 2009. "Social and Public Experiments and New Figurations of Science and Politics in Postcolonial Africa." *Postcolonial Studies* 12 (4): 423–440.

Rottenburg, Richard, Sally Engle Merry, Sung-Joon Park, and Johanna Mugler, eds. 2015. *The World of Indicators: The Making of Governmental Knowledge through Quantification.* New York: Cambridge University Press.

Salamone, Frank. 1977. "The Methodological Significance of the Lying Informant." *Anthropological Quarterly* 50 (3): 117–124.

Sambakunsi, Rodrick, Moses Kumwenda, Augustine Choko, Elizabeth L. Corbett, and Nicola Ann Desmond. 2015. "Whose Failure Counts? A Critical Reflection on Definitions of Failure for Community Health Volunteers Providing HIV Self-Testing in a Community-Based HIV/TB Intervention Study in Urban Malawi." *Anthropology and Medicine* 22 (3): 234–249.

Samsky, Ari. 2012. "Scientific Sovereignty: How International Drug Donation Programs Reshape Health, Disease, and the State." *Cultural Anthropology* 27 (2): 310–332.

Sana, Mariano, and Alexander Weinreb. 2008. "Insiders, Outsiders, and the Editing of Inconsistent Survey Data." *Sociological Methods and Research* 36 (4): 515–541.

Sangaramoorthy, T., and A. Benton. 2012. "Enumeration, Identity, and Health." *Medical Anthropology* 31 (4): 287–291.

Scheper-Hughes, Nancy. 1990. "Three Propositions for a Critically Applied Medical Anthropology." *Social Science in Medicine* 30 (2): 189–197.

Scheper-Hughes, Nancy. 1997. "Demography without Numbers." In *Anthropological Demography: Toward a New Synthesis*, edited by David I. Kertzer and Tom Fricke. Chicago: University of Chicago Press.

Schumaker, Lyn. 2001. *Africanizing Anthropology: Fieldwork, Networks, and the Making of Cultural Knowledge in Central Africa.* Durham, NC: Duke University Press.

Scott, James. 1998. *Seeing Like a State: How Certain Schemes to Improve the Human Condition Have Failed.* New Haven, CT: Yale University Press.

Sedgwick, Eve. 2003. *Touching, Feeling: Affect, Pedagogy, Performativity.* Durham, NC: Duke University Press.

Segone, Marco, ed. 2004. *Bridging the Gap: The Role of Monitoring and Evaluation in Evidence-Based Policy Making.* New York: UNICEF.

Setel, Philip W. 2000. *A Plague of Paradoxes: AIDS, Culture, and Demography in Northern Tanzania.* Chicago: University of Chicago Press.

Sgaier, Sema K., Jason B. Reed, Anne Thomas, and Emmanuel Njeuhmeli. 2014. "Achieving the HIV Prevention Impact of Voluntary Medical Male Circumcision: Lessons and Challenges for Managing Programs." *PLOS Medicine*, May 6. https://doi.org/10.1371/journal.pmed.1001641.

Shapin, Steven. 1989. "The Invisible Technician." *American Scientist* 77 (6): 554–563.

Shapin, Steven. 1994. *A Social History of Truth: Civility and Science in Seventeenth Century England.* Chicago: University of Chicago Press.

Shapin, Steven, and Simon Schaffer. 1985. *Leviathan and the Air-Pump: Hobbes, Boyle, and the Experimental Life.* Princeton, NJ: Princeton University Press.

Shubber, Zara, Sharmistha Mishra, Juan F. Vesga, and Marie-Claude Boily. 2014. "The HIV Modes of Transmission Model: A Systematic Review of Its Findings and Adherence to Guidelines." *Journal of the International AIDS Society* 17 (1): 18928.

Simpson, Audra. 2016. "Consent's Revenge." *Cultural Anthropology* 31 (3): 326–333.

Singer, Eleanor, and C. Ye. 2013. "The Use and Effects of Incentives in Surveys." *Annals of the American Academy of Political and Social Science* 645 (1): 112–141.

Smith, Daniel Jordan. 2008. *A Culture of Corruption: Everyday Deception and Popular Discontent in Nigeria.* Princeton, NJ: Princeton University Press.

Smith, Tom W. 2002. "Developing Comparable Questions in Cross-National Surveys." In *Cross-Cultural Survey Methods,* edited by Janet A. Harkness, Fons J. R. van de Vijver, and Peter P. Mohler. New York: Wiley.

Soreide, Tina, Arne Tostensen, and Ingvild Skage. 2012. *Hunting for Per Diem: The Uses and Abuses of Travel Compensation in Three Developing Countries.* Oslo: Norad.

Spagat, Michael. 2010. "Ethical and Data-Integrity Problems in the Second *Lancet* Survey of Mortality in Iraq." *Defence and Peace Economics* 21 (1): 1–41.

Star, Susan Leigh, and James R. Griesemer. 1989. "Institutional Ecology, 'Translations' and Boundary Objects: Amateurs and Professionals in Berkeley's Museum of Vertebrate Zoology, 1907–39." *Social Studies of Science* 19: 387–420.

Star, Susan Leigh, and Martha Lampland. 2008. "Reckoning with Standards." In *Standards and Their Stories,* edited by Martha Lampland and Susan Leigh Star. Ithaca, NY: Cornell University Press.

Stecklov, Guy, and Alex Weinreb. 2010. "Improving the Quality of Data and Impact-Evaluation Studies in Developing Countries." Washington, DC: Inter-American Development Bank.

Stecklov, Guy, Alex Weinreb, and Calogero Carletto. 2015. "Can Gifting Improve Survey Data Quality in Developing Countries?" Annual Meeting of American Population Association, San Diego, CA, April 30.

Stevenson, Lisa. 2014. *Life beside Itself: Imagining Care in the Canadian Arctic.* Berkeley: University of California Press.

Stewart, K., and N. Sewankambo. 2010. "Okukkera Ng'omuzungu (Lost in Translation): Understanding the Social Value of Global Health Research for HIV/AIDS Research Participants in Uganda." *Global Public Health* 5 (2): 164–180.

Strathern, Marilyn. 1988. *The Gender of the Gift: Problems with Women and Problems with Society in Melanesia.* Berkeley: University of California Press.

Street, Alice. 2014. *Biomedicine in an Unstable Place: Infrastructure and Personhood in a Papua New Guinea Hospital.* Durham, NC: Duke University Press.

Sudman, Seymour, and Norman M. Bradburn. 1974. *Response Effects in Surveys: A Review and Synthesis.* Chicago: Aldine.

Sullivan, Noelle. 2016. "Hosting Gazes: Clinical Volunteer Tourism and Hospital Hospitality in Tanzania." In *Volunteer Economies: The Politics and Ethics of Voluntary Labour in Africa,* edited by Ruth Price and Hannah Brown. Melton, U.K.: James Currey.

Swartz, Alison. 2013. "Legacy, Legitimacy and Possibility: An Exploration of Community Health Worker Experience across the Generations in Khayelitsha, South Africa." *Medical Anthropology Quarterly* 27 (2): 139–154.

Swidler, Ann, and Susan Cotts Watkins. 2007. "Ties of Dependence: AIDS and Transactional Sex in Rural Malawi." *Studies in Family Planning* 38 (3): 147–162.

Swidler, Ann, and Susan Cotts Watkins. 2009. "Teach a Man to Fish: The Doctrine of Sustainability and Its Effects on Three Strata of Malawian Society." *World Development* 37 (7): 1182–1196.

Szreter, Simon, Hania Sholkamy, and A. Dharmalingam. 2004. "Contextualizing Categories: Toward a Critical Reflexive Demography." In *Categories and Contexts: Anthropological and Historical Studies in Critical Demography*, edited by Simon Szreter, Hania Sholkamy, and A. Dharmalingam. New York: Oxford University Press.

Tarver, James D. 1996. *The Demography of Africa*. Westport, CT: Praeger.

Taussig, Michael. 2009. *What Color Is the Sacred?* Chicago: University of Chicago Press.

Tendani, R. 2002. " 'Vampires' Strike Malawi Villages." BBC *News*, December 23. http://news.bbc.co.uk/2/hi/africa/2602461.stm.

Thomas, Deborah. 2011. *Exceptional Violence: Embodied Citizenship in Transnational Jamaica*. Durham, NC: Duke University Press.

Thompson, Charis. 2005. *Making Parents: The Ontological Choreography of Reproductive Technologies*. Cambridge, MA: MIT Press.

Thoreson, Ryan R. 2014. "LGBT Human Rights Advocacy and the Partnership Principle." In *Transnational LGBT Activism: Working for Sexual Rights Worldwide*. Minneapolis: University of Minnesota Press.

Thornton, Rebecca L. 2008. "The Demand for, and Impact of, Learning HIV Status." *American Economic Review* 98 (5): 1829–1863.

Tichenor, Marlee. 2017. "Data Performativity, Performing Health Work: Malaria and Labor in Senegal." *Medical Anthropology* 36 (5): 436–448.

Tilley, Helen. 2007. "Africa, Imperialism and Anthropology." In *Ordering Africa: Anthropology, European Imperialism, and the Politics of Knowledge*, edited by Helen Tilley and Robert J. Gordon. Manchester: Manchester University Press.

Tilley, Helen. 2011. *Africa as a Living Laboratory: Empire, Development, and the Problem of Scientific Knowledge*. Chicago: University of Chicago Press.

Tilley, Helen. 2016. "Medicine, Empires, and Ethics in Colonial Africa." AMA *Journal of Ethics* 18 (7): 743–753.

Timmermans, Stefan. 2015. "Trust in Standards: Transitioning Clinical Exome Sequencing from Bench to the Bedside." *Social Studies of Science* 45 (1): 77–99.

Timmermans, Stefan, and Marc Berg. 2003. *The Gold Standard: The Challenge of Evidence-Based Medicine*. Philadelphia: Temple University Press.

Timmermans, S., and S. Epstein. 2010. "A World of Standards but Not a Standard World: Toward a Sociology of Standardization." *Annual Review of Sociology* 36: 69–89.

Titmuss, Richard. (1970) 1997. *The Gift Relationship: From Human Blood to Social Policy*. New York: New Press.

Tomlinson, Deborah, Carl L. von Baeyer, Jennifer N. Stinson, and Lillian Sung. 2010. "A Systematic Review of FACES Scales for the Self-Report of Pain Intensity in Children." *Pediatrics* 125 (5).

Tousignant, Noemi. 2013. "Broken Tempos: Of Means and Memory in a Senegalese University Laboratory." *Social Studies of Science* 43 (5): 729–753.

Townsend, Nicholas, Sangeetha Madhavan, Mark Collinson, and Michael Garenne. 2006. "Collecting Data on Intra-household Relationships in the Agincourt Health and Population Survey." In *African households: Censuses and Surveys*, edited by Etienne van de Walle. New York: Routledge.

Trouillot, Michel-Rolph. 2003. *Global Transformations: Anthropology and the Modern World*. London: Palgrave Macmillan.

True, Gala, Leslie B. Alexander, and Kenneth A. Richman. 2011. "Misbehaviors of Front-Line Research Personnel and the Integrity of Community-Based Research." *Journal of Empirical Research on Human Research Ethics* 6 (2): 3–12.

Tsing, Anna. 2004. *Friction: An Ethnography of Global Connection*. Princeton, NJ: Princeton University Press.

Turner, Victor. 1969. *The Ritual Process: Structure and Anti-Structure*. Ithaca, NY: Cornell University Press.

UNAIDS. 2013. "Epidemiological Fact Sheet on HIV/AIDS, Malawi." New York: UNAIDS.

UNDP. 2015. "Human Development Report, 2015, Malawi." New York: United Nations Development Program.

UNICEF. 2001. "A Report on an Initiative for Improving the Situation of Girls in Malawi in the Context of Cultural and Traditional Values and Practices." New York: United Nations Children's Fund.

Union of African Population Studies (UAPS). 2017. "Home." http://uaps-uepa.org/en/home/.

University of Pennsylvania Population Studies Center (UPPSC). 2017. "Research themes." Retrieved from: https://www.pop.upenn.edu/research/themes.

Usten, T. Bedirhan, Somnath Chatterji, Abdelhay Mechbal, and Christopher J. L. Murray. 2005. "Quality Assurance in Surveys: Standards, Guidelines and Procedures." In *Household Sample Surveys in Developing and Transition Countries*. New York: United Nations Statistics Division.

Vail, Leroy, and Landeg White. 1991. *The Creation of Tribalism in Southern Africa*. Berkeley: University of California Press.

van den Broeck, J., S. A. Cunningham, R. Eeckels, and K. Herbst. 2005. "Data Cleaning: Detecting, Diagnosing, and Editing Data Abnormalities." *PLoS Medicine* 2 (10): e267.

van de Ruit, Catherine. 2012. "The Institutionalization of AIDS Orphan Policy in South Africa." PhD diss., University of Pennsylvania.

van de Walle, Etienne. 1968. "Characteristics of African demographic data." In *The Demography of Tropical Africa*, edited by William Brass, Ansley J. Cole, Paul Demeny, Don F. Heisel, Frank Lorimer, Anatole Romaniuk, and Etienne van de Walle. Princeton, NJ: Princeton University Press.

van de Walle, Etienne. 1993. "Recent Trends in Marriage Ages." In *Demographic Change in Sub-Saharan Africa*, edited by Karen A. Foote, H. Hill, and Linda G. Martin. London: Academy.

van de Walle, Etienne. 2006. "Introduction." In *African Households: Censuses and Surveys.* New York: Routledge.

Vaughan, Megan. 1982. " 'Better, Happier and Healthier Citizens': The Domasi Community Development Scheme, 1949–54." Unpublished manuscript, Malawiana collection, University of Malawi.

Vaughan, Megan. 1991. *Curing Their Ills: Colonial Power and African Illness.* Palo Alto, CA: Stanford University Press.

Vemuri, Murali Dhar. 1994. "Data Collection in Census: A Survey of Census Enumerators." *Economic and Political Weekly*, December 17–24.

Verran, Helen. 2013. "Numbers Performing Nature in Quantitative Valuing." *NatureCulture* 2: 23–37.

Vertesi, Janet. 2012. "Seeing Like a Rover: Visualization, Embodiment, and Interaction on the Mars Exploration Rover Mission." *Social Studies of Science* 42 (3): 393–414.

Vian, Taryn, Candace Miller, Zione Themba, and Paul Bukuluki. 2012. "Perceptions of Per Diems in the Health Sector: Evidence and Implications." *Health Policy and Planning* 28 (3): 237–246.

Wagner, Roy. 1981. *The Invention of Culture.* Chicago: University of Chicago Press.

Waller, Lloyd George. 2013. "Interviewing the Surveyors: Factors Which Contribute to Questionnaire Falsification (Curbstoning) among Jamaican Field Surveyors." *International Journal of Social Research Methodology* 16 (2): 155–164.

Walt, Gill. 1994. "How Far Does Research Influence Policy?" *European Journal of Public Health* 4: 233–235.

Wangel, Anne-Marie. 1995. "AIDS in Malawi—a Case Study: A Conspiracy of Silence?" Master's thesis, London School of Tropical Medicine.

Watkins, Susan Cotts. 1993. "If All We Knew about Women Was What We Read in *Demography*, What Would We Know?" *Demography* 30 (4): 551–577.

Watkins, Susan Cotts, and Ann Swidler. 2009. "Hearsay Ethnography: Conversational Journals as a Method for Studying Culture in Action." *Poetics* 37 (2): 162–184.

Watkins, Susan Cotts, and Ann Swidler. 2012. "Working Misunderstandings: Donors, Brokers, and Villagers in Africa's AIDS Industry." *Population and Development Review* 38: 197–218.

Watkins, Susan Cotts, Ann Swidler, and Crystal Biruk. 2011. "Hearsay Ethnography: A Method for Learning about Responses to Health Interventions." In *Handbook of the Sociology of Health, Illness, and Healing*, edited by Bernice A. Pescosolido, Jack K. Martin, Jane D. McLeod, and Anne Rogers. New York: Springer.

Weheliye, Alexander G. 2014. *Habeas Viscus: Racializing Assemblages, Biopolitics, and Black Feminist Theories of the Human.* Durham, NC: Duke University Press.

Weiner, Annette. 1976. *Women of Value, Men of Renown.* Austin: University of Texas Press.

Weinreb, A. 2006. "The Limitations of Stranger-Interviewers in Rural Kenya." *American Sociological Review* 71 (6): 1014–1039.

Weinreb, Alex, S. Madhavan, and P. Stern. 1998. "The Gift Received Must Be Repaid: Respondents, Researchers and Gifting." Paper presented at Annual Meeting of the Eastern Sociological Association, Philadelphia, March 27.

Weinreb, Alexander A., and Mariano Sana. 2009. "The Effects of Questionnaire Translation on Demographic Data and Analysis." *Population Research and Review* 28 (4): 429–454.

Wendland, Claire. 2008. "Research, Therapy, and Bioethical Hegemony: The Controversy over Perinatal AZT Trials in Africa." *African Studies Review* 51 (3): 1–23.

Wendland, Claire. 2010. *A Heart for the Work: Journeys through an African Medical School.* Chicago: University of Chicago Press.

Wendland, Claire. 2012. "Moral Maps and Medical Imaginaries: Clinical Tourism at Malawi's College of Medicine." *American Anthropologist* 114 (1): 108–122.

Wendland, Claire. 2016. "Estimating Death: A Close Reading of Maternal Mortality Metrics in Malawi." In *Metrics: What Counts in Global Health,* edited by Vincanne Adams. Durham, NC: Duke University Press.

West, Anna. 2016. "Body Politics in the Postcolony: Global Health and Local Governance in Rural Malawi." PhD diss., Stanford University.

West, Paige. 2006. *Conservation Is Our Government Now: The Politics of Ecology in Papua New Guinea.* Durham, NC: Duke University Press.

Weston, Kath. 2008. "Real Anthropology and Other Nostalgias." In *Ethnographica Moralia: Experiments in Interpretive Anthropology,* edited by Neni Panourgiá and George E. Marcus. New York: Fordham University Press.

White, Bob W., and Kiven Strohm. 2014. "Ethnographic Knowledge and the Aporias of Intersubjectivity." HAU 4 (1).

White, Luise. 2000. *Speaking with Vampires: Rumor and History in Colonial Africa.* Berkeley: University of California Press.

WHO. 2011. "Standards for Ethics Review of Health-Related Research with Human Participants." Geneva: World Health Organization.

Whyte, S. R., M. A. Whyte, L. Meinert, and J. Twebaze. 2013. "Therapeutic Citizenship: Belonging in Uganda's Mosaic of AIDS Projects." In *When People Come First: Anthropology and Social Innovation in Global Health,* edited by J. Biehl and A. Petryna. Princeton, NJ: Princeton University Press.

Wirtz, Andrea L., Vincent Jumbe, Gift Trapence, Dunker Kamba, Eric Umar, Sosthenes Ketende, Mark Berry, Susanne Stromdahl, Chris Beyrer, and Stefan D. Baral. 2013. "HIV among MSM in Malawi: Elucidating HIV Prevalence and Correlates of Infection to Inform HIV Prevention." *Journal of the International AIDS Society* 16 (4).

Wool, Zoe. 2015. *After War: The Weight of Life at Walter Reed.* Durham, NC: Duke University Press.

Wroe, Daniel. 2012. "Donors, Dependency, and Political Crisis in Malawi." *African Affairs* 111 (442): 135–144.

Yanagisako, Sylvia Junko. 1979. "Family and Household: The Analysis of Domestic Groups." *Annual Review of Anthropology* 8: 161–205.

Yansaneh, Ibrahim S. 2005. "Overview of Sample Design Issues for Household Surveys in Developing and Transition Countries." In *Household Sample Surveys in Developing and Transition Countries.* New York: United Nations Statistics Division.

Zeleza, Paul Tiyambe. 2002. "The Politics of Historical and Social Science Research in Africa." *Journal of Southern African Studies* 28 (1): 9–23.

Zuberi, T. 2005. "Building Regional Data Archives: The African Census Analysis Project (ACAP)." Paper presented at the IUSSP XXV International Population Conference, Tours, France, July 18.

Zuberi, Tukufu, and Martin W. Bangha. 2006. "The History and Future of African Census Analysis Project (ACAP)." Paper presented at Information Systems in Demography and in Social Sciences, Louvain-la Neuve (Belgium), November 29–December 1.

Zuberi, Tukufu, Amson Sibanda, Ayaga Bawah, and Amadou Noumbissi. 2003. "Population and African Society." *Annual Review of Sociology* 29: 465–486.

ARCHIVAL AND OTHER UNPUBLISHED SOURCES

Centre for Social Research (CSR) Documentation Unit

CSR/16/82. "Centre for Social Research, University of Malawi. The First Three Years, 1979–1982."

Malawi National Archives (MNA)

Central African Archives (CAA). S1/1382/29. "Correspondence Related to Increasing the Customs Duty on Soap."

CAA. S2/14/32. "Nyasaland Soap Industry."

CAA. 1935. S1/168/35. "Notes on the conference, 15–17 April, 1935, Salisbury between Governors of Northern Rhodesia and Nyasaland."

CAA. 1936. S1/9861A/25. "Research Conference Proceedings, Coordination of General Medical Research in East African Territories, Nairobi, January 20–22, 1936.

CAA. M2/14/1. "Medical Surveys by Medical Officers and Sub-assistant Surgeons." Subsection of file: "An Account of a Medical Survey of an Isolated Community by T. A. Austin."

CAA. 1939. NC 1/26/13. "A Letter from the District Commissioner of Kota Kota to the Senior Provincial Commissioner, October 20, 1939."

M2/4/2. 1931. "Letters from Livingstonia Mission to Director of Medical and Sanitation Services, 1930–1931."

M2/14/1. 1935. "Medical Surveys by Medical Officers and Sub-assistant Surgeons, 1934–1935."

NSZ 1/5/1. 1938. District Commissioners' Conference at Nyambadwe, minutes, October 7–8.

S1/986 (A11)/25. 1952. Nyasaland Medical Department (NMD). "Health Survey for the Year 1952."

Other

"Minutes." Minutes of a meeting of members of the National Research Council, November 18, 2005, made available to the author.

"The General Laws and Liberties of the Massachusetts Colony: Revised and Reprinted by Order of the General Court Holden at Boston. May 15th, 1672." 1672. Cambridge [MA]: Printed by Samuel Green, for John Usher of Boston.

circumcision, female, 182–83, 234n12
circumcision, male, 62, 175–76, 177, 179, 226n23, 234n5; HIV transmission and, 179–80; sexually active status and, 182
clean data, 24; clean questionnaires and, 134–35; demography and, 55, 120; fieldwork and, 132; handling of, 145–46; informed consent and, 127; interviewers' role in, 144; standards for, 35, 132–33; survey design and, 50, 120; survey projects and, 203; threats to, 133; transactions and, 101–2, 125; writing and, 149. *See also* data cleaning; data quality; raw data
Cohn, Bernard, 15
collaboration: data and, 5, 6; fieldwork and, 44; local, 40–41; in MAYP (pseud.), 39; as performance, 43; unequal, 40–44, 198, 209
College of Medicine Research and Ethics Committee (COMREC), 39
Colonial Development and Welfare Act (1940), 23
colonialism: African mind, conceptions of, 231n3; biopower and, 21; censuses under, 23, 147; development under, 210–11; survey-based research and, 210
Colvin, Christopher J., 214
community-based organizations (CBOs), 186–87
Community Based Rural Land Development Project, 118
conservation laws: free labor and, 122–23
consultancies, 42–44, 96, 175, 198; material stakes in, 175; remuneration for, 94, 195–96
contraception: Gambian women and, 54
cooked data, 4–5, 135, 139–40, 214. *See also* clean data; data quality; raw data
cooking data, 1, 29, 132, 200–201; age recall and, 142; anthropology and, 27; in beans exercise, 138; creativity and, 8; curbstoning, 223n2; fieldwork and, 38; interviewers and, 60; in Malawi, 1, 3; policy and, 169; probing as, 180; rhetoric of, 99. *See also* clean data; data quality; raw data

Council for International Organizations of Medical Science (CIOMS), 103
critical demography, 65. *See also* demography
critical development studies, 210; local knowledge and, 83
critical global health studies, 201, 203–4, 210; evidence and, 172; anthropological method and, 202, 215
critical medical anthropology, 6
culture: anthropology and, 19; data collection and, 64; demography and, 19, 56; global health and, 178; invention of, 79–80; progress and, 79; as site of contestation, 184–85; survey research and, 64; as traditional, 79

data: accuracy of, 135–36, 144, 231n2; and Africa, 24–27; as collaborative, 5, 6; conventional wisdom and, 181; errors, sources of, 135; ethnographic, 213; ethnography of, 3–4; as evidence, 169–71, 173, 200; as facts, 17; as inherently cooked, 139–40; invention of, 1; limitations of, 224n8; local knowledge and, 83; as manufactured artifact, 5; objectivity and, 7; policy and, 191; production of, 8, 34–35, 68; quality of, 33–34; raw information and, 145; reliability of, 135–36, 144; sharing of, 197; standardization of, 26–27, 145–46; as term, 223n3; as translation, 133; uncertainty and, 47. *See also* clean data; data quality; raw data
data cleaning, 135, 166–67; callbacks and, 146; of raw data, 166. *See also* cooking data
data collection, 2 fig. 1.1, 200, 223n23; age falsification and, 142; boundaries and, 75; costs of, 7; creativity and, 8; culture and, 64; data quality and, 28; discourse of, 3–4; ethics of, 104, 125; fieldwork, 6–7; infrastructure of, 33; local knowledge in, 70–71, 83; lying and, 146–47, 232n10; in Malawi, 1, 3, 223n1; politics and, 11, 34, 36; sampling and, 45, 154–55; social bound-

aries of, 75; social relations and, 163; standardization and, 7, 28, 74; standards for, 131, 134; training and, 147; as transactional, 7, 101–2, 127; translation and, 34, 98. *See also* fieldwork; survey projects

data quality, 33–34; attrition and, 155, 159; data collection and, 28; fieldwork and, 38, 135–36; gifting and, 109–10; of LSAM (pseud.), 133; in research projects, 145; sampling and, 154–55; survey design and, 59, 200; survey projects and, 24–27; surveys and, 45, 132–33; translation and, 48, 64; validity and, 58

Deane, Phyllis, 25

demographers, 11–12, 223n4. *See also* demography

Demographic and Health Surveys (DHS) program, 23, 224n10

demography: as acultural, 64–65; anthropology and, 15, 18–22, 26, 65, 202, 207, 211, 215; biopolitics and, 20; clean data and, 55, 120; cultural imperialism and, 21; culture and, 19, 56; discourse of, 9, 33, 223n4; fertility and, 19; fieldwork in, 36–37; institutionalization of, 22; knowledge production and, 22, 44; language of, 45; numbers and, 15–16, 20; objectivity and, 19; pictographic scales in, 52–55; as positivist, 19; postmodernism and, 22; standards of, 3; translation and, 47–49; uncertainty and, 15–16

Demography (journal), 173

Demography of Tropical Africa, The (van de Walle), 231n7

development: anthropology and, 210; bloodsucker rumors and, 118; colonial, 210–11; compensation for, 121–22; population studies and, 22–23; rhetoric of, 175; unpaid labor and, 121

DevInfo, 233n2

Ebola epidemic, 201

El-Badry, M. A., 232n13

Emanuel, Ezekiel J., 107

English: fluency in, 90, 229n25

enumeration, 120–21; critiques of, 45–46; facts and, 168; household as unit of, 56–57; technologies of, 155

enumeration areas, 130–31, 230n1

epistemology: ethnography and, 204; evidence and, 168; of local knowledge, 83; translation and, 64. *See also* knowledge production

Epstein, Steven, 82

Erikson, Susan L., 26

Esacove, Anne, 224n8

ethics: anthropology and, 124; of data collection, 104, 125; of gifting, 102, 109; of human subjects research, 120, 127–28; informed consent and, 28, 103–5, 229n1; of research projects, 102, 116–17, 125; of research transactions, 121, 124; survey design and, 103–4

ethnography: of data, 3–4; epistemology and, 204; of global health, 69, 213, 215; knowledge production and, 206; LSAM (pseud.) and, 224n8

evidence: authority of, 170, 173; as cooked, 199; critical global health studies and, 172; data as, 169–71, 173, 200; epistemology and, 168; etymology of, 172; ghost numbers and, 184; in global health, 168, 172, 185; local knowledge and, 184; numbers as, 168, 170–72, 186, 189–91, 199; policy and, 191–92, 196, 198; postcolonial hierarchies and, 175; quantitative data and, 170–71; as social artifact, 196; validity of, 170

family planning, 22, 233n3

Fassin, Didier, 213

Feierman, Steven, 196

Ferguson, James, 65, 121, 201

field: boundaries of, 206–7; construction of, 38, 69; as data container, 37; office and, 76–77; as purview of anthropology, 37–38, 206; as space of difference, 77; survey design and, 36, 63

fieldwork, 6–7; academia and, 36–37; as adventure, 77–78; callbacks in, 81–82, 145–47;

HIV transmission and, 173–74, 176, 181–85, 235nn14–15; policy and, 186, 192; rhetoric of, 176, 186. *See also* HIV/AIDS; human rights
health research: politics of, 14
Healy, Kieran, 212
Hemmings, Colin, 212
HIV/AIDS: cultural practices and, 10, 169, 173–80, 181–85, 229n22, 234n10, 235nn14–15; data collection and, 3; discourse of, 224n9; evidence-based policy and, 168; lying and, 232n10; in Malawi, 5, 10, 12–14, 173–74; male circumcision and, 179–80; among MSM, 169, 187–88; prevention strategies for, 171, 173–76, 183, 194; risk factors for, 181–84; in sub-Saharan Africa, 12–14, 169; survey taking and, 13; testing for, 112–13, 119; traditional healers and, 67
HIV Modes of Transmission Model, 181
Hodzic, Saida, 199
Holland, Dana, 41–42, 44
homophobia: emotional politics of, 189; in Malawi, 188–89
households, 56–57; anthropological critique of, 56; as category, 65; as heuristic tool, 65; names and, 57; as unit of enumeration, 56–57; sampling of, 154; in surveys, 9, 56, 152, 154; as western category, 58
human rights: cultural practices and, 172, 185; governance and, 21; LGBT persons and, 188
human subjects research: coercion in, 122; ethics of, 120, 127–28. *See also* informed consent
Hunter, Mark, 105
Hutchinson, Sharon, 110

informed consent, 120; clean data and, 127; ethics and, 28, 103–5, 229n1; subjectivity and, 104. *See also* human subjects research
initiation ceremonies, 87, 163, 177, 179–80, 182–83, 185
Integrated Public Use Microdata Series, 233n2

International Conference on Population and Development, 233n3
International Family Planning Perspectives (journal), 173
International Union for the Scientific Study of Population, 172
interviewer effects, 147–54; ethnic, 232n11; probing and, 150–52; racial, 232n11; sex and, 232n11; vignettes and, 150–51
interviewers: callbacks and, 146–47; clean data and, 144; cooking data and, 60; creative labor of, 62; interview questionnaires, 147–48; penmanship of, 152, 154, 232n13; precarity of, 97–98; reliability and, 60, 61; training of, 141, 147; wages for, 143. *See also* fieldworkers

Jerven, Morten, 25, 120
Justice, Judith, 210, 211

Kaufulu, Moses Mphatso, 180, 234n4
King, Gary, 58
King, Nicholas B., 21
Kingori, Patricia, 115, 117, 210
knowledge: performance of, 170; policy and, 174–75; statistics as, 170; trust and, 84. *See also* epistemology; local knowledge
knowledge production: demography and, 22, 44; and ethnography, 206; fieldwork and, 71
Knowledge Transition Platform, 196
Kuczynski, Robert René, 23
kulowa kufu, 176, 234n4

Lampland, Martha, 26
Latour, Bruno, 46, 56
Lekgoathi, Sekibakiba, 98
Lévi-Strauss, Claude, 4, 5
Likoma Network Survey, 226n16
local knowledge: boundary work and, 49, 83; commodification of, 98; constructed nature of, 87; credibility of, 184–85; critical development studies and, 83; data collection and, 70–71, 83; epistemology of, 83; evidence and, 184; in fieldwork, 68;

raw data, 4, 29; cleaning of, 166; editing of, 6; as fiction, 164–65, 168, 200, 214; policy and, 172. *See also* clean data; data

Read, Margaret, 210–11, 213

research: collaboration in, 198; dissemination of, 186–87, 195–96, 236n31; impact on field, 212; as productive, 215–16. *See also* research projects; survey projects

research fatigue, 101–2

research participants: coercion of, 101, 103–5, 107–8; compensation for, 106–7, 121

research participation: as "eating money," 116–17; ethics of, 125; HIV testing and, 119; refusal of, 112–14, 115, 119, 121, 159; time costs of, 115, 116. *See also* gifting; soap

research projects: as contact zones, 89; data quality in, 145; ethics of, 120, 116–17, 125; gifting in, 89–91, 115, 127, 229n3; human subjects in, 102; labor migration and, 72, 94, 155–59; local collaborators in, 40–41; local knowledge in, 98–99; in Malawi, 40–44; refusal to participate in, 112–14, 115, 119, 121, 159; reporting back to field, 208–9; sampling in, 232n15; scouts, use of, 87, 126, 159–60, 233n20; social capital and, 89, 91–93; social hierarchies within, 96–98; training sessions for, 148; transactions in, 110–11, 115, 121–22, 124, 229n7; trust and, 85; unequal collaboration in, 40–44, 198, 209. *See also* research; survey projects

Riedmann, Agnes, 21, 121

Riles, Annelise, 198

Rosenberg, Daniel, 223n3

samples: attrition of, 159; bounding of, 155, 157, 162–63; as category, 65; investment in, 133; as political units, 155; social relations with, 163–64

sampling, 161–62; data collection and, 45, 154–55; data quality and, 154–55; of households, 154; of population, 155; in research projects, 132, 232n15

Sariola, Salla, 210

Schumaker, Lyn, 80

science and technology studies, 6

science studies, 65

Scott, James, 20–21, 131, 155

Sedgwick, Eve, 202, 213

Shapin, Steven, 84

Simpson, Audra, 207

soap: as "clean" gift, 106–7, 109; cultural meaning of, 105; economic status and, 108; as ethical gift, 119, 120, 122; gifting of, 17, 32, 100–106, 108–9, 130; hierarchies of, 229n4; as human right, 112; imperialism and, 107–8; imposters and, 162; modernity and, 108, 109; as remuneration, 114, 162; as unjust gift, 111, 123

social capital: of fieldworkers, 89–90; financial capital and, 91–92, 93; research projects and, 89, 91–93

standardization: of data, 26–27, 145–46; data collection and, 7, 28, 74; of gifting, 107; v. improvisation, 3

statistics: hegemony of, 191; as knowledge, 170; numbers and, 5; policy and, 5, 192; as "science of the state," 20

Studies in Family Planning (journal), 173

subjectivity: informed consent and, 104; translation and, 64

survey design, 20, 27, 226n18; clean data and, 50, 120; data quality and, 59, 200; ethics and, 103–4; the field and, 36, 63; households in, 56; local expertise and, 50–51; local knowledge and, 82, 180; of LSAM (pseud.), 136, 172; as negotiation, 46; representation in, 46; research ethics and, 103–4; steps instrument in, 50–53, 51 fig. 1.1, 52 fig. 1.2; thermometer instrument in, 53, 54, 55 fig. 1.3; translation and, 34, 54, 62–64, 136. *See also* surveys

survey projects, 201; attrition in, 155; bloodsuckers and, 117–19; clean data and, 203; culture and, 64; data quality and, 24–27; discursive effects of, 172; gifting in, 101; imposters in, 161; infrastructure of, 32–33; local collaboration in, 40–41; of LSAM (pseud.), 10, 112, 233n3; lying in, 161–62, 232n10; sampling and, 132; social bound-